Endoscopic Surgery of Nose and Paranasal Sinuses

and Related Topics

for Postgraduate Students and ENT Practitioners

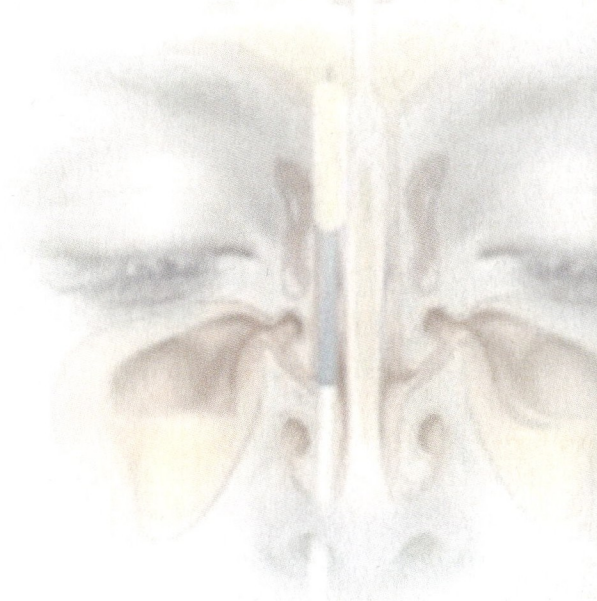

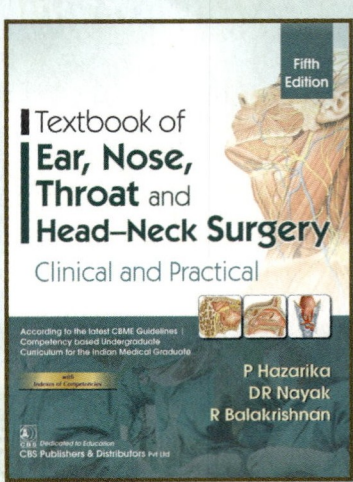
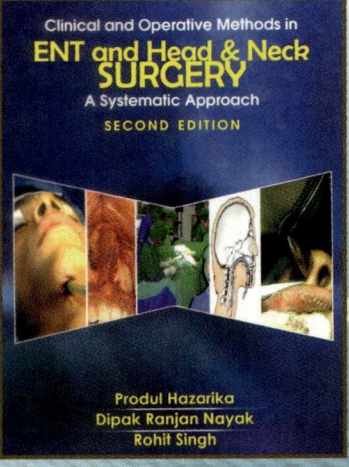
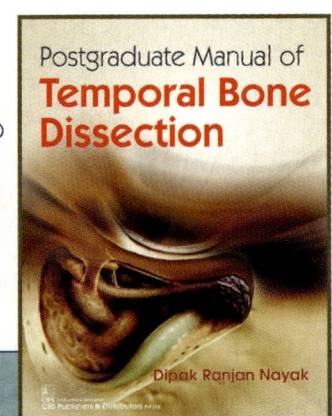

Endoscopic Surgery of Nose and Paranasal Sinuses and Related Topics

for Postgraduate Students and ENT Practitioners

Chief Editor

Dipak Ranjan Nayak MBBS, MS, FICS, Fellow of UICC
Professor and Former Head

Associate Editors

Balakrishnan Ramaswamy MS, DNB (ORL)
Professor and Former Head

Rohit Singh MS (ORL)
Associate Professor

Department of Otorhinolaryngology–Head and Neck Surgery
Kasturba Medical College, Manipal Academy of Higher Education, Manipal

Guest Editors

Prepageran Narayanan FRCS (Edin)
Consultant Otorhinolaryngologist and
Skull Base Surgeon
Professor, Department of Otorhinolaryngology
Faculty of Medicine, University of Malaya
Kuala Lumpur, Malaysia

Produl Hazarika DLO, MS, FRCS
Former Professor and Head
Department of Otorhinolaryngology–Head and Neck
Surgery
Kasturba Medical College, Manipal
Consultant ENT Surgeon
Nemcare Hospital, Guwahati, Assam

P Satyanarayana Murthy MS, DLO
Former Professor
Department of Otorhinolaryngology–Head and Neck
Surgery
Kasturba Medical College, Manipal

Dean and Professor
Dr P Siddhartha Institute of Medical Sciences and
Research Center
Chinnaautapalli, Gannavaram, AP

Kailesh Pujary MS (ORL), DNB
Professor and Head
Department of Otorhinolaryngology–Head and Neck
Surgery
Kasturba Medical College, Manipal

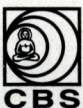

CBS

CBS Publishers & Distributors Pvt Ltd

New Delhi • Bengaluru • Chennai • Kochi • Kolkata • Lucknow • Mumbai
Hyderabad • Jharkhand • Nagpur • Patna • Pune • Uttarakhand

Endoscopic Surgery of
Nose and Paranasal Sinuses
and Related Topics
for Postgraduate Students and ENT Practitioners

ISBN: 978-93-90709-57-1

Copyright © Editors and Publisher

First Edition: 2022

Published by Satish Kumar Jain and produced by Varun Jain for

CBS Publishers & Distributors Pvt Ltd

4819/XI Prahlad Street, 24 Ansari Road, Daryaganj, New Delhi 110 002, India.
Ph: 011-23289259, 23266861, 23266867
Fax: 011-23243014
Website: www.cbspd.com
e-mail: delhi@cbspd.com; cbspubs@airtelmail.in.

Corporate Office: 204 FIE, Industrial Area, Patparganj, Delhi 110 092
Ph: 011-4934 4934   Fax: 011-4934 4935
e-mail: publishing@cbspd.com; publicity@cbspd.com

Branches

- **Bengaluru:** Seema House 2975, 17th Cross, K.R. Road, Banasankari 2nd Stage, Bengaluru 560 070, Karnataka, India
  Ph: +91-80-26771678/79   Fax: +91-80-26771680   e-mail: bangalore@cbspd.com
- **Chennai:** 7, Subbaraya Street, Shenoy Nagar, Chennai 600 030, Tamil Nadu, India
  Ph: +91-44-26680620, 26681266   Fax: +91-44-42032115   e-mail: chennai@cbspd.com
- **Kochi:** 42/1325, 1326, Power House Road, Opp KSEB, Power House, Ernakulum Kochi 682 018, Kerala, India
  Ph: +91-484-4059061-65,67   Fax: +91-484-4059065   e-mail: kochi@cbspd.com
- **Kolkata:** 147, Hind Ceramics Compound, 1st Floor, Nilgunj Road, Belghoria, Kolkata-700056, West Bengal, India
  Ph: +91-9096713055/7798394118, 9836841399   e-mail: kolkata@cbspd.com
- **Lucknow:** Basement, Khushnuma Complex, 7 Meerabai Marg (Behind Jawahar Bhawan),Lucknow-226001, UP, India
  Ph: +0522-4000032   e-mail: tiwari.lucknow@cbspd.com
- **Mumbai:** PWD Shed, Gala no 25/26, Ramchandra Bhatt Marg, Next to JJ Hospital Gate no. 2, Opp. Union Bank of India, Noorbaug, Mumbai-400009, Maharashtra, India
  Ph: 022-66661880/89   e-mail: mumbai@cbspd.com

Representatives

• Hyderabad	0-9885175004	• Jharkhand	0-9811541605	• Nagpur	0-9421945513
• Patna	0-9334159340	• Pune	0-9623451994	• Uttarakhand	0-9716462459

Printed at   Nutech Print Services, Faridabad, Haryana, India

Foreword

Over the last two decades, endoscopic sinus surgery has received increasing interest from the otorhinolaryngologists, ophthalmologists as well as neurosurgeons across the globe. This has also led to a significant surge in the literature search on this topic. The book titled *Endoscopic Surgery of the Nose and Paranasal Sinuses and Related Topics* by Dr Dipak Ranjan Nayak provides a comprehensive reference starting from the anatomy and basic steps of endoscopic sinus surgery to the most advanced techniques of pituitary surgery. The list of contributors is impressive with excellent expertise in their respective fields. The text is wide ranging and covers all the aspects needed for mastering the art of endoscopic sinus surgery. This book would be a useful addition to the armamentarium of any surgeon interested in endoscopic sinus surgery. This book is a valuable contribution to the literature. Wish you all an enjoyable reading.

Adj Prof Dr Satish Kumar Jain MBBS, MS
Senior Consultant
ENT, Head & Neck Cancer and Skull Base Surgeon
Jain ENT Hospital
Jaipur, Rajasthan

Contributors

INTERNATIONAL

Arun Kumar FRCS (UK), FAA (USA)
Manipal Hospitals Klang
Klang, Selangor, Malaysia

Jaspal Singh Sahota MS (ORL)
Vice-Chancellor
Manipal University College
Malaysia

Prepageran Narayanan FRCS (Edin)
Consultant Otorhinolaryngologist and
Skull Base Surgeon
Professor
Department of Otorhinolaryngology
Faculty of Medicine
University of Malaya
Kuala Lumpur, Malaysia

Revadi Govindaraju
MS (ORL and Head-Neck Surgery) (Malaya)
Senior Lecturer and Consultant Otolaryngologist
Head and Neck Surgeon, Department of ENT
Faculty of Medicine, University of Malaya
Kuala Lumpur, Malaysia

Tang Ing Ping MS (ORL & Head-Neck Surgery) (Malaya)
Consultant Otorhinolaryngologist and
Skull Base Surgeon, Associate Professor
Department of Otorhinolaryngology
Faculty of Medicine, University of Malaya
Kuala Lumpur, Malaysia

Vicknes Waran Mathaneswaran
FRCS (Edin), FRCS (Neurosurgery)
Consultant Neurosurgeon
Department of Neurosurgery
Faculty of Medicine, University of Malaya
Kuala Lumpur, Malaysia

NATIONAL

Aditi Ravindra MBBS
Resident
Department of Otorhinolaryngology–Head and
Neck Surgery
Kasturba Medical College, Manipal

Ajay Bhandarkar MS (ORL)
Associate Professor
Department of Otorhinolaryngology–Head and
Neck Surgery
Kasturba Medical College, Manipal

Akshay Krishnamurthy MBBS
Resident
Department of Otorhinolaryngology–Head and
Neck Surgery
Kasturba Medical College, Manipal

Aniketh Venkataram MS, MCh (Plastic)
Consultant Plastic Surgeon
The Venkat Center
Vijaynagar, Bengaluru

Architha Menon MS (ORL)
Senior Resident
Department of ENT
Bangalore Medical College
Bengaluru

Asheesh Dora MS
Assistant Professor
Department of ENT
Pratima Medical College
Karimnagar

Balakrishnan Ramaswamy MS, DNB (ORL)
Professor and Former Head
Department of Otorhinolaryngology–Head and
Neck Surgery
Kasturba Medical College, Manipal

Billakanti Prakash Babu MD (Anat)
Associate Professor
Department of Anatomy
Kasturba Medical College, Manipal

Chinmay Sundar Ray MS (ORL), FICS
Associate Professor
Department of ENT
PRM Medical College
Baripada Mayurbhanj, Odisha

Deepak Nayak M MD (Path), DCP
Associate Professor
Department of Pathology
Kasturba Medical College, Manipal

Dipak Ranjan Nayak MS (ORL), FICS, UICC Fellow
Professor and Former Head
Department of Otorhinolaryngology–Head and
Neck Surgery
Kasturba Medical College, Manipal

Devaraja K MS (ORL), Head and Neck Fellow (AIIMS)
Assitant Professor
Department of Otorhinolaryngology–Head and
Neck Surgery
Kasturba Medical College, Manipal

Deeksha Rao MS (ORL)
ENT Consultant
The Venkat Center
Vijaynagar, Bengaluru

K Deepak Murty MS (ORL)
Consultant ENT Specialist
Manipal Hospital, Panji, Goa

Kabikant Samantray MS (ORL)
Professor
Department of ENT
Kalinga Institute of Medical Sciences
Bhubaneswar, Odisha

Kailesh Pujary MS (ORL), DNB
Professor and Head
Department of Otorhinolaryngology–Head and
Neck Surgery
Kasturba Medical College, Manipal

Krushna Chandra Mallick
Professor
Department of ENT
SLN Medical College, Koraput, Odisha

Lokadolalu Chandracharya Prasanna MD (Anat)
Professor and Head
Department of Aanatomy
Kasturba Medical College, Manipal

N Apoorva Reddy MS (ORL)
Head and Neck Oncology Fellow
HCG, Bengaluru

Nikitha Periaswamy MS (ORL)
Consultant
Vega ENT Hospital
RS Puram, Coimbatore
Tamil Nadu

Nithu Mathew MS
Assitant Professor
Department of Otorhinolaryngology–Head and
Neck Surgery
Kasturba Medical College, Manipal

P Satyanarayan Murthy MS, DLO
Former Professor
Department of Otorhinolaryngology–Head and
Neck Surgery
Kasturba Medical College, Manipal
Dean and Professor
Dr P Siddhartha Institute of Medical Sciences and
Research Center
Chinnaautapalli, Gannavaram, AP

Prerit Rao MS (ORL)
Senior Resident
Department of Otorhinolaryngology–Head and
Neck Surgery
Kasturba Medical College, Manipal

Produl Hazarika DLO, MS, FRCS
Former Professor and Head
Department of Otorhinolaryngology–Head and
Neck Surgery
Kasturba Medical College, Manipal
Consultant ENT Surgeon
Nemcare Hospital, Guwahati, Assam

Poorvi Sharma MS
Assistant Professor
Department of Otorhinolaryngology–Head and
Neck Surgery
Kasturba Medical College, Manipal

Rohit Singh MS (ORL)
Associate Professor
Department of Otorhinolaryngology–Head and
Neck Surgery
Kasturba Medical College, Manipal

Rudranarayan Biswal MS
Former Professor and Head
SCB Medical College, Cuttack and KIMS,
Bhubaneswar

Shamma Shetty MS (ORL)
Assistant Professor
Department of Otorhinolaryngology–Head and
Neck Surgery
Kasturba Medical College, Manipal

Sneha Guruprasad Kalthur MD (Anat)
Professor and Former Head
Department of Anatomy
Kasturba Medical Colleg, Manipal

Subrat Behera MS (ORL)
Professor
Department of ENT
SCB Medical College, Cuttack

Suraj Nair MS (ORL), DNB (ENT-HNS)
Fellowship in Head and Neck Oncology
(Ahmedabad)
ENT Consultant, Holy Cross Hospital
Thane, Mumbai

Suresh Pillai DNB (ORL)
Professor
Department of Otorhinolaryngology–Head and
Neck Surgery
Kasturba Medical College, Manipal

Swetapadma Nayak MBBS
Resident
Department of ENT
SCB Medical College, Cuttack

Tulasi Karanth MS (ORL)
Senior Resident
Department of Otorhinolaryngology–Head and
Neck Surgery
Kasturba Medical College, Manipal

Preface

Functional endoscopic sinus surgery is now a well-established technique for the management of chronic rhinosinusitis, initially described by late Prof W Messerkliger (Austria) in 1978 and later popularized by late Prof H Stammberger (Austria) and Prof D Kennedy (USA). There has been tremendous expansion in the field of endoscopic surgery of the nose, paranasal sinuses and skull base with application in the field of neurosurgery and head and neck oncology since then. Invasive fungal sinusitis has become a new challenge, especially with Covid-19 associated mucormycosis. At present, there are very few books/manuals to cater to the needs of the postgraduate students in this field. There are many books which are too advanced for a postgraduate trainee in India and are also expensive. Looking at the current status, we decided to come out with the concept of having a concise manual encompassing most of the topics in this field entitled *Endoscopic Surgery of Nose and Paranasal Sinuses and Related Topics*. This edition consists of 25 chapters including basic sciences related to the field of anatomy, physiology, anatomical abnormalities, pathophysiology, endoscopic diagnosis and indications, instruments, disinfection and sterilization, anesthesia, technique of functional endoscopic sinus surgery including minimal invasive technique and advanced, balloon sinuplasty, endoscopic management of nasopharyngeal cancer, CSF rhinorrhea, endoscopic pituitary surgery, draf procedures, endoscopic medial maxillectomy and anterior skull base surgery, endonasal approach to orbit. A lot of stress have been given on in depth anatomy and development, applied physiology of nose and paranasal sinuses including mucociliary clearance and pathophysiology in a concise manner for better understanding of the reader. The book also covers other related topics on nasal allergy, DCR, allergic fungal sinusitis and rhinoplasty, etc. and a comprehensive chapter on nasopharyngeal angiofibroma. The book has been formatted with a scope for further improvement with future expansion in knowledge and advancing technology. There are eminent international contributors from Malaysia. The chapter "Endoscopic pituitary surgery" is written by Dr Govindraju, Dr Tang, Prof Waran and Prof Prepageran. Chapter on "Endoscopic management of nasopharyngeal cancer" is written by Prof Sahota and Dr Arun Kumar. Prof R Balakrishnan has written the chapter "Endoscopic endonasal approach to the orbit" and Dr Venkataram and Dr Deeksha Rao have written the chapter "Basics of rhinoplasty" as the main national contributors besides others. Surgical videos on **pituitary surgery** by Prof Prepageran and **endoscopic lothrop procedure** by Prof Nayak have been provided with link. The Foreword to the book has been written by one of the most dynamic endoscopic sinus, skull base and head and neck surgeons of India Adj Prof Dr Satish Kumar Jain.

Dipak Ranjan Nayak

Acknowledgements

This book would not have been completed without the blessings of our great teachers and the mentors. We would like to thank all our great teachers and mentors including Prof MC Sahoo, Late Prof G Behera (Cuttack), and Prof P Hazarika, Prof PSN Murthy and Late Prof Rajamma Rajan (Manipal), who have given us the foundation to grow and develop our skill and knowledge.

We are grateful to our founder beloved President of MAHE, Dr Ram Das M Pai, Pro-Chancellor, Prof HS Ballal, Vice-Chancellor, Lt Gen Prof MD Venkatesh, Dean of KMC, Manipal, Prof Sarath Rao, Head, Department of Otorhinolaryngology–Head and Neck Surgery, Prof Kailesh Pujary, who kindly permitted us to carry on the work on this book in this institution lacking which, we fear, it would not have been possible to bring this work to light.

We deeply appreciate Adj Prof Dr Satish Kumar Jain, Senior Consultant, ENT–Head and Neck Cancer and Skull Base Surgeon, Jain ENT Hospital Jaipur, for writing the Foreword to this book. He has tremendous contribution in inspiring many young ENT enthusiasts to take up interest in endoscopic surgery of nose, paranasal sinuses and skull base through his mesmerizing surgical skills.

We are grateful to all our guest editors Prof Prepageran Narayanan, Prof P Hazarika, Prof PSN Murthy, and Prof Kailesh Pujary for their valuable contributions in editorial assistance.

We are extremely thankful to all our authors from Malaysia, especially Prof Prepageran, a renowned otolaryngologist and skull base surgeon, for agreeing to be one of the guest editors and taking an active part in initiating and completing the chapter on "Pituitary surgery" along with his colleagues, Dr Revadi Govindaraju, Dr Tang Ing Ping and Prof Vicknes Waran. Dr Revadi has been very kind enough in helping and completing this chapter as a key author, through timely communication and answering to all the queries. Prof Jaspal Singh Sahota and Dr Arun Kumar are the alumni of KMC, Manipal, and have contributed to the chapter on "The role of nasal endoscopy in the management of nasopharyngeal cancer". We thank all of them for their contribution. We are thankful to all our Indian authors and co-authors including Dr. Aniketh Venkataram and Dr Deeksha Rao for chapter "Basics of rhinoplasty". Dr Deeksha has taken a keen interest in allergic rhinitis and her contribution is key to that chapter. We are also thankful to all our co-authors for various chapters including Prof P Hazarika, Prof PSN Murthy, Prof K Pujary, Prof LC Prasanna, Prof K Samantaray, Prof S Guruprasad, Prof Pillai, Prof RN Biswal, Prof Behera, Prof KC Mallick, Dr Deepak Nayak (Pathology), Dr Bhandarkar, Dr Prakash Babu, Dr Deepak Murty, Dr Devaraja, Dr CS Ray, Dr Shetty, Dr Sharma, Dr Mathew, Dr Nair, Dr Reddy, Dr Dora, Dr Periaswamy, Dr S Nayak, Dr Menon, Dr Karanth, Dr Rao, Dr Krishnamurty, and Dr Ravindra. All the contributors deserve applaud for whatever contribution they have made, whether it is big or small, without which it would not have been possible to finish this stupendous task on time.

We thank all our faculties for their contribution and constructive criticism. A lot of people have helped in various ways while preparing the manuscript. They are our past and present postgraduate students. We thank Dr Nishanth, Dr Nikhil, Dr Abhinay, Dr Prashant, Dr Pooja, Dr Reshmi, Dr Nithu, Dr Jalwa, Dr Aditi, Dr Ishan Sardesai, Dr Faria, Dr Tejashwi, Dr Vidhi,

Dr Shyam, Dr Mihika, Dr Aiswarya, Dr Majitha, Dr Akshaya K, Dr Akshay P, Dr Jigisha for their timely help.

Special thanks to Dr Swetapadma Nayak for doing a tireless proofreading and also contributing to key illustrations.

We would be failing in our duty if we do not appreciate the contributions of our parents. Special thanks to our spouse and children for their help and guidance. We sincerely thank Mr Bhaskar, Mr Sudhakar, for their assistance in operating room, Mrs Latha for secretarial assistance, Mr Sitharam, Mrs Mangala, Mr Shreekant our OPD technicians, Mrs Baby, OPD sister, Mrs Usha our OT sister and all other non-teaching staff of the department for their kind help.

Finally we would like to thank all our patients, those who have undergone endoscopic surgery of the nose and paranasal sinuses. Without their participation, this book would not have been possible.

Dipak Ranjan Nayak
Balakrishnan Ramaswamy
Rohit Singh

Contents

Surgical Anatomy—Nose and Paranasal Sinuses

DR Nayak, R Balakrishnan, GK Sneha, B Prakash Babu, S Nayak

The surgical anatomy of the nasal cavity and paranasal sinuses are complex and variable. The anatomical variations in the lateral wall may lead to impairment of drainage leading to chronic sinusitis. Nasal endoscopy and advent of multidetector computed tomography (MDCT) have paved the way in understanding this complex anatomy. A precise understanding of the three-dimensional anatomy of lateral nasal wall, sphenoethmofrontal sinuses and their vital relations to adjacent structures including skull base and cadaveric dissections is mandatory. Moreover, with expansion in indications for endoscopic surgeries in this region and beyond, a detail knowledge and understanding of this complex anatomy and associated landmarks are the key to become a successful endoscopic sinus and skull base surgeon. Vital structures like the orbit, cranial cavity, optic nerve, internal carotid artery, etc. lie in close relation to the sphenoethmofrontal sinuses, usually separated by a thin bone; making them vulnerable to injury during an endoscopic sinus surgery.

The exact orientation of various intranasal and extranasal structures with respect to their location, attitude and interrelation can be studied only by repeated cadaveric dissections. Strong knowledge of anatomy and its variation plays a pivotal role in diagnosis and endoscopic approaches to surgeries like septoplasty, septorhinoplasty, adenoidectomy, hypophysectomy, excision of benign tumour like glioma, medial maxillectomy, etc.

The introduction of nasal and sinus endoscopy, better imaging techniques and study of whole organ mounted sections has helped us to understand better the microarchitectural anatomy of sphenoethmoids and their vital relations.

SKELETAL FRAMEWORK OF EXTERNAL NOSE (Figs 1.1 and 1.2)

It consists of bony and cartilaginous supportive framework.

Bony part consists of the following (Fig. 1.1).
1. Paired nasal bone
2. Paired frontal process of the maxilla
3. Nasal process of the frontal bone.

Nasal bone articulates with the nasal process of the frontal bone superiorly, frontal

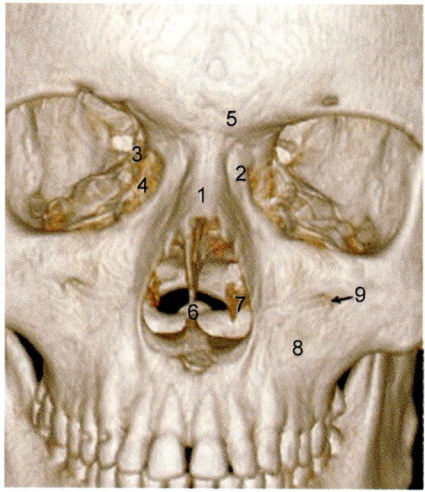

Fig. 1.1: Bony skeletal framework of external nose and orbit: (1) Nasal bone, (2) Frontal process of maxilla, (3) Lamina papyracea, (4) Lacrimal bone, (5) Nasal process of frontal bone, (6) Nasal septum, (7) Concha, (8) Canine fossa, (9) Infraorbital foramen

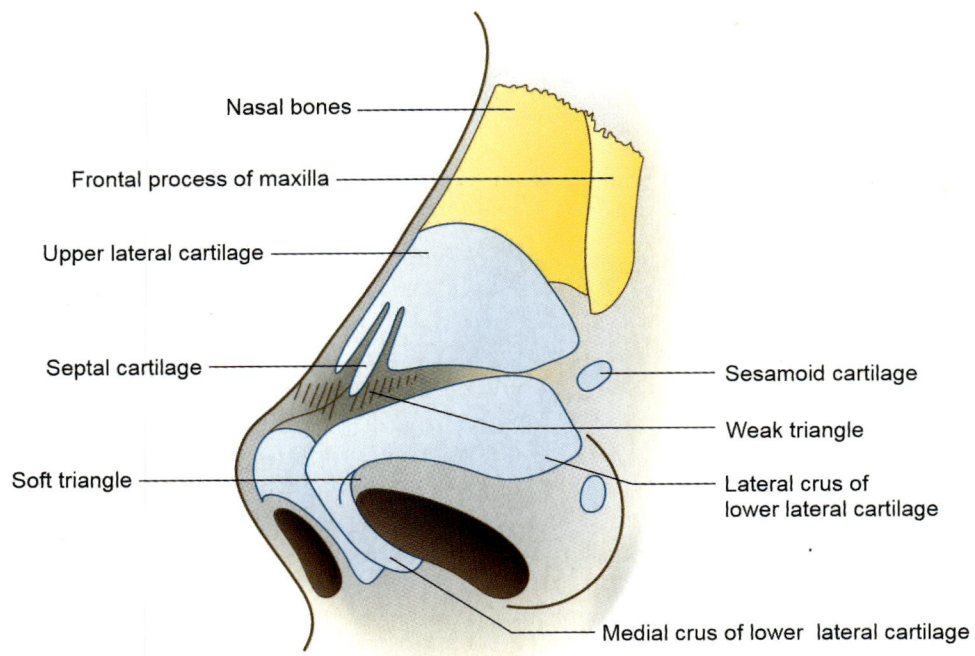

Fig. 1.2: Skeletal framework of external nose

process of the maxilla laterally, inferiorly with the upper lateral cartilage and medially with nasal bone of the other side. The junction between the two nasal bones forms the bridge of the nose (Oneal and Beil 2010).

Cartilaginous part is made up of the following cartilages (Coverse 1955).
1. Paired upper lateral cartilage.
2. Paired lower lateral cartilage (alar cartilages)
3. Sesamoid cartilage
4. Anterior part of the septal cartilage.

The upper lateral cartilage is triangular in shape and is attached above with the frontal process of maxilla and inferior margin of nasal bone. Medially it is continuous with the septal cartilage and in fact is a triangular flat expansion of the septal cartilage forming the middle third of the nose.

The lower lateral cartilage or the alar cartilage forms the lower third of the nose and is responsible for maintaining the projection and shape of the tip. It consists of slender medial crus and wider lateral crus. The two medial crurae support the columella. Each lateral crus forms the ala of the nose. The projection between the medial and lateral crurae of the cartilage supports the tip of the nose, which forms the dome.

The minor sesamoid cartilages are present between the upper and lower nasal cartilages.

The nasal cartilages are made up of hyaline cartilage. Nasal bones and cartilages are connected to each other by periosteum and perichondrium, which is continuous. The upper and lower lateral cartilages prevent the collapse of the vestibule during inspiration.

The skin covers the skeletal framework of the external nose, which is continuous with the skin of the columella and vestibule of the nose.

NASAL CAVITY

Knowledge of the interior of nasal cavity to human being dates back to ancient civilization when the nose was predominantly associated with the sense of smell. The earliest record of an anatomical observation is in the papyrus of Ebers and Egyptian tomb inscriptions, dated well before 1500 BC, where the nose was used as a route for extracting the contents of the cranial vault as part of the mummification process, thereby avoiding any facial disfigurement. This implies an intimate knowledge of the intricate relationship between the roof of the ethmoids and the brain (Kaluskar 1997). The nasal cavity is divided into right and left nasal cavities by the nasal septum. Each nasal cavity has a medial and a lateral wall, a roof and a floor cottle. The anterior most part of the nasal cavities lined by the skin is called the vestibule of the nose. Rest of the nasal cavities is lined by the respiratory epithelium below and olfactory epithelium above (dangerous area of nose). Each nasal cavity is approximately 5–7 cm in length and 5 cm in height. It is narrow transversely, measuring approximately 1.5 cm at the floor and 1–2 mm at the roof.

VESTIBULE

It is the entrance of the nasal cavity from the nostrils and is lined by skin containing hair follicles. It forms the part of the dangerous area of face because of the presence of the retrograde venous drainage through ophthalmic veins (without valves), which can lead to complications like cavernous sinus thrombosis. The vestibule is demarcated from the nasal mucosa by the limen nasi, which corresponds to the superior margin of the lower lateral cartilage (Oneal, et al 1999).

COLUMELLA

It is the part between the two nasal vestibules and forms the caudal end of the nasal septum. It is formed by the medial crurae of the two lower lateral cartilages. The lower lateral cartilages and the caudal end of the septum supports the tip of the nose. Injury of any form to either caudal septum or lower lateral cartilages will change the shape of the tip.

Framework of the Nasal Cavity

In an articulated skull, the following bones/cartilages bind each nasal cavity.

1. **The floor is formed by:**
   a. Palatine process of the maxilla.
   b. Horizontal process of the palatine bone.

2. **The roof consists of:**
   a. Cribriform plate of the ethmoid.
   b. Nasal process of the frontal bone.
   c. Body of the sphenoid.

3. **The medial wall is formed by:**
   a. Cartilaginous nasal septum
   b. Bony nasal septum
   c. Membranous columella.

4. **Lateral wall consists of:**
   a. Medial wall of the maxilla
   b. Inferior concha
   c. Middle and superior concha of the ethmoid bone.

MEDIAL WALL (NASAL SEPTUM)

This is formed by bony and cartilaginous framework and is lined by the mucoperiosteum and the mucoperichondrium, respectively. This forms the bulk of the nasal septum. The small caudal part is membranous (columella) and is lined by skin. The superior part of nasal septum located above the inferior turbinates and extending up to the anterior part of the middle turbinates is termed as septal swell body. Histologically, it contains glandular structures with lesser vascularity than inferior turbinate (Wexler, et al 2006).

Following structures form the bony nasal septum (Figs 1.3 and 1.4).

Major contribution from:
- Perpendicular plate of ethmoid
- Vomer
- Palatine crest
- Maxillary crest

Small contribution from:
- Nasal spine of the frontal bone
- Rostrum of the sphenoid
- Anterior nasal spine of the maxilla

The **cartilaginous** part of the nasal septum is formed by quadrangular cartilage with contributions from upper and lower lateral cartilages (Converse 1955).

Membranous columella: It is the membranous part of the septum between the medial crus of the lower lateral cartilage and the quadrangular cartilage. It is lined by skin. It

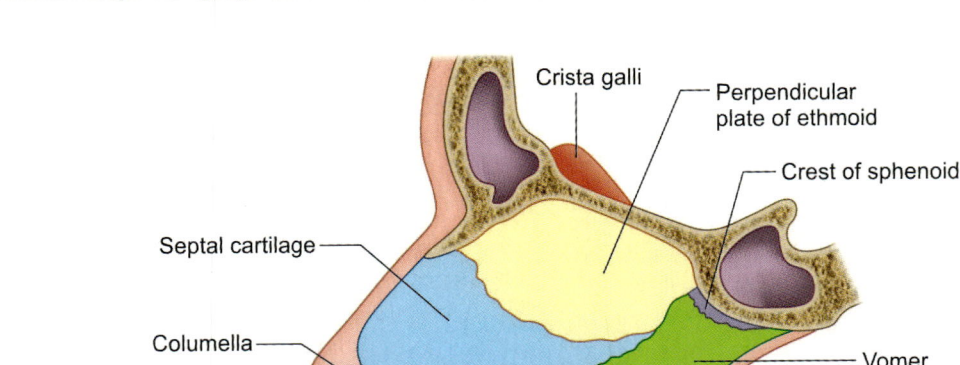

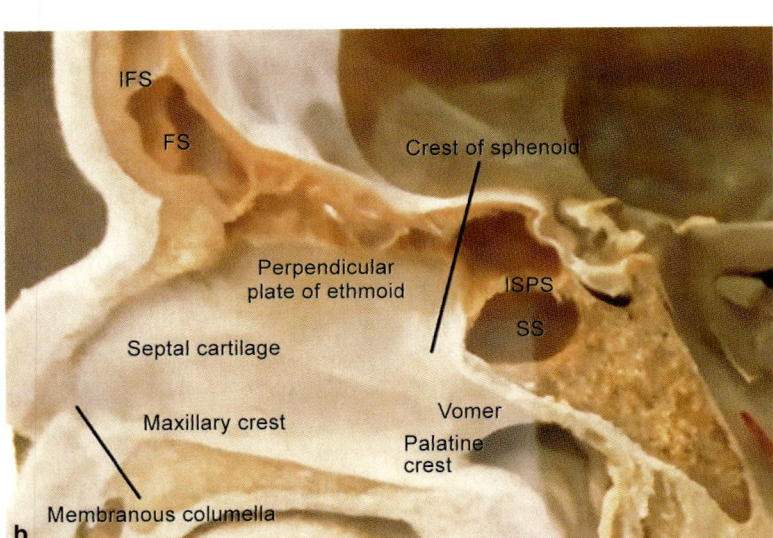

Fig. 1.3: a. Bony and cartilaginous part of the nasal septum; **b.** Various parts of nasal septum and frontal sinus (FS), interfrontal septum (IFS), intersphenoidal septum (ISPS), sphenoid sinus (SS)

does not have much relevance with respect to endoscopic sinus surgery, except that a deviated septum can be associated with caudal dislocation of the septum. Injury to caudal septum and medial crus can change the shape of the nasal tip.

Roof: The roof of nasal cavity is curved with concave surface downwards. The middle part is formed by the cribriform plate of ethmoid and is nearly horizontal. The anterior and posterior parts are sloping. The anterior part is formed by the nasal part of frontal bone, the nasal bone.

The posterior part consists of the anterior and inferior surfaces of the body of the sphenoid and the bones in contact with these surfaces (Oneal, et al 1999).

Lateral Wall of the Nasal Cavity

Compared to the simple medial wall, the lateral wall is complicated in its anatomy. It bounds most of the paranasal sinuses and receives the openings from these sinuses (Figs 1.4 and 1.5).

The external nares lead to the skin lined part of the lateral nasal wall, the vestibule. This

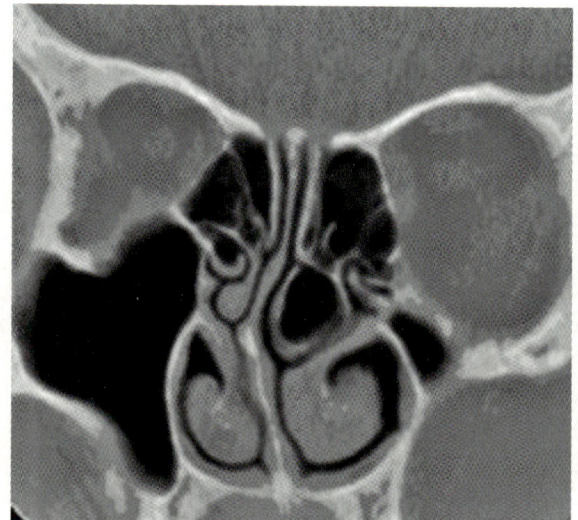

Fig. 1.4a: CT scan of the nose and paranasal sinus

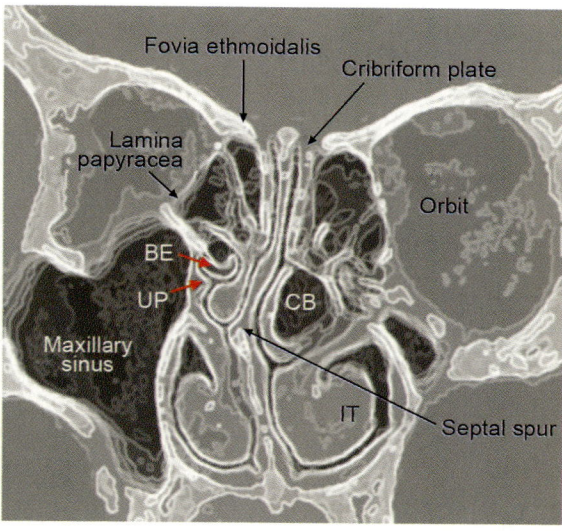

Fig. 1.4b: Same CT restructured showing the details—uncinate process (UP), bulla ethmoidalis (BE), pneumatized middle turbinate or concha bullosa (CB), inferior turbinate (IT)

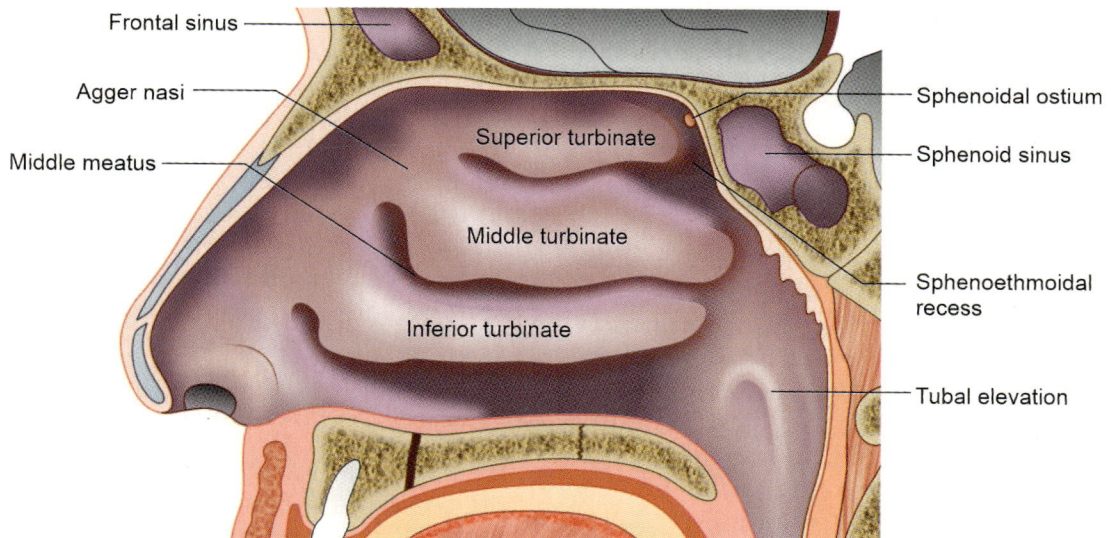

Fig. 1.5a: Anatomy of the lateral nasal wall

corresponds to the ala of the nose and is separated from the rest of the lateral wall (lateral wall proper) by a ridge, limen nasi or limen vestibuli which is formed by the lower end of upper lateral cartilage.

The lateral wall proper, lined by mucosa, bears 3 or 4 nasal conchae or turbinates, which are delicate projecting scrolls of bone covered by mucous membrane (Fig. 1.5a and b).

These are named from below to upwards— inferior, middle and superior conchae. The fourth one, the supreme concha, is present unilaterally or bilaterally in 60% of cases. This is the smallest of all and is usually a mere ridge. The air spaces beneath and lateral to the conchae are termed meati which are named according to turbinates to which they are related, viz. inferior, middle and superior meati. The supreme meatus when present is

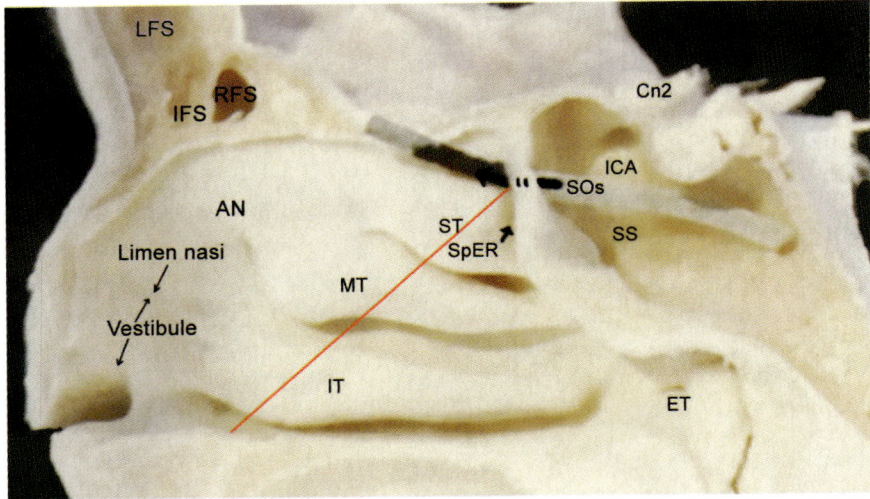

Fig. 1.5b: The vestibule, limen nasi, agger nasi (AN), inferior turbinate (IT), middle turbinate (MT), superior turbinate (ST), arrow leading to opening of sphenoid sinus (SOs), sphenoethmoidal recess (SpER), left frontal sinus (LFS) connected through interfrontal septum (IFS) with right frontal sinus (RFS), interior of sphenoid sinus (SS), bulging of internal carotid artery (ICA) and optic nerve (Cn2) and optic carotid recess appearing as a depression between the two, eustachian tube (ET), the red line denotes the distance between anterior nasal spine to sphenoid ostium to be 7 cm

usually a barely perceptible furrow below supreme concha. The part of the nasal cavity above the uppermost concha and below the body of sphenoid bone is the sphenoethmoidal recess. The sphenoid ostium is about 7 cm from anterior nasal spine (Fig. 1.5b).

All the anterior group of sinuses, viz. the frontal, anterior and middle ethmoid and maxillary sinuses drain into the middle meatus. The posterior group of sinuses, i.e. the posterior ethmoid and sphenoid drain above the middle turbinate. The sphenoid sinus drains into the sphenoethmoidal recess and the posterior ethmoids into the superior or supreme meatus (Figs 1.5 and 1.6).

Both inferior and middle conchae begin anteriorly approximately at the level of the vertical plane of the forehead and extend one below the other almost to the choana.

Anterior to these two conchae, the lateral wall of nose above the limen nasi is more delicately marked, i.e.

1. About halfway between the anterior end of the middle concha and the dorsum of the nose is a slight projection, the agger nasi (Fig. 1.5b). It is derived from the Latin word *agger* meaning mound (Wormald

2005). It is said to be the remnant of additional concha found in lower animals, but is more important in man as it marks the location of anterior most of the anterior ethmoid cells called agger nasi cells. It is situated in the lacrimal bone and is present anterior and superior to the anterior buttress of the middle turbinate. It is the most prominent and constant ethmoidal cell, which is characterized as a bulge in the lateral nasal wall in over 90% of CT scans studied (Womald 2005). The uncinate process and the agger nasi cell are derived from 1st ethmoturbinal. During the process of development, the descending part of the first ethmoturbinal persists as the uncinate process, while the ascending portion regressed as the agger nasi cell (Daniel, et al 2003).

2. The passageway above the agger nasi, the olfactory sulcus, leads to the olfactory area (dangerous area of nose).

3. Below and posterior to the agger nasi, it leads to the middle meatus proper through a shallow depression known as atrium of the middle meatus. This is situated above and anterior to the attached end of inferior turbinate.

The superior concha, about half the length of the other two, begins at about the middle of these. The three conchae converge somewhat towards each other posteriorly and the remaining part of the nasal cavity behind their posterior ends is the nasopharyngeal meatus. This opens into the nasopharynx through the choana. Sphenopalatine foramen is situated in the nasopharyngeal meatus, just midway between posterior ends of middle and superior turbinates. The vessels and nerves here can be traced towards the foramen and their vanishing point helps to locate the foramen.

Inferior Nasal Concha (Fig. 1.6) and Inferior Meatus

Inferior nasal concha is an independent bone covered with thick mucous membrane which contains a vascular, cavernous plexus.

It is so arched that the inferior meatus is narrow anteriorly and posteriorly, but is both wider and higher at the junction of anterior and middle one-third of inferior turbinate. Here the attachment of inferior turbinate curves sharply, called the genu of inferior turbinate.

The nasolacrimal duct opens into the inferior meatus, in its most cephalic part, under the genu of inferior turbinate and is about 15–20 mm from limen nasi and 30–40 mm from the anterior nares. Nasolacrimal duct dysfunction rarely results from surgery of inferior meatus, just under the genu.

The nasolacrimal duct rarely opens lower in the inferior meatus and in such cases the orifice is slit-like, as the duct runs obliquely through the mucous membrane. Here it is usually protected by a fold of mucous membrane, the plica lacrimalis or the valve of Hasner.

Middle Nasal Concha (Fig. 1.6) and Middle Meatus

The lateral wall of nasal cavity above the inferior turbinate is basically formed by the ethmoid labyrinth. Middle nasal concha is a part of the ethmoid labyrinth.

The attachment of middle turbinate to the lateral wall has 2 slopes, the ascending and the descending rami which meet at an angle, the genu of middle turbinate. The genu is situated anteriorly. The highest part of the middle meatus lies below the genu and is known as the frontal recess (Holinshead).

The insertion of the middle turbinate into the lateral wall is called axilla. Creating a flap

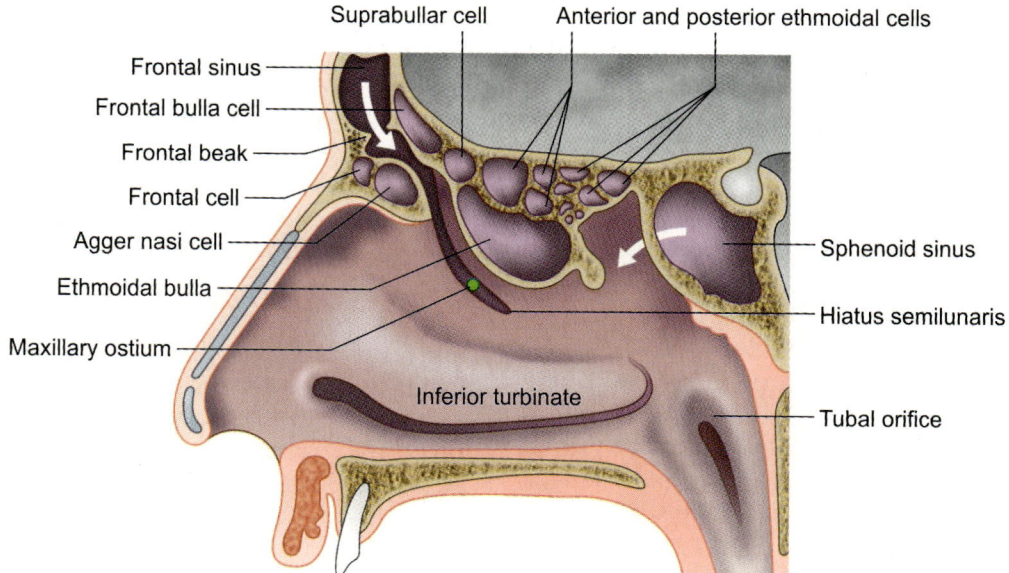

Fig. 1.6a: Endoscopic anatomy of the lateral nasal wall and middle meatus

Labels:
Suprabullar cell
Anterior and posterior ethmoidal cells
Frontal sinus
Frontal bulla cell
Frontal beak
Frontal cell
Agger nasi cell
Ethmoidal bulla
Maxillary ostium
Inferior turbinate
Sphenoid sinus
Hiatus semilunaris
Tubal orifice

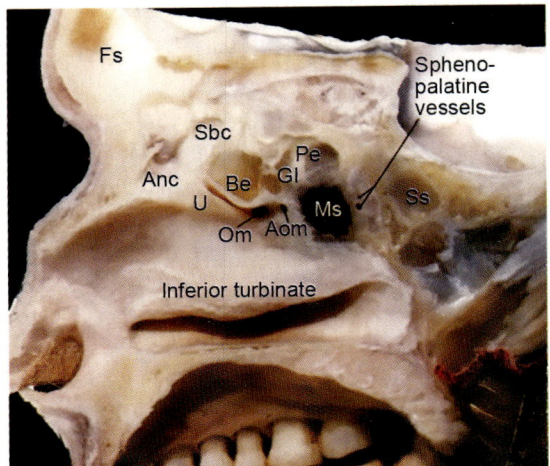

Fig. 1.6b: Structures in the lateral wall parasagittal cut through middle meatus in cadaveric specimen: Frontal sinus (Fs), agger nasi cell (Anc), uncinate process (U), opened bulla ethmoidalis (Be), suprabullar cell (Sbc), posterior ethmoid (Pe), ground lamella (Gl), maxillary ostium (Om), accessory maxillary ostium (Aom), maxillary sinus cavity (Ms) after removal of posterior medial wall

in this region (axillary flap) can overcome the problem in accessing the frontal recess and the frontal sinus (Wormald, 2002). The middle turbinate has three attachments: 1. Junction of cribriform plate and the fovea ethmoidalis, 2. Lamina papyracea, 3. Posterior ethmoid.

The prominent structures in the middle meatus from the anterior to posterior are the uncinate process, the hiatus semilunaris and the bulla ethmoidalis.

The uncinate process is a crescent-shaped ledge of bone, part of the ethmoid, and its posterior free and sharp margin form the anterior margin of a semilunar opening, the hiatus semilunaris. The bulla ethmoidalis, a term introduced by Zukerkandl in 1893, is a rounded projection of the middle meatus, contains one or more ethmoid cells with their delicate walls. These cells are known variously as middle ethmoid or bullar cells. Some consider it as a part of anterior ethmoid. About 30% of ethmoidal bulla poorly pneumatizes and are termed as Torus ethmoidalis (Lang 1988).

The recess above the bulla is called suprabullar recess. This is found when the the

ethmoidal bulla does not reach the skull base and when the dorsal border of bulla does not reach the middle turbinate it is called the retrobullar recess. Part of middle meatus posterosuperior to bulla and anterior to the posterior part of middle turbinate is called sinus lateralis.

The hiatus semilunaris leads to a groove between the uncinate process and bulla and presents as a sagittally oriented cleft (Figs 1.6b and 1.7b). It acts as an entrance to a curved channel known as ethmoidal infundibulum, a term used by Boyer in 1805, which is an upstream of maxillary sinus like a narrow funnel (Messerklinger, 1979). The ethmoidal infundibulum from the hiatus semilunaris extends downwards and forwards and varies in depth from 0.5 to 10 mm (average 5 mm) and therefore the upwardly projecting uncinate process varies in its height. Removal of uncinate process during endoscopic sinus surgery (ESS) exposes the infundibulum (infundibulotomy).

Boundaries of ethmoidal infundibulum (Fig. 1.8): It is a three-dimensional space and is bounded as follows:

- *Anteriorly and superiorly:* Frontal process of maxilla.
- *Anteromedially and anteroinferiorly:* Uncinate process, and the mucosa lining over it.
- *Posteriorly:* Bulla ethmoidalis.
- *Medially:* Communicates with middle meatus through the hiatus semilunaris, which forms the super medial boundary.
- *Laterally:* Lamina papyracea and the lacrimal bone superiorly and the maxillary fontanelle inferiorly.

The relationship of infundibulum to frontal recess is determined by the attachment of the uncinate process. Based on the attachment superiorly with different situations, the uncinate process can be divided as (Fig. 1.7a) depending on the drainage of the frontal sinus (Bolger and Stamburger 1995) although five types have been described by some authors due to combination of primary types. Type-1 comprises 33%, type-2 (10%) and Type-3 attachment or with combinations comprises 57% (Zhang, et al 2016):

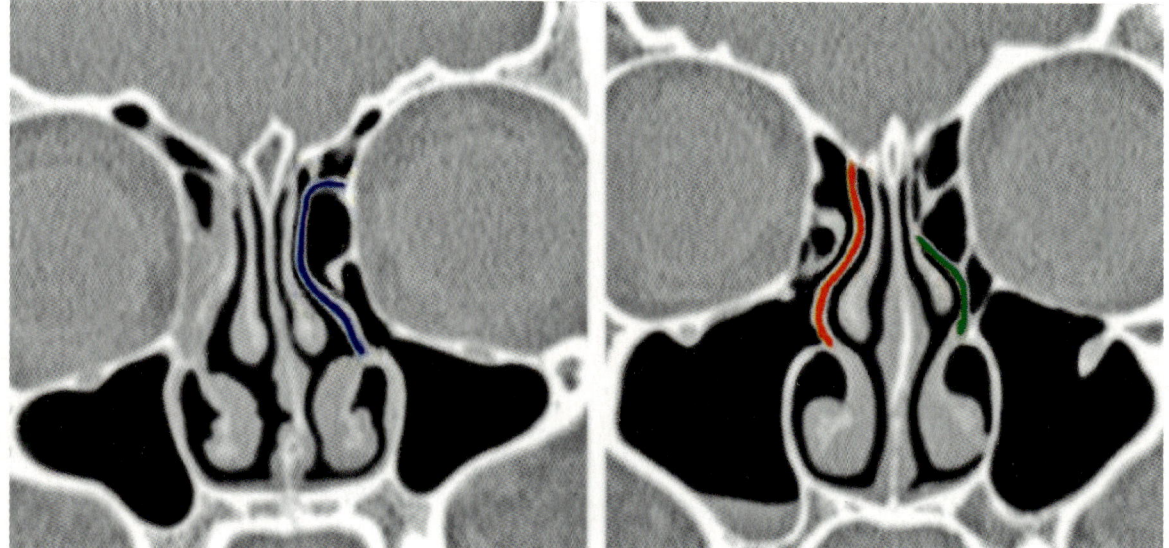

Fig. 1.7a: CT scans showing different types of uncinate process: Type-1 (•), Type-2 (•), Type-3 (•)

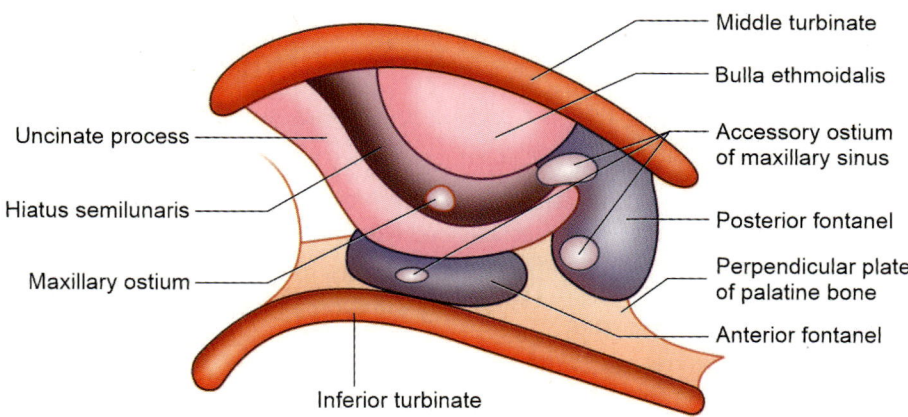

Middle turbinate

Bulla ethmoidalis

Uncinate process

Accessory ostium
of maxillary sinus

Hiatus semilunaris

Posterior fontanel

Maxillary ostium

Perpendicular plate
of palatine bone

Anterior fontanel

Inferior turbinate

Fig. 1.7b: Anatomy of the middle meatus

- Type-1: If inserts at the lamina papyracea
- Type-2: If inserts at the skull base
- Type-3: If inserts at the middle turbinate.

The posteroinferior one-third of the infundibulum receives the natural ostium of the maxillary sinus which is formed by part of the maxillary fontanelle (Fig. 1.7b).

The term **frontal recess** was first used by Killian in 1898. A true frontonasal duct does not exist. Mosher described connection between frontal sinus and anterior ethmoid as a recess. The frontal recess is bounded laterally by the lamina papyracea, medially by the vertical lamella of middle turbinate, anteriorly the agger nasi cell and posteriorly the ethmoidal bulla cells. Van Alyea found the relationship of anterior ethmoidal cells to frontal recess besides agger nasi and termed these cells frontal cells. Agger nasi cell can vary in size and thus can affect the drainage pathway within the frontal recess. Zhang, et al (2006) observed by using spiral CT of skulls and cadaver sectioning, and confirmed that the agger nasi cell was medially, superiorly

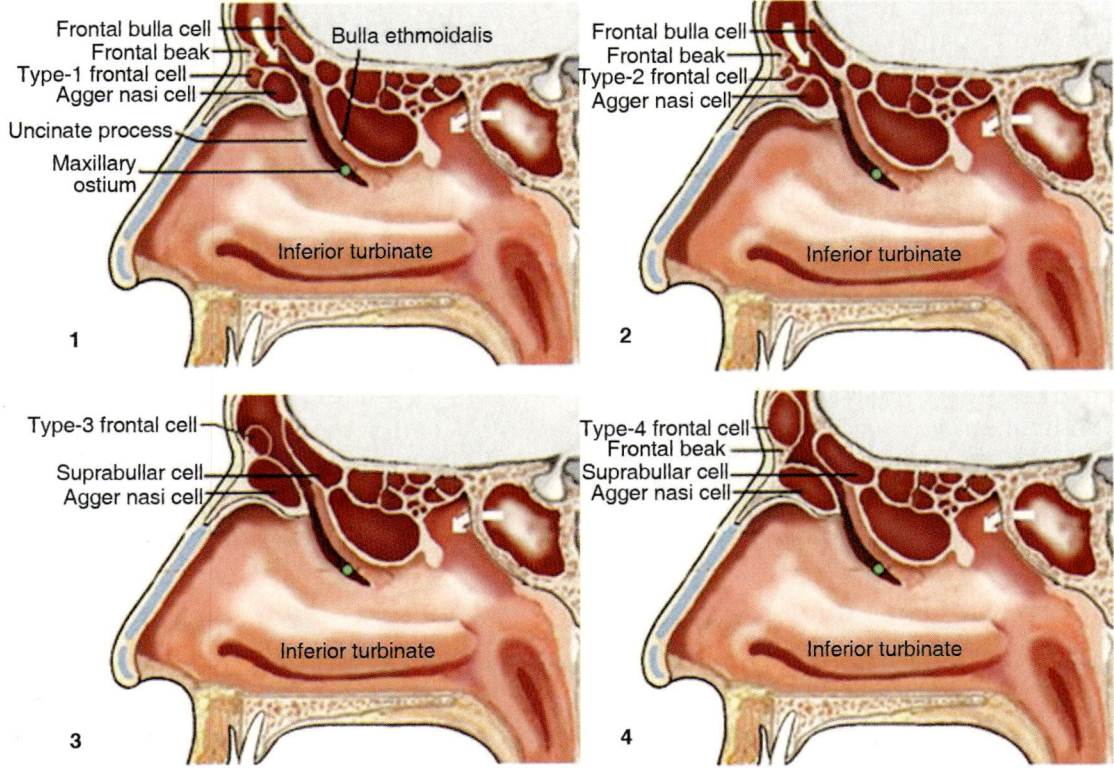

Fig. 1.7c: Four types of frontal cells: **1.** Type-1, **2.** Type-2, **3.** Type-3, **4.** Type-4, classified by Kuhn in1996

and inferiorly bounded by the uncinate process. Nearly 90% of the uncinate processes attached to the lamina papyracea. Kuhn (1996) classified frontal cells into four different types, the modification of this includes (Fig. 1.7c):

- **Type-1:** Single cell above the agger nasi
- **Type-2:** Tier of cells above the agger nasi
- **Type-3:** Cells extending cephalad into the frontal sinus through the ostium but not extending 50% beyond the vertical height.
- **Type-4:** Frontal cell that extends more than 50% beyond the vertical height.

Frontal bulla cell: Cell that extends from the suprabullar area and extends into the frontal sinus along the posterior wall. Wormald, et al (2016) call it as **suprabullar frontal cell.**

Because of the variation in the development of the agger nasi and the frontal cell, the frontal recess surgery is quite challenging and the surgeon needs to have a thorough knowledge and prior radiological evaluation should be done before carefully uncapping

these cells to clear the disease from the frontal recess and the frontal sinus.

Anatomy of drainage pathway anterior group of sinuses: The medial wall of maxillary sinus is partially membranous in the posterior part of middle meatus between the uncinate process, inferior concha and palatine bone, where the bone is dehiscent. This is divided into anterior and posterior fontanelles by the ethmoidal process of the inferior turbinate (Fig. 1.7b). The maxillary sinus opens at the junction of anterior and posterior fontanelles. At the fontanelle, the maxillary sinus mucosa and nasal mucosa are coated with no intervening bone. Any dehiscence in the fontanelle presents as an accessory ostium, thus creating an additional opening into the infundibulum.

Posteriorly and inferiorly, the infundibulum becomes continuous with the middle meatus. Myerson demonstrated that the constant guide to cannulation of maxillary ostium is the angle formed by divergence of the uncinate process and bulla from one another in the posterior part of infundibulum.

The frontal sinus drains either directly or indirectly through the anterior ethmoidal cells into the infundibulum through frontal recess into the middle meatus medial to the infundibulum through the anterior ethmoid cells (Figs 1.7a and d). The frontal ostium is situated between frontal beak anteriorly and skull base posteriorly and is the narrowest area between frontal sinus and frontal recess. The drainage of frontal sinus into the infundibulum is dependent on the three types of superior attachement of the uncinate process. In type 1, it drains medial to the infundibulum and thus directly to the middle meatus, while in type 2 and 3, frontal sinus drains into the infundibulum. Thus frontal sinusitis in type 2 and 3 can cause secondary maxillary sinusitis (Stammberger and Bolger 1995).

The anterior ethmoid cells drain either into the infundibulum (at the frontoethmoidal recess) or anterior to it through the uncinate process (frontal recess of middle meatus).

The middle ethmoid cells open upon or above the bulla (suprabullar recess).

The opinion regarding the location and configuration of maxillary sinus ostium varies with different pioneers.

Myerson (1932) imagined a three-dimensional relationship of maxillary ostium. He opined that the internal ostium leads into a tubular intranasal channel of varying configuration depending on the development of uncinate process and bulla. He recognized that the ostium is located immediately below the orbital floor and the lamina papyracea, and penetrating the lateral wall of infundibulum superior to ostium during surgery can violate the orbit.

Van Alyea (1936) found maxillary ostium situated posteriorly in the infundibulum in two-thirds of cases, in the middle in one-fourth of cases and in the anterior in 70% of cases. He found that the ostium was easily accessible for cannulation in only 40% of specimens.

When viewed from inside the antrum, the internal ostium is situated just 2–3 mm below the junction of medial wall and roof of the sinus, roughly half distance between anterior and posterior walls and about 4 cm from the floor of the antrum. When peered through the ostium towards the nasal cavity, uncinate process is seen anterosuperiorly and bulla posterosuperiorly.

The accessory sinus ostium when present is usually situated posterior to the natural ostium, even though endoscopically due to illusory effect, it appears inferior to natural ostium. Van Alyea found accessory ostium in 23%, Myerson in 31%, Schaeffer in 43%, and Neivert in 25% of specimens.

Thus from the functional standpoint, the infundibular space represents the confluence of drainage from frontal, anterior and middle ethmoidal and maxillary sinuses. The infundibulum like the stem of a funnel collects the drainage from the anterior group of sinuses and opens into the middle meatus through the hiatus semilunaris. All these microchannels are situated in the anterior and middle ethmoid sinuses and hence any anatomical and pathological variation here causes diseases in dependent sinuses (Fig. 1.8).

Noting this clinical significance, Naumann in 1965 described the anterior ethmoid-middle meatus complex as ostiomeatal unit (Fig. 1.8).

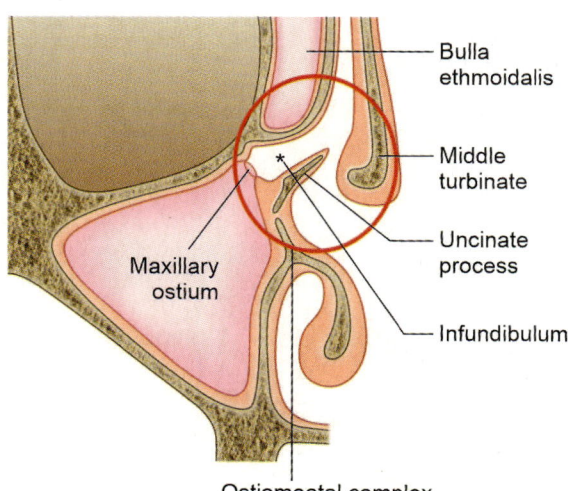

Ostiomeatal complex

Fig. 1.8: The cross-sectional anatomy of ostiomeatal complex

Osteology of Lateral Nasal Wall

Mainly formed by two bones:

1. Ethmoid labyrinth
2. Inferior nasal concha

Other bones participating:

1. Medial wall of maxillary antrum
2. The lacrimal bone
3. Nasal bone
4. Frontal process of maxilla
5. Palatine bone (vertical lamina)

PARANASAL SINUSES

Berenger del Carpi, an anatomist in 16th century, gave clear indication about the existence of the paranasal sinuses (Lund, et al 2002). They are air-filled spaces in the skull bones and are lined by mucosa, which drains into the nasal cavity by the mucociliary drainage. They are 8 in number, 4 on each side, namely the frontal, ethmoidal, maxillary and sphenoidal sinuses. The 4 pairs of paranasal sinuses are lined by ciliated, pseudostratified columnar epithelium. Goblet cells are interspersed among the columnar cells. The mucosa is attached directly to the bone. Involvement of the surrounding bone and further extension

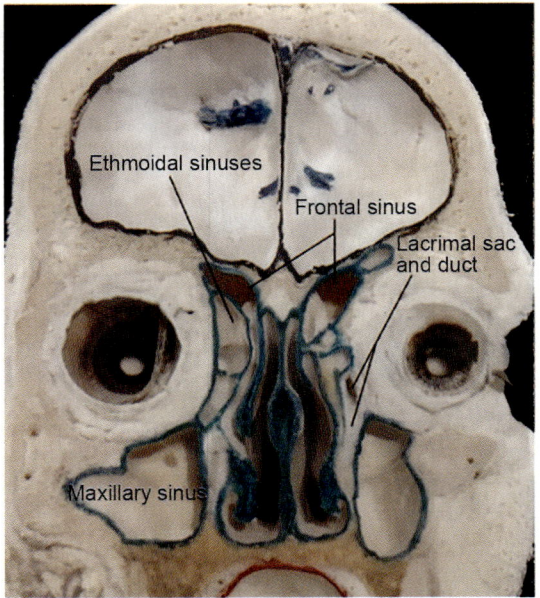

Fig. 1.9: Position of the anterior group of sinuses in the skull

of the infection into the orbital and intracranial compartments occur in inadequately treated patients and in specific types of sinusitis such as fungal sinusitis (Fig. 1.9).

Functionally there are two groups:

1. *Anterior group:* These drain into the middle meatus.
   a. Frontal sinus
   b. Maxillary sinus
   c. Anterior ethmoidal sinus
2. *Posterior group:* These drain into the superior meatus/sphenoethmoidal recess.
   a. Posterior ethmoidal sinus
   b. Sphenoid sinus.

MAXILLARY SINUS (ANTRUM OF HIGHMORE)

Nathaniel Highmore (1651) was first to recognize and describe precisely the maxillary antrum. This is a three-sided pyramidal in shape. In an adult, its capacity is approximately 15 ml (Fig. 1.10).

Base (medial wall) corresponds to the lateral wall of nasal cavity in relation to the middle and inferior turbinates. The ostium of the maxillary sinus opens in the medial wall into the middle meatus between the uncinate process and the bulla ethmoidalis as described under lateral wall of the nasal cavity.

Apex is directed towards zygomatic process.

The three walls of this pyramid are:

a. *Anterolateral wall* covered by the periosteum, soft tissue and skin of the cheek. It is relatively thinner in the canine fossa and is present lateral to the canine eminence. This site is used for approaching the maxillary sinus in Caldwell-Luc operation. This wall has an opening called infraorbital foramen, which is situated about 1 cm below the infraorbital margin. Infraorbital nerve and vessels emerge through this foramen.

b. *Superior wall (roof of antrum)* is formed by orbital plate. This is covered by the orbital periosteum. At its midpoint in its inferior aspect is a groove, through which the infraorbital nerve and vessels pass before emerging out of the infraorbital foramen.

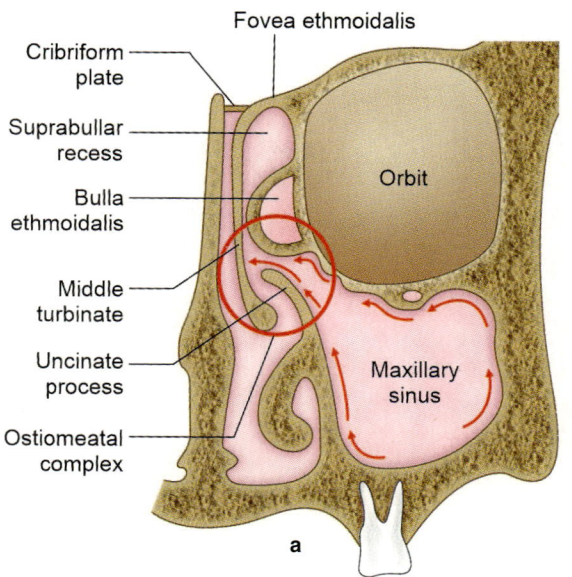

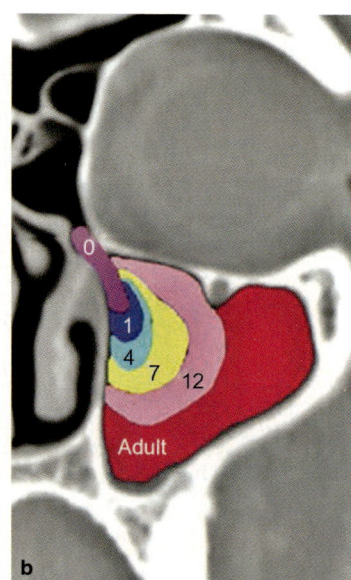

Fig. 1.10: a. Relations of maxillary sinus with respect to orbit, ethmoids and ostiomeatal complex; **b.** Development of maxillary sinus in relation to age—from birth (0) to 12 years of age

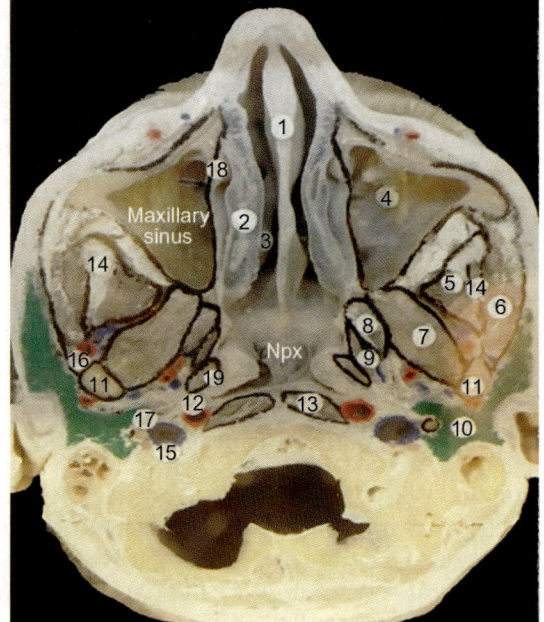

Fig 1.10c: Relationship of the maxillary sinus: (1) Nasal septum, (2) inferior turbinate, (3) middle turbinate, (4) infraorbital nerve and vessels, (5) temporalis muscle, (6) messeter, (7) lateral pterygoid, (8) tensor veli palatini, (9) eustachian tube, (10) parotid gland, (11) mandibular condyle, (12) internal carotid artery, (13) prevertebral muscles, (14) coronoid process, (15) internal jugular vein, (16) external carotid artery, (17) CN IX, X, XI, (18) nasolacrimal duct, (19) levator veli palatini

c. **Posterior wall** is formed by a thin plate of bone and is related to pterygopalatine fossa, which consists of third part of internal maxillary artery, vidian nerve and the sphenopalatine ganglion. Posteromedially the bone is attached to pterygoid plates with a dehiscence called the sphenopalatine foramen. This opens into the lateral wall of the nose just behind the posterior end of the middle turbinate. This foramen transmits the sphenopalatine vessels and the nerves. Knowing various relations to this wall is extremely important for endoscopic surgical approaches to pterygopalatine fossa, pterygoid recess, sphenoid, nasopharynx and middle cranial fossa.

Floor is formed by alveolar and palatine process of the maxilla and is variable with age. It lies at or above the floor of the nasal cavity in a child while it lies at a lower level in an adult (Fig. 1.10b).

FRONTAL SINUS

It is pyramidal in shape and its volume, size and shape is variable and can often be rudimentary. The two frontal sinuses are often asymmetrical in shape. Bony septa may partially subdivide it into one or more compartments. Its average capacity is about

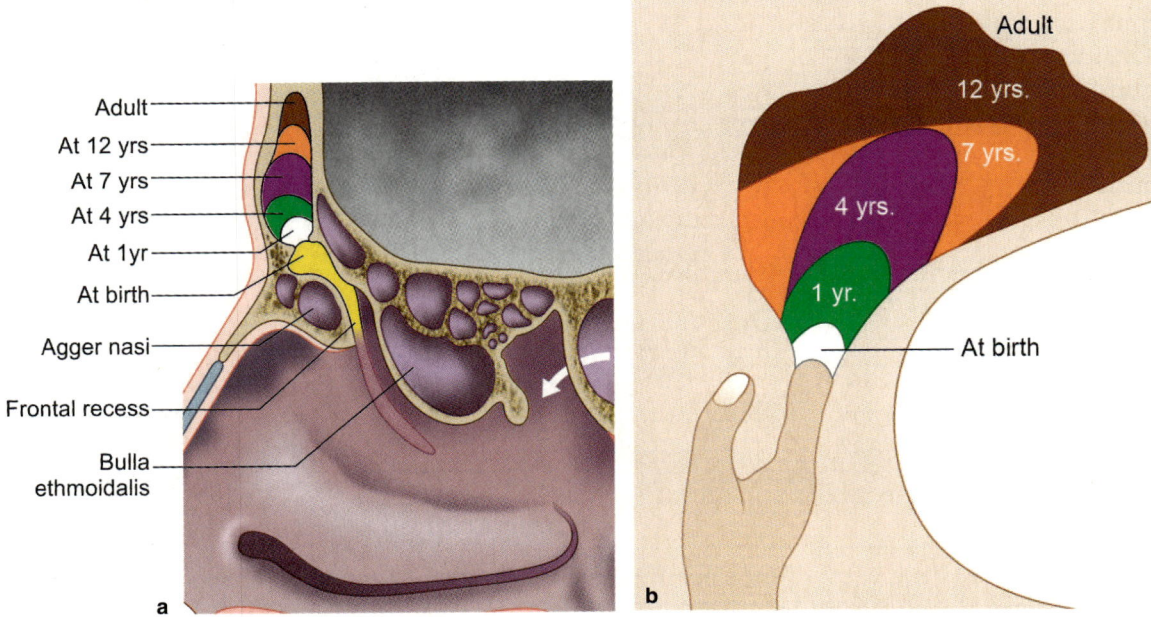

Fig. 1.11: Size and extent of the frontal sinus at various age

7 ml in adults. It is not present at birth and it usually develops after the age of about 5 years as an extension of the anterior ethmoidal air cell. The age-wise expansion of frontal sinus is depicted in Fig. 1.11.

Development of this sinus varies markedly. It develops as one of the several outgrowths from the region of the frontal recess similar to the anterior ethmoidal cells. In fact some regard it as an anterior ethmoid cell that has invaded the frontal bone.

Several sinuses may occur on one or both sides, lying one lateral to other or one behind the other. These sinuses may either drain one into the other or drain separately.

Frontal bulla is cells that pneumatize from the anterior ethmoid into the frontal sinus. Two features distinguish a frontal bulla from a Kuhn type-3 cell:

- It is pneumatized from the region above the ethmoid bulla and along the skull base into the frontal sinus.
- Its posterior wall is formed by the skull base. Its anterior wall directly faces the interior of the frontal sinus.

Frontal bullae may narrow the frontal recess from the posterior side. When combined with agger nasi and Kuhn cells, they may contribute to the obstruction of ventilation and drainage (Leunig, 2008).

Important relations of frontal sinus are the anterior cranial fossa and the orbit. The bone separating the sinus from the above is usually thin and thus an operative perforation can easily occur.

Frontonasal Connections (Frontal Recess)

It is a space posterior to nasal process of frontal bone (frontal beak) to which frontal sinus drains (Wormald, et al. 2016). The drainage of frontal sinus is highly variable and depends on its development, i.e. whether it originates in frontal recess directly or from one or more anterior ethmoid cells (frontal cells) arising in frontal pits (discussed in detail under **ethmoidal sinuses**).

According to Kasper's investigations, the frontal sinus drained into the frontoethmoidal recess directly in 4% of cases and indirectly through the infundibular anterior ethmoidal cells in 34% of cases. In 62%, it drained via the anterior ethmoidal cell into the area below the genu of middle turbinate either anterior, posterior or superior to the frontoethmoidal recess also known as frontal recess, the term first used by Killian in 1903, which is now considered as a key area for surgical approach to frontal sinus (Lee, et al 2004).

Van Alyea opined that anatomical variations such as frontal bulla and blockage of middle meatus caused by impingement of middle turbinate head against lateral wall were the commonest causes of chronic frontal sinusitis. Zhang, et al (2006) found in their study, the interaction between the upper portion of the uncinate process and the agger nasi cells to be important for understanding the anatomy of the frontal recess drainage pathway. Frontal recess is a highly complex space with variable anatomy depending on pneumatization of various cells surrounding this space including agger nasi, frontal cells, suprabullar cells, frontal bullar cells, supraorbital cells and interfrontal cells (Walter, et al 2004). The anatomy of frontal sinus and the recess is like an hourglass with the narrowest part being the ostium. It is bounded mainly by agger nasi cell anteriorly, middle turbinate medially, orbit laterally while posterior boundary depends on the upper attachment of bulla (Daniel, et al 2003).

Position and Relations of Frontal Sinus

- It is situated between the inner and outer table of the frontal bone. It occupies variable amount of frontal bone.
- Floor is formed by orbital roof. As it is relatively thin, it is used as a surgical approach.
- Medially it is separated from the other frontal sinus by a thin interfrontal septum.
- Posterior wall is related to anterior cranial fossa.
- Anterior wall is covered by periosteum and skin of the forehead (Fig. 1.12).

ETHMOIDAL SINUSES

It is well developed in children and it occupies the medial wall of the orbit and upper third of the lateral wall of the nose. It consists of 7 to 15 cells on each side and is divided into two groups based on their drainage. The ethmoidal air cells are small and do not have regular disposition, symmetry or fixed number.

These are situated within the ethmoid labyrinth and separates the nasal cavity from orbit. The ethmoid labyrinth is roughly pyramid shaped with the base posteriorly in relation to sphenoid and apex anteriorly limited by the frontal process of maxilla and nasal process of frontal bone.

It is about 4–5 cm long (anteroposterior), 2.5–3 cm high and about 0.5 cm wide anteriorly and 1.5 cm posteriorly. Thus as a whole, the ethmoid labyrinth forms a thin plate broader posteriorly and thinner anteriorly.

Superiorly, the labyrinthine roof is thicker and is called fovea ethmoidalis. This is limited anteriorly by the inferior wall of frontal sinus and posteriorly by the sphenoidal bone. Superior wall of ethmoid labyrinth/the ethmoidal roof is formed by fovea ethmoidalis and is related to the anterior cranial fossa (ACF). The fovea slopes medially and downward. Its medial part is thinner and may be easily injured. The fovea is at a higher level than the cribriform plate, especially in its lateral part.

Laterally, it is related to the orbit and the lacrimal sac and is separated by a papery thin bone called lamina papyracea.

Posterolaterally, it is related to the sphenoid sinus. The posterior ethmoid cells may extend lateral to the sphenoid sinus where it is related to the optic nerve. These cells are called Onodi's cells.

Medially, the ethmoid labyrinth is related to nasal cavity.

The lateral wall of the ethmoidal labyrinth is attached to several bones that are related to the optic nerve, orbit and the lacrimal sac. They are extremely important to the surgeon as they can be injured or can be surgically approached through this wall. They include frontal bone lying anteriorly and above, lacrimal bone (OS unguis) anteriorly and below. Immediately posterior to these two structures is the lamina papyracea (OS planum) above that separates the orbit and the medial wall of maxilla and the vertical lamina of the palatine bone below.

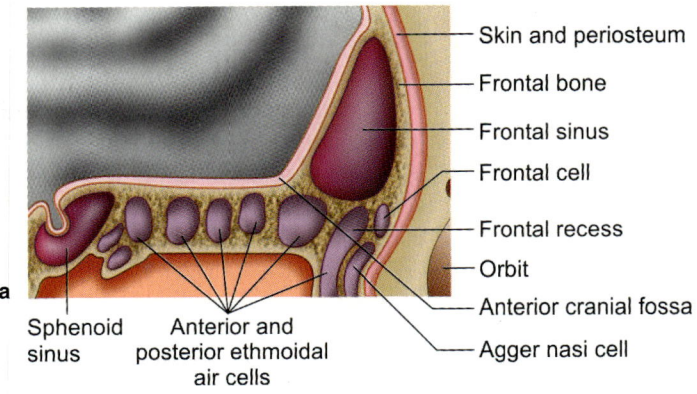

Skin and periosteum
Frontal bone
Frontal sinus
Frontal cell
Frontal recess
Orbit
Anterior cranial fossa
Agger nasi cell

a

Sphenoid sinus

Anterior and posterior ethmoidal air cells

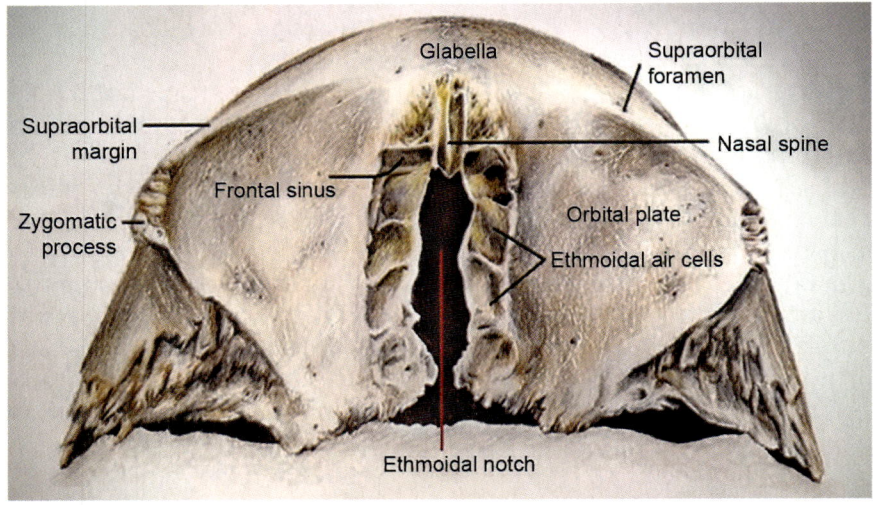

Glabella
Supraorbital foramen
Supraorbital margin
Nasal spine
Frontal sinus
Orbital plate
Zygomatic process
Ethmoidal air cells
Ethmoidal notch

b

Fig. 1.12: a. Relation of the frontal sinus and ethmoids; **b.** Relations of ethmoid and orbit shown in a cadaveric specimen (coronal section)

Inferiorly ethmoid has no wall. Its lower limits are marked by the opening of middle meatus and can, therefore, be considered the horizontal plane passing along the lower margin of middle turbinate.

The medial wall of ethmoid labyrinth consists above of a continuous lamina called turbinate lamina and below of ridges called turbinates (middle, superior and supreme) and corresponding meat.

The medial wall has five principal lamellae which penetrate into the labyrinth towards the lateral wall. They are: 1. Uncinate process, 2. bulla, 3. middle turbinate, 4. superior turbinate and 5. supreme turbinate (Fig. 1.13b).

The more delicate secondary lamellae are placed irregularly between the primary ones, giving rise to multiple ethmoid cells.

1. **Uncinate process lamella** is crescent shaped, curves downwards and backwards with the concave free sharp margin facing upwards. It is inserted obliquely into the external wall forming a part of the infundibular canal. The lower free edge is secured from front to back to the frontal process of maxilla, lacrimal bone and maxillary sinus medial wall immediately above the attachment of inferior turbinate.

The uncinate process lamella posteriorly terminates in a partially membranous wall of maxilla (fontanelle) where it splits onto several slender extensions which reinforce the membranous wall.

2. **Bullar lamella:** Few millimeters behind and above the uncinate process is a second arched lamella which forms a dome-shaped

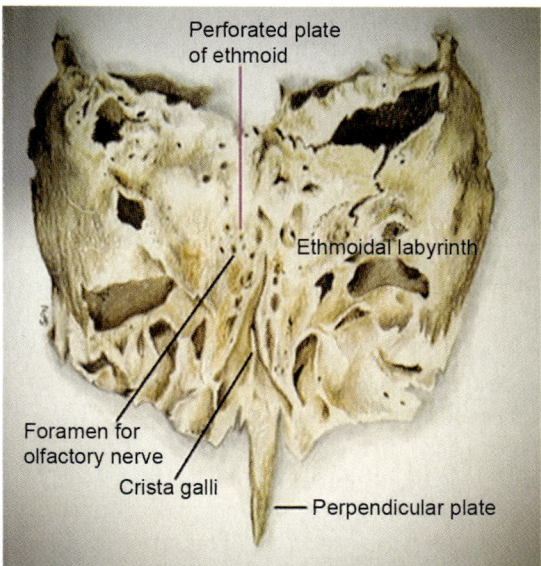

Fig. 1.13a: Ethmoid bone

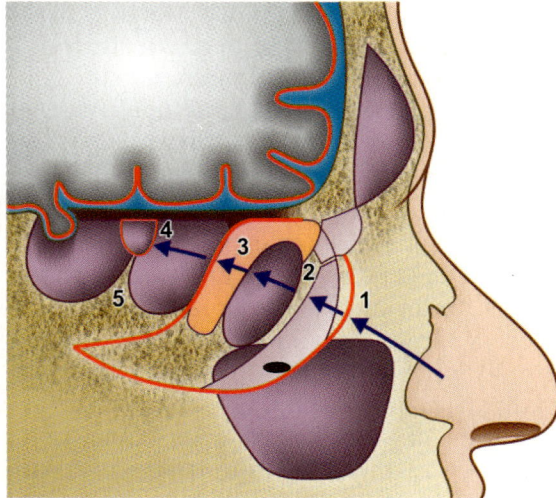

Fig. 1.13b: Five principal lamellae of the medial wall of ethmoid

protuberance called the bulla ethmoidalis. This lamella is applied laterally on the papyraceous lamina. Posteriorly, it is attached to the front of the middle turbinate lamella, forming a sulcus, the suprabullar sulcus.

3. *Middle turbinate lamella* is the least variable. It consists of two parts: One lateral (lamina basilaris) and another medial (lamina recurvata), perpendicular to each other. The lamina basilaris (ground lamella) forming the posterior part of

middle turbi-nate runs obliquely downwards and back-wards from the anterior ethmoid roof to a small crest of palatine bone (vertical branch) near sphenopalatine foramen, towards the lateral surface of the labyrinth (lamina papyracea). The lamina basilaris separates the middle and posterior ethmoidal cells.

The lamina recurvata forming the anterior part of middle turbinate ascends upwards lining the ethamoid air cells medially and is attached to the roof of ethmoid at the junction of fovea with the cribriform plate.

The lamina recurvata thus forms the anterior part of the turbinate lamina. The middle turbinate thus has two attachments:

- To the lamina papyracea via basal lamina.
- To the ethmoid roof (junction of fovea and cribriform plate) via lamina recurvata.

4. *The superior turbinate lamella* (present in 85% of cases). This divides the posterior ethmoidal cells into two groups—one above and one below the lamella.

5. *Lamella of the sphenoid sinus:* The ethmoids during their development have a tendency to grow steadily in all directions beyond the confines of ethmoid until deterred by hard compact bone. The cells which reside within the ethmoid bone are termed intramural cells and those outside are called extramural cells. Thus the ethmoid cells may invade the supraorbital plate of frontal bone, infraorbital plate of maxilla, the middle turbinate (concha bullosa), the sphenoid and lacrimal bone. The frontal sinus is considered by some as part of ethmoid which has invaded the frontal sinus.

The extent of pneumatization of ethmoid has definite implication in an endoscopic sinus surgery.

The *anterior group of cells*, according to Bagatella and Guirado (1983), consists of 2–10 cells, their number being inversely proportional to their size. They are topographically divided into four subgroups from front to back as:

1. *Preinfundibular cell* (0–1) or agger nasi cell: Derived form the latin word '*nasal*

mound' is the remnant of 1st ethmoturbinal. The agger nasi cell is first to pneumatize in newborn, is bounded anteriorly by frontal process of maxilla, anterolaterally by nasal and lacrimal bones, laterally by lamina papyracea, superiorly by frontal sinus and inferiorly by uncinate process depending on pneumatization (Yanagisawa and Joe 1999).

2. *Lateral infundibular cells* (0–2) situated lateral to infundibulum, between the frontal process of maxilla, floor of frontal sinus and lacrimal bone. In over pneumatized state, these can invade the above bones. These cells are consistent with frontal and lacrimal cells. These cells are situated above the agger cell hence called **supra-agger frontal cell** (Wormald 2016).

3. *Postinfundibular cells* (0–2) situated posterior to infundibulum and anterior to bulla, between the papyraceous lamina and the floor of frontal sinus. These cells are suprabullar and frontal bulla cells. These cells are also called **suprabullar frontal cells** (Wormald, et al 2016).

4. *The bullar cells* (2–5): These are suprabullar cells a subset of variably present frontal recess cells and frontal bullar cells that extends into the frontal sinus along its posterior table.

The **posterior ethmoidal cells** are of two types:

1. *Intramural cells*, which are located within the ethmoid bone.

2. *Extramural cells*, which are located in the adjacent bones like maxilla and sphenoid bones, like Haller cells, Onodi cells.

The posterior ethmoidal cells are situated behind the level of the basal lamella and above the horizontal attachment of the middle turbinate to the lateral nasal wall. The posterior ethmoid cells are large and more rectangular in shape with their lateral wall in close contact with optic nerve. At a lower level, the sphenoid rostrum, protrudes into the posterior ethmoid cells at the midline like the nose cone of a rocket. Thus here the sphenoid ostium is surrounded by the posterior ethmoidal cells.

Here, the surgeon, who tries to enter the sphenoid through the posterior ethmoid, has to be cautious not to mistake the junction the sphenoid rostrum and roof of posterior ethmoid cells for the anterior sphenoidal wall. If mistaken, a craniotomy could be performed.

SPHENOIDAL SINUS

The sphenoid bone is situated in the posterior part of the nasal cavity and separates it from the anterior and middle cranial cavity. It has a body and two wings (greater and lesser) on either side giving the appearance of a bat. The sphenoid sinus is situated in the body of sphenoid. The sinuses of the two sides are divided by an asymmetrically placed median intersphenoidal septum. The sphenoid sinus drains into the sphenoethmoidal recess. It is related to a number of important structures because of its situation in the skull.

This sinus appears and begins to grow only after 3rd year and actually excavate the body of sphenoid. The degree of pneumatization of this sinus is highly variable. Its capacity is said to vary from 0.5 to 30 ml (average 7.5 ml).

The sinus either may be limited to the body of sphenoid, or it may extend to other parts of sphenoid, namely the greater and lesser wings, anterior clinoid process, pterygoid process, etc. and also to the basilar portion of the occipital bone. As the degree of pneumatization increases, the surrounding vital relations like optic nerve, ICA, maxillary nerve, etc. are brought more into the sinus cavity producing corresponding bulges into the cavity. ESS in such state is more dangerous.

The sphenoid sinus opens into the sphenoethmoidal recess (Fig. 1.6) usually through the posterior wall of the recess. Occasionally, it may open through the lateral wall of the recess. Anatomical variations can have an impact on approaching the pituitary through transphenoidal route. The type of sphenoid sinus can be classified into three groups in adults (Fig. 1.14a):

1. Conchal (area below the sella is solid block of bone without air cavity)

2. Presellar (moderate air cavity with no sellar indentation)

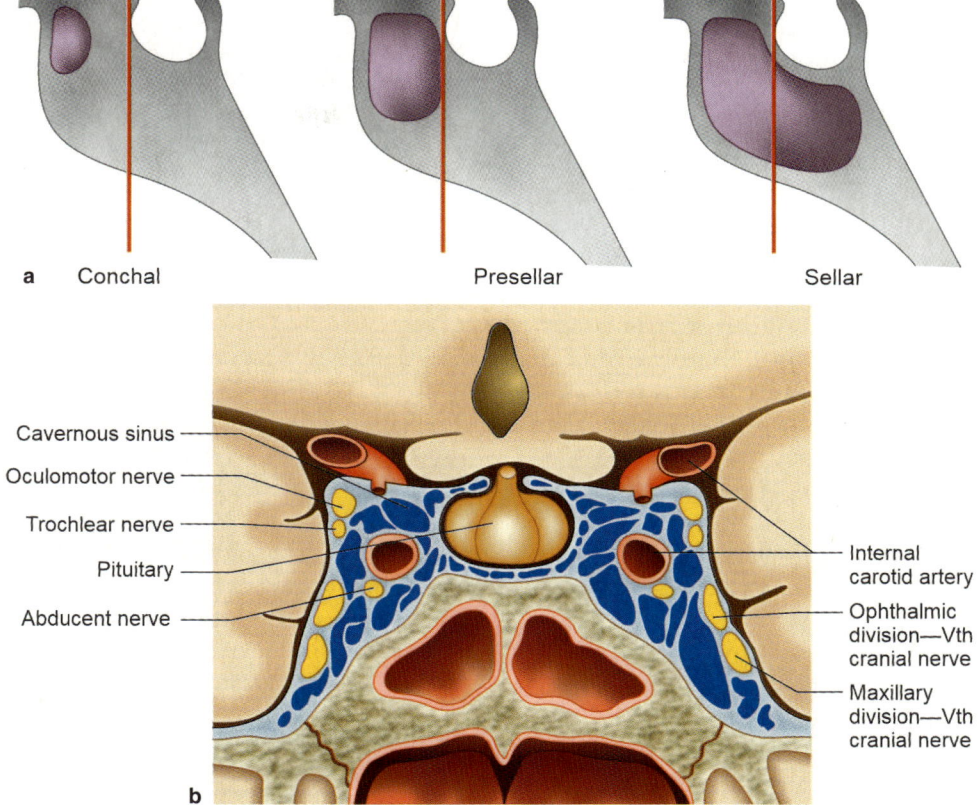

a   Conchal   Presellar   Sellar

Cavernous sinus
Oculomotor nerve
Trochlear nerve
Pituitary
Abducent nerve

Internal
carotid artery

Ophthalmic
division—Vth
cranial nerve

Maxillary
division—Vth
cranial nerve

b

Fig. 1.14: a. Pneumatization of sphenoid sinus; **b.** Relations of the sphenoid sinus and contents of the cavernous sinus

3. Sellar (well-pneumatized sphenoid cavity with full indentation of sella)

Relations (Fig. 1.14b)

Superiorly

1. Pituitary gland bulges into the sphenoid sinus posterosuperiorly. This is often used as a surgical approach (transsphenoidal hypophysectomy).
2. Optic chiasma
3. Olfactory tract
4. Frontal lobe of the brain

Anteriorly

1. Sphenopalatine foramen
2. Sphenoidal crest
3. Nasal cavity

Inferiorly

1. Nasopharynx and choana

2. Vidian nerve is situated inferolaterally and its position helps in vidian neurectomy.

Posteriorly

1. Basilar artery
2. Brainstem

Laterally

1. Cavernous sinus and its contents (III, IV, V and VI cranial nerves).
2. Internal carotid artery

Vital Relations of Sphenoethmoidal Sinuses

Orbit

The ethmoid labyrinth is separated from the orbit by only a thin bone 'the lamina papyracea'. Apart from this, the lamina may have natural dehiscences especially in the two cranial quarters. This permits infection to spread from ethmoids to orbit (5.6% in Kozlov's series and 14/1188 skulls in Zuckerlandl's series had natural dehiscences).

The inferomedial aspect of lamina papyracea forms the lateral boundary of ethmoid infundibulum in close relation to the maxillary sinus ostium.

Thus an attempt to perform middle meatal antrostomy superior to the natural ostium violates the orbit.

A previous ethmoid surgery is likely to have distorted the nasal anatomy, and also could have caused dehiscence in the lamina, thus making prone to orbital injury during ESS (Fig. 1.15).

Injury to the lamina at the plane of anterior ethmoid artery could cause injury to medial and superior rectus causing diplopia.

Optic Nerve

This lies in close apposition to the lateral aspect of posterior ethmoid and sphenoid. The optic canal varying in length from 5.5 to 11.5 mm (av 9.22 mm) runs between the two roots of the lesser wing of sphenoid after coming in relation to posterior ethmoid.

Its distal opening termed the optic ring borders the most posterior ethmoid cells in about 50% of cases, on the sphenoid sinus in

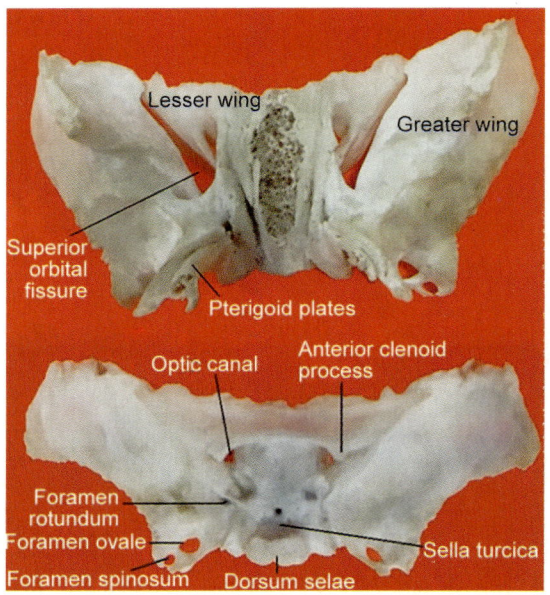

Fig. 1.15b: Sphenoid bone as seen from below: Sphenoid bone anterior wall with conchal type rudimentary sphenoid sinus open through anterior wall and posterior wall and above (cranial aspect)

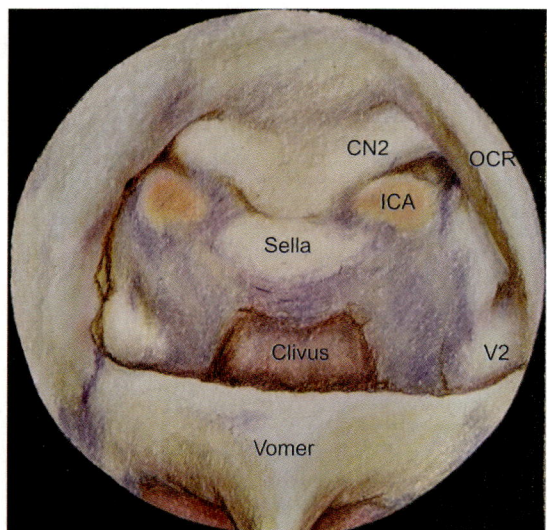

Fig. 1.15c: Interior of right sphenoid sinus endoscopic visualization through the ostium showing optic nerve (CN2), internal carotid artery (ICA), optic carotid recess (OCR) and maxillary nerve (V2)

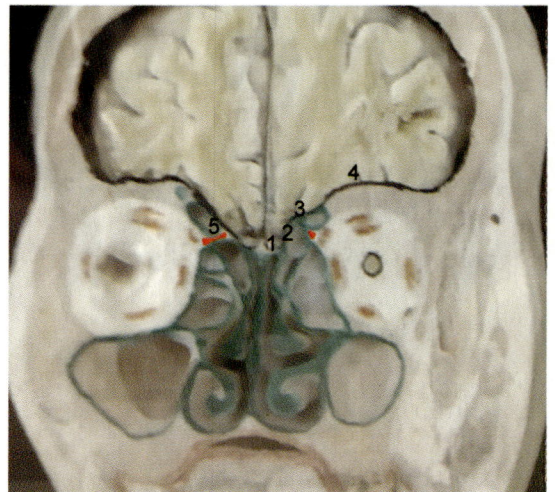

Fig. 1.15a: Relation of ethmoid and orbit in cadaveric specimen: 1—Cribriform plate, 2—lateral lamella, 3—fovea ethmoidalis, 4—orbital plate and 5—anterior ethmoidal artery

25% and on the partition separating the two sinuses in other 25% of cases. Thus, in nearly 75% of cases, the optic nerve is not only in close relationship with sphenoid sinus, but also with the ethmoid sinus as well. In 25% of

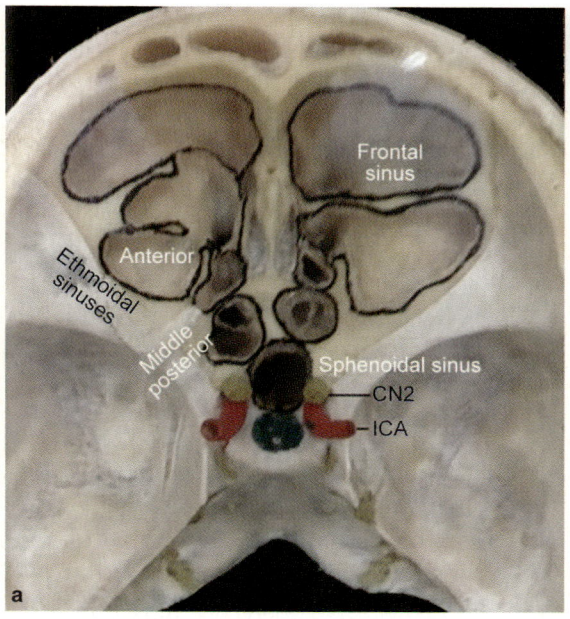
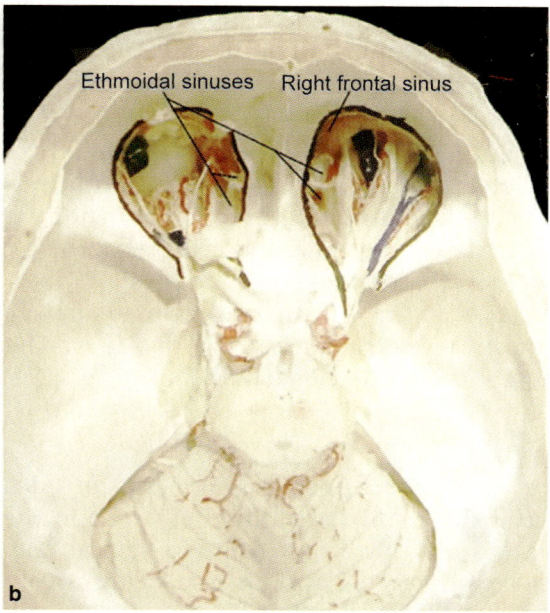

Fig. 1.16: a. Vital relations of sphenoid and ethmoids, orbital contents, optic nerve (CN2) and internal carotid artery (ICA) shown in cadaveric specimen with well-pneumatized frontal and ethmoid sinuses; **b.** Less pneumatized frontal and ethmoid sinuses. Note the orbital apex is directly related to middle cranial fossa

cases, the nerve is almost completely surrounded by an air space (Fig. 1.16).

During its course, the optic nerve produces against the superolateral wall of sphenoid, a bulge called optic bulge (Fig 1.5b) which is more pronounced in over pneumatized sphenoid cells. Such eminence was missing in only one of the 50% specimens investigated by Fuji, *et al*. They found that 78% of specimens had less than a 0.5 mm thickness of bone separating the nerve from sinus and dehiscence were present in 4%. Similar findings were observed by Maniscalco and Habal (1978), Meloni, *et al*. observed optic eminence with extremely thin bone in 70% patients by axial CT scans.

Internal Carotid Artery (ICA)

Similar to optic nerve, the internal carotid artery can also produce bulges into the sphenoid sinus between the bulging optic nerve and ICA, there is a recess called optic carotid recess (Fig. 1.5b).

Van Alyea found 65% of arteries bulging into the sinus. In 14% the whole serpentine course of vessel could be tracked along the lateral sinus wall. Renn and Rhoton (1975) reported carotid prominence in 71% of specimens. In 66%, the thickness of bone separating the artery from sinus was less than 1 mm and dehiscence was noticed in 4%. According to Fuji, *et al*., the bony layer separating was thinner than 0.5 mm in 88% of specimens and dehiscence found in 8%. Teatani, *et al*. observed carotid prominence in 72% of axial CT scans.

Lacrimal Sac and Nasolacrimal Duct

The medial wall of lacrimal sac roughly corresponds to the atrium of the middle meatus. The anterior ethmoid cells may invade the lacrimal bone and in such conditions the lacrimal sac is vulnerable to injury by an ESS which is very rare.

The **nasolacrimal duct** runs from the lacrimal fossa downwards but slightly backwards and laterally and lies in a bony wall (nasolacrimal canal) between the maxillary sinus and nasal cavity. In the canal, the duct is closely fused to the periosteum.

Whitnall found close contact between anterior ethmoidal cells and upper half of lacrimal fossa in all 100 orbits he examined, and in more than half of these, the fossa was directly related to these cells. The lower half of the fossa was found, in every instance, directly related to the middle meatus.

The nasolacrimal duct may be injured during a middle meatal antrostomy when the ostium is enlarged anteriorly with a backbiting forceps. The duct lies 8–17 mm (av 10 mm) anterior to the ostium and approximately 5 mm from the anterior border of the membranous anterior fontanelle.

Anterior Ethmoidal Artery

The anterior and posterior ethmoidal arteries leave the orbit through their respective foramina in the frontoethmoid suture line, approximately 24 and 36 mm, respectively from anterior lacrimal crest. The arteries cross across the sinus having a brief intracranial course and enter the nose through their own foramina just below the cribriform plate.

During the intracranial course, at the skull base, the anterior ethmoidal artery runs in a partial or complete bony conduit at the junction of anterior and middle ethmoid cells, usually being attached to the ethmoidal roof by a bony septum.

This artery is a useful landmark during FESS as it indicates the level of fovea and thus the superior limit of ethmoidectomy. The artery is likely to be injured during ESS.

Anterior Cranial Fossa

The cribriform plate and the fovea separate the anterior cranial fossa from nasal cavity and ethmoids, respectively.

The cribriform plate is the most dependent portion of the anterior cranial fossa and forms the roof of the nasal cavity. It is perforated by nerve filaments of the olfactory nerve. Anteriorly the middle turbinate is attached to it by means of the planum recurvatum. This attachment is at the junction of fovea and cribriform plate.

The fovea ethmoidalis is the roof of the ethmoid labyrinth and lies at a higher level than cribriform plate. The former sharply dips down medially and gets attached to the latter. The medial aspect of fovea is very thin and can be easily damaged.

The surface of fovea is undulating and descends 15° from the horizontal as it passes posteriorly.

The level of cribriform plate is marked by the mid-pupillary line externally and by level of ethmoid foramina within the orbit.

The fovea ethmoidalis was found to be 4–7 mm higher than the level of cribriform plate in about 70%. Based on this depth, Keros (1962) described the olfactory fossa into three types: Type-I (0–3 mm), Type-II (4–7 mm), and Type-III (8–16 mm). Also the two cribriform plates could be found at different levels. During ethmoidectomy, staying lateral to the middle turbinate will prevent violation of cribriform plate. Traction to the mid-turbinate during nasal procedures may injure the cribriform plate.

Bone defects in the fovea have been reported. Kozlov observed them in 8.5% of 70 cadaver dissections. The dura is closely applied to the roof of the ethmoid and hence CSF leak easily occurs by injury to fovea. During ethmoidectomy, identify the fovea a yellowish bone. Anterior ethmoidal artery also suggests the level of fovea. Staying below this level helps in prevention of injury to fovea. At the region of anterior ethmoidal artery, the fovea was found to be 10 times thinner than the neighbouring roof (Stammberger).

Blood Supply of the Paranasal Sinuses

Infraorbital and superior dental arteries derived from the internal maxillary artery supply maxillary sinus.

Branches of the anterior and posterior ethmoidal artery supply ethmoidal and frontal sinuses.

Sphenoid sinus is supplied by pharyngeal branch of the internal maxillary artery.

Development of the Nose and Paranasal Sinuses

Nose develops from a number of mesenchymal processes surrounding the primitive stomodeum. The frontonasal process arises between the central aspect of the forebrain and the epithelial roof of the mouth. A highly specialized ectodermal tissue called olfactory placode develops during the 6th week of intrauterine life, on each side of ventral surface of the frontonasal elevation. This divides it into median and lateral nasal processes. The olfactory placode sinks in to form the olfactory pit (Fig. 1.17).

The extension of the mesenchyme from the median process gives rise to premaxillary process of the developing mouth. This subsequently also forms the upper lip and medial crus of the lower lateral cartilage. In the mean time, another mesenchymal process,

the maxillary process, develops from the dorsal end of the mandibular arch and this fuses with the lateral nasal process, the two being separated by the nasomaxillary groove. Ectoderm along the boundaries of these two processes remains, giving rise to the nasolacrimal ridge from which the nasolacrimal duct arises later. The lateral nasal process forms the nasal bones, the upper lateral cartilages and the lateral crus of the lower lateral cartilages. The median maxillary process fuses with the median nasal elevation leading to the formation of the primitive external nares. From this, a deepening pit in the mesenchyme produces the nasal cavity. The primitive nose

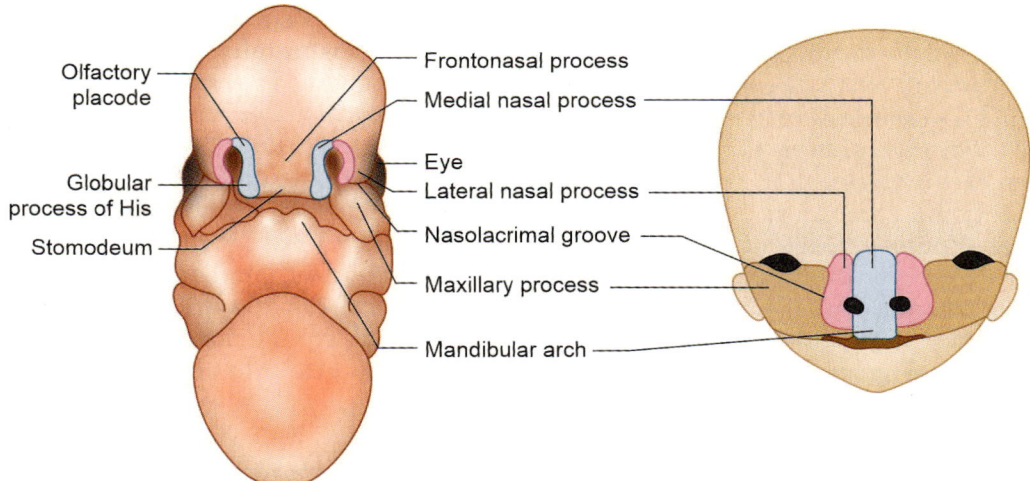

Fig. 1.17a: Embryo showing early stage (5 weeks) of development of nose, nasal and related structures and development at 10th week of gestation

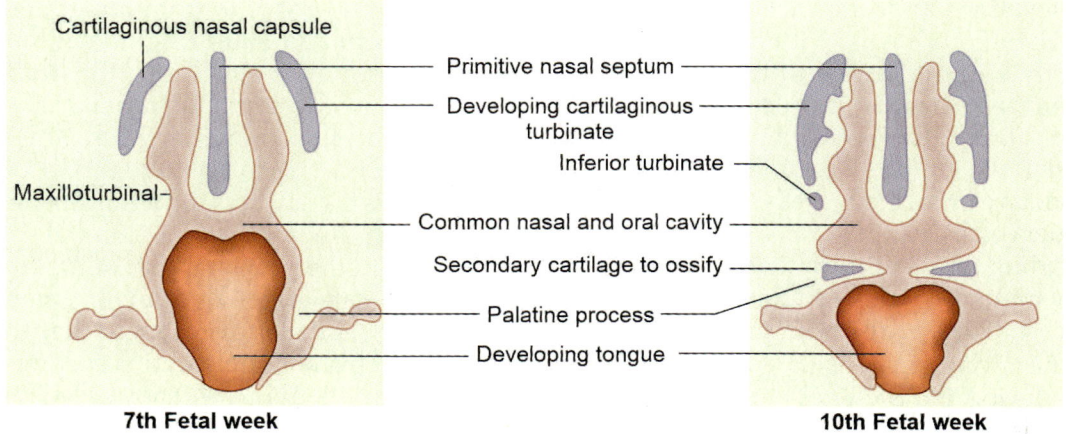

7th Fetal week   **10th Fetal week**

Fig. 1.17b: Development of nasal septum

and mouth are separated by the bucconasal membrane, which disappears later to facilitate communication posteriorly through a primitive choana. This is situated just behind the primitive palate. Failure to canalise leads to choanal atresia. Initially the external nares are widely separated but later come closer as the frontonasal process reduces gradually.

The precartilaginous nasal septum is formed from the frontonasal process. The cartlaginous extension to this nasal septum from the body of the sphenoid bone forms the primary cartilage of this primitive nasal septum. The primitive nasal septum is initially entirely cartilaginous. The superior portion undergoes ossification to form the perpendicular plate of the ethmoid. The premaxillary and the maxillary proceses establish the continuity with the primitive nasal septum, thus defining the two primitive nasal cavities. On each side of the anterior nasal septum, an invagination of the ectoderm represents the vomeronasal organ which is vestigial in human being. The vomer ossifies in the connective tissue covering the residual posterior inferior cartilage from two centres, which unites below the cartilage creating a deep grove in which the the developing septal cartilage (quadrilateral cartilage) lodges. As the growth continues, the bony lamellae fuse and the cartilage gets absorbed. At puberty, the lamellae are almost completely united with the everted alae. An anterior groove remains suggestive of the vomer's bilamellar origin. On the lateral wall of the nose, a series of elevations appears (three ethmoturbinals and maxilloturbinals) within the nasal cavity at 6th week of intrauterine life, which ultimately forms the turbinates. The ossification of the nose and nasal cavity starts during 5th month of fetal life, including the previous cartilaginous areas of the turbinates. Influenced by various transcriptional factors, including Sox, cells differentiate further into the various cell types including the respiratory mucosa (Park, et al 2006).

The development of the sinuses arise rather late during the prenatal period. The frontal sinus is the last to develop. In the first and second months of intrauterine life, the main features of the nasal cavities are defined. The paranasal sinuses arise as localized epithelial invaginations or recesses of the nasal mucosa, after the second month. These recesses become the ostia of the various sinuses. The maxillary sinus and sphenoidal sinus arise as mucosal recess during the 3rd prenatal month. The invagination developing from the hiatus semilunaris forms the future maxillary sinus. The maxillary sinus is present at birth and most of the growth occurs in first 8 years and the maximal size is reached by 16 years of age (Fig. 1.11). The age related size of the sinus can be best studied by CT scan (Lorkiewicz-MuszyMuszynskaska, et al 2015). In contrast to the paranasal sinuses, which develop into existence postnatally, the ethmoid exists before birth and is simply ventilated afterward. The cartilaginous forerunner of the ethmoid starts to develop from the beginning of the 8th week of embryonic life, in parallel with the olfactory region of the nasal cavity (Muller and O'Rahilly 2004). The ethmoidal cells originate during the 5th and 6th months of the IUL from the middle and superior meatus into anterior and posterior groups. They are divided into anterior and posterior groups respectively based on their origin. The frontal sinus (Fig. 1.11) develops after birth with a lot of variation due to different source of origin like either direct extension of the frontal recess into the frontal bone, in which case the frontal sinus drainage pathway is through a distinct ostium (primary frontal sinus ostium) or if it is from the ethmoidal infundibulum and takes origin from one or more anterior ethmoidal cells, the drainage pathway is restricted to the frontonasal duct. The growth of surrounding ethmoidal cells can encroach upon the proximal part of the frontal sinus to compress the nasofrontal duct. The growth of surrounding ethmoidal cells can encroach the proximal part of the frontal sinus and can affect the development of frontal sinus and may even exceed the growth of primary frontal sinus and sometime can present as a bullous presentation called frontal bulla {Fig 1.7c (2)}.

ORBITAL ANATOMY

The orbits divide the upper facial skeleton from the middle face. They are conical in shape and surround the organs of vision (Turvey and Golden 2012). The orbit is closely related to the paranasal sinuses. Each orbit is composed of **seven bones** including ethmoid, sphenoid, maxilla, zygomatic, frontal, lacrimal and palatine bone. The ethmoid sinus is separated from the orbit by a papery thin plate of bone called lamina papyracea. The lateral wall of the sphenoid sinus is closely related to the orbital apex and the optic nerve. Frontal sinus is related to the roof of the orbit and if over-pneumatized, the frontal sinus may even form the entire roof of the orbit. The roof of the maxillary sinus forms the floor of the orbit. Any inflammatory, traumatic or neoplastic lesion of the paranasal sinuses may complicate the orbit and similarly an orbital lesion may present in or could be surgically accessed through the sinuses. Moreover, the orbital anatomy is important for endoscopic sinus surgeon to perform endoscopic dacryocystorhinostomy. It is important to note that the lateral orbital wall and orbital apex are related to the middle cranial fossa (MCF) and the orbital roof is related to the anterior cranial fossa (Fig. 1.16b).

Orbit is a quadrilateral pyramid with its base facing forwards, laterally and slightly inferiorly. The average volume of orbit is 30 ml, of which 70% is occupied by retrobulbar structures. Orbit is made up of **seven bones**, namely sphenoid, lacrimal, palatal, maxillary, ethmoid, frontal, and zygomatic. It has also **seven important contents**, namely the globe (7 ml), extraocular muscles (EOM), optic nerve, cranial nerves III, IV, V and VI, blood vessels, lacrimal gland and sac, orbital fat. The intraorbital muscles are also seven in number except sphincter oculi muscles. There are also seven orbital nerve which passes through the superior orbital fissure except the optic nerve, that passes through optic canal (Rai and Rattan 2012).

The orbit consists of four walls (Fig. 1.18):
- Medial
- Lateral
- Superior (roof)
- Inferior (floor)

Medial Wall

- It is composed of
  - Frontal process of maxilla
  - Lacrimal bone
  - Lamina papyracea of ethmoid
  - Body of sphenoid
- At the frontoethmoid suture, where the medial wall meets the roof, foramina for anterior and posterior ethmoidal vessels and nerves are located.
- Ethmoid foramina are also indicators of level of cribriform plate.

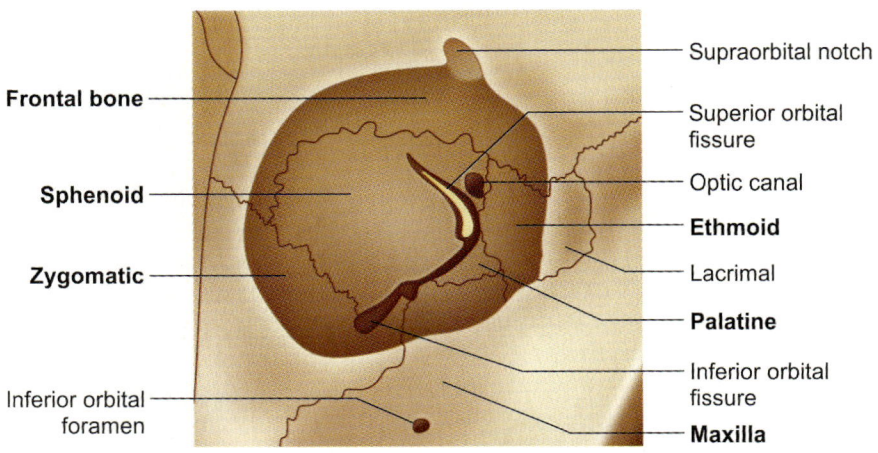

Fig. 1.18: Orbital anatomy

- Rule of 24-12-6 (Rontal, *et al.*)
  - Distance from anterior lacrimal crest to anterior ethmoid foramen—24 mm
  - Distance from anterior to posterior ethmoid foramen—12 mm
  - Distance from posterior ethmoid foramen to optic canal—6 mm
  - Lacrimal fossa for lacrimal sac lies between anterior and posterior lacrimal crests
- As the medial wall is thin in parts and could be dehiscent, there is risk for orbital cellulitis, from spread of paranasal sinus infection or mucocele.

Lateral Wall

- Greater wing of sphenoid
- Orbital surface of zygoma
- Zygomatic process of frontal bone:
  - Posterior boundaries of lateral wall could be taken as the superior and inferior orbital fissures.
  - **Superior orbital fissure** is about 28 mm from the frontozygomatic suture at the orbital rim.
  - Optic nerve lies 8 mm behind the medial edge of the superior orbital fissure (SOF).
  - SOF extends posteriorly to the cavernous sinus.
  - Lateral wall is encountered in:
    - Orbital decompression
    - Lateral craniotomy
    - Infratemporal fossa surgery
    - Lateral orbitotomy
    - Exploration of fractures

Superior Wall (Roof)

- Triangular in shape and consists of:
  - Orbital plate of frontal bone
  - Lesser wing of sphenoid
- In the superomedial area of roof, 5 mm posterior to the orbital rim is the trochlea—a connective tissue sling anchoring the tendinous part of the superior oblique muscle to the orbit. Avoid injury to trochlea during surgery to prevent vertical diplopia.

- Supraorbital notch/foramen in the superior orbital margin transmitting supraorbital vessels and nerves.
- Superior wall is encountered in:
  - Frontal sinus trephination
  - External frontoethmoidectomy
  - Orbital decompression
  - Orbital fracture repair
  - Orbital clearance/exenteration
  - Faciocranial resection

Inferior Wall (Floor)

- Composed of:
  - Orbital plate of maxilla (Fig. 1.19)
  - Zygomatic orbital plate (anterolaterally)
- The infraorbital canal which transmits infraorbital nerve and artery is the thinnest and hence weakest part of the floor. It leads to the infraorbital foramen.
- Anteromedially just behind the orbital rim is a shallow depression for the origin of the inferior oblique muscle. Disruption of IO causes vertical diplopia.
- Floor is separated from lateral wall by inferior orbital fissure. It transmits infra-orbital nerve and artery, inferior ophthal-mic vein and anterior/posterior superior alveolar nerves.
- It is encountered in:
  - Orbital decompression

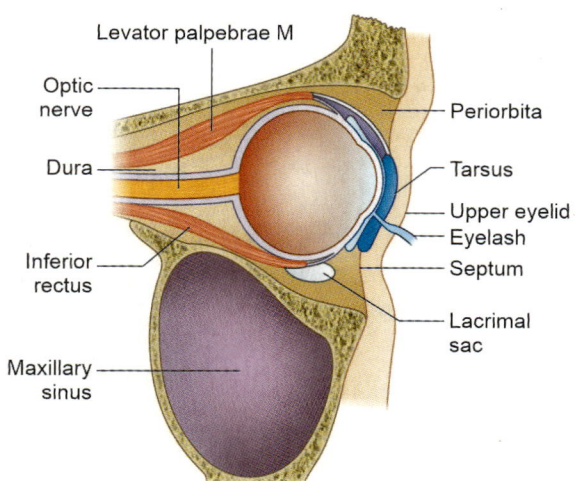

Fig. 1.19: Orbit and related structures

– Repair of orbital floor fractures
– Maxillectomy

Inferior orbital fissure: The lateral wall and floor of the orbit are separated posteriorly by this fissure. It dirrectly communicates with the MCF. Zygomatic branch of maxillary nerve and ascending branch of pterygopaltine ganglion pass through the fissure. Other structures which pass are inferior division of ophthalmic veins and infraorbital vessels.

Periorbita

• It is the periosteum lining the bony walls.
• It is continuous with the dura mater at the optic foramen and superior orbital fissure.
• Inferiorly and medially, it splits to line the fossa and to invest the lacrimal sac.
• Superiorly, it forms the pulley of the superior oblique tendon.
• Septa pass from the periorbita to divide the orbital fat into lobules.

Orbital Septum/Palpebral Fascia

• It is a fibrous sheet that stretches across the entrance of the orbit and is continuous with the periorbita at the rim.
• It is related to the posterior aspect of orbicularis oculi muscle.
• In the upper lid, it unites with the levator aponeurosis and in the lower lid, it fuses with the tarsus and sheath of the inferior rectus.

Bulbar Fascia/Tenon's Capsule

Fibrous sheath surrounding the globe, except the cornea that facilitates eye movement.

Muscular Fascia

• Made up by the fusion of the fibrous sheaths of the EOM.
• Surgical space between the periosteum and the muscular fascia—peripheral space.
• Surgical space deep to the muscular fascia, within the muscle cone—central space.

Orbital Vessels

• Main blood supply to orbit—ophthalmic artery branch of internal carotid artery. It enters through optic foramen.
• Anterior/posterior ethmoid arteries are branches from the ophthalmic artery.
• Parts of inferior orbit are supplied by the infraorbital artery, branch of internal maxillary artery.
• The superior ophthalmic vein and superior branch of inferior ophthalmic vein drain into cavernous sinus through superior orbital fissure.
• Inferior branch of inferior ophthalmic vein communicates with pterygoid plexus by passing through inferior orbital fissure.

APPLIED ANATOMY OF NASOLACRIMAL SYSTEM (Fig. 1.20)

The lacrimal apparatus consists of the following structures:
• Lacrimal gland
• Lacrimal canaliculi
• Lacrimal sac
• Nasolacrimal duct.

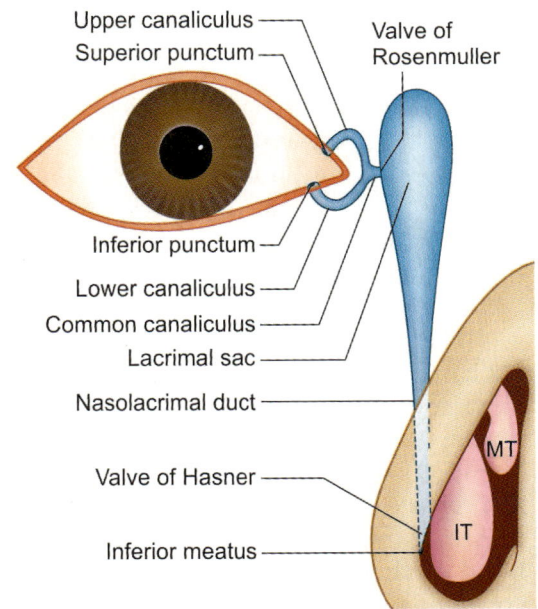

Fig. 1.20: The drainage of lacrimal secretions to inferior meatus (IT–inferior turbinate, MT–middle turbinate)

The lacrimal sac rests on a depressed area on the medial aspect of inferior orbital rim called lacrimal fossa formed by the maxillary and lacrimal bones. The fossa has two crests. The anterior lacrimal crest is a part of lacrimal bone and posterior lacrimal crest belongs to lacrimal bone. Medial to the anterior lacrimal crest on the frontal process of maxilla is a groove called sutura longitudinalis imperfecta of Weber that carries two twigs of infraorbital artery supplying the bone and nasal mucosa and can cause bleeding unless anticipated during dacryocystorhinostomy.

The nasolacrimal system consists of two systems:

A. Secretory System

- Basic secretors
  - Goblet cells in conjunctiva
  - Accessory lacrimal glands of subconjunctiva of upper lid
  - Tarsal meibomian glands
- Reflex secretors, lacrimal gland in the lacrimal fossa in the lateral orbit superiorly and anteriorly.

B. Excretory System

- In each eyelid, there is an opening located medially at the margin called punctum which leads to the respective canaliculus
- Canaliculus has two components as follows:
  - Vertical component—2 mm in length
  - Horizontal component—8 mm in length
    They joint together to form common canal that empties into lacrimal sac through valve of Rosenmuller that consists of mucosal fold and is related to orbicularis oculi.
- Lacrimal sac is situated in lacrimal fossa situated in anterior part of medial orbital wall.
- Lacrimal sac empties into nasolacrimal duct (NLD) which measures about 12 mm in length. Although the maxillary line and the head of the middle turbinate are often considered useful guides to the position of the ipsilateral NLD, their spatial relationship to the NLD is not consistent (Ali, et al.

2014). The duct has a valve in the distal end called valve of Hasner. It is not exactly a true valve but rather surrounded by cavernous space of the inferior turbinate (Bloching 2007) canaliculi and sac are lined by stratified squamous epithelium.

BIBLIOGRAPHY

1. A Leunig, B Sommer, CS Betz, F Sommer. Surgical anatomy of the frontal recess—is there a benefit in multiplanar CT-reconstruction? Rhinology, 2008; 46, 188–194.
2. Ali MJ, Nayak JV, Vaezeafshar R, Li G, Psaltis AJ. Anatomic relationship of nasolacrimal duct and major lateral wall landmarks: Cadaveric study with surgical implications. Int Forum Allergy Rhinol. 2014 Aug;4(8):684–8. doi: 10.1002/alr.21345.
3. Benjt JP, Cuilty-Siller C, Kuhn FH. The frontal cell as a cause of frontal sinus obstruction. Am J Rhinol, 1994; 8:185–191.
4. Bent JP, Cuilty-Siller C, Kuhn FA: The frontal cell as a cause of frontal sinus obstruction; Laryngoscope, 1996; 106:1119–25.
5. Bloching MB. Disorders of the nasal valve area; GMS Current Topics in Otorhinolaryngology—Head and Neck Surgery 2007, Vol. 6, p 1–13 ISSN 1865–1011.
6. Daniels DL, Mafee MF, Smith MM, Smith TL, Naidich TP, Brown WD, et al. The frontal sinus drainage pathway and related structures. Am J Neuroradiol 2003; 24: 1618–27.
7. F Meloni, R Mini, S Rovasio, F Stomeo and GP Tetani. Anatomic variations of surgical importance in ethmoid labyrinth and sphenoid sinus. A study of radiological anatomy. Surgical and Radiological Anatomy 1992; Vol. 14; pp. 65–70.
8. Fuji K, Chambers A, Rhoton J. Neurosurgical relationships of the sphenoid sinus: A microsurgical study. J Neurosurg 1979; 50:31–39.
9. Hayek G, Mercier PH, Fournier HD. Anatomy of the Orbit and its Surgical Approach; Advances and Technical Standards in Neurosurgery, Vol. 31, p 35–71, 2006.
10. Hollinshead WH. Anatomy for Surgeons, 2nd ed. Vol. 1. The Head and Neck. New York: Harper and Row, 1968.
11. Hollinshead WH. The head and neck. In: Hollinshead WH. Anatomy for Surgeons. 2nd ed., vol. 1. New York: Harper and Row, 1968.

12. Kaluskar SK. Endoscopic Sinus Surgery—Practical Approach; Springer-Verlag London 1997, ISBN 978-1-4471-0919-8

13. Kasper KA. Nasofrontal connections: a study of one hundred consecutive dissections. Arch Otolaryngol 1936;23:322–43.

14. Kennedy DW, Zinreich SJ, Rosenbaum AE, Johns ME. Functional endoscopic sinus surgery. Theory and diagnostic evaluation. Arch Otolaryngol 1985;111:576–82.

15. Keros P. On the practical value of difference in the level of lamina cribrosa of the ethmoid. J Laryngol Rhinol Otol 1962; 41:808–13.

16. Kozlov VS. Anatomical of the endonasal opening of the cells of the ethmoid labyrinth. Vestn Otorhinolaryngology 1975; 37:76–79.

17. Lang J. Klinische Anatomie der Nase, Nasenhöhle und Nebenhöhlen. Thieme, Stuttgart, New York, 1998.

18. Lang J. Clinical Anatomy of Nose, Nasal cavity and Paranasal Sinuseses. Stuttgart, New York: Thieme; 1989.

19. Lund V. Evolution of surgery on maxillary sinus for chronic rhinosinusitis. Laryngoscope 2002 Mar;112(3):415–19.

20. Maniscalco JE, Habal MB. Microanatomy of the optic canal. J Neurosurgery 1978.

21. Martin C, Costa e Silva IE, Campero A, et al. Microsurgical Anatomy of Orbit: Rule of seven; Anatomy Research International Volume, 2011, Article ID 468727, doi:10.1155/2011/468727.

22. Müller F, O'Rahilly R. Olfactory structures in staged human embryos. Cells Tissues Organs 2004;178(2):93–116.

23. Myerson. The natural orifice of maxillary sinus, Anatomical studies. Archives of Otolaryngology 1932; Vol. 5, pp. 80–91.

24. Naumann H. Pathologische Anatomie der Chronischen Rhinitis und Sinusitis. In: Proceedings VIII International Congress of Otorhinolaryngology. Amsterdam: Excerpta Medica; 1965. p. 80.

25. Neivert H. Surgical anatomy of the maxillary sinus. Laryngoscope 1930;40:1–4.

26. Park KS, Wells JM, Zorn AM, Wert SE, Whitsett JA. Sox17 influences the differentiation of respiratory epithelial cells. Dev Biol 2006; 294: 192–202. DOI: 10.1016/j.ydbio.2006.02.038.

27. Peter J Wormald. Anatomy, Three-dimensional Reconstruction and Surgical Technique, 2nd edition, Thieme Medical Publication, 2002.

28. Renn WH, Rhoton AL. Microsurgical anatomy of the sellar region. The J Neurosurg 1975; 43:288–98.

29. Rontal E, Rontal M, Guilford FT. Surgical anatomy of the orbit. Ann Otol 1979;88:382–386.

30. Scheaffer JP. Paranasal Sinuses, Nasolacrimal Passage Ways and Olfactory Organ in Man. Philadelphia. Blakiston, 1920.

31. Stammberger H. Endoscopic endonasal surgery. Concepts in treatment of recurring rhinosinusitis. Part I. Anatomic and pathophysiologic considerations. Otolaryngol, Head and neck Surgery 1986;94:143–155.

32. Tetani G, Simonet G, Solvini U, et al. Computed tomography of ethmoid labyrinth and adjacent structure. Normal anatomy and most common variants. Ann Otolaryngology 1987;96:239–250.

33. Turvey TA, Golden BA. Orbital anatomy for the surgeon. Oral Maxillofac Surg Clin North Am 2012 November; 24(4): 525–536. doi:10.1016/j.coms.2012.08.003.

34. Van Alyea OE. Nasal Sinuses. An Anatomical and Clinical Consideration. 2nd edition, Baltimore (MD) William Wilkins, 1951.

35. Van Alyea, OE. The Ostium maxillary anatomic study of its surgical accessibility. Archives of Otolaryngology 1936; Vol. 24, pp. 553–559.

36. Wormald P-J. Endoscopic sinus surgery. Anatomy of the Frontal Recess and Frontal Sinus. New York: Thieme; 2005.

37. Zuckerkandl E. Normale und pathologische Anatomie der Nasenhöhle und ihrer pneumatischen Anhänge, vol 1, 2. Braumüller, Wien Leipzig

38. Zuckerkandl E. Die Untere Siebbeinmuschel (mittelere nosenmuschel) normal and pathological, Bd1, Bd2 Wein and Leipzeg 1993.

39. Lorkiewicz-Muszyåska, ska D, Kociemba W, Rewekant A, et al. Development of maxillary sinus from birth to age 18. Postnatal growth pattern. Int J Pediatr Otorhinolaryngol 2015 Sep; 79(9):1393–400.

40. Zhang L, Han L, Ge W, et al. Anatomical and computed tomographic analysis of the interaction between the uncinate process and the agger nasi cell. Acta Otolaryngologica 2016; 126,8:845–52.

41. Rontal E, Rontal M, Guilford FT. Surgical anatomy of the orbit. Ann Otol Rhinol Laryngol 1979; 88:382–86.

42. Converse JM. The cartilaginous structures of the nose. Ann Otol Rhinol Laryngol 1955 Mar; 64(1):220–29.

43. Oneal RM, Beil RJ. Surgical anatomy of the nose. Clin Plast Surg 2010 Apr;37(2):191–211.

44. Wexler DB, Braverman I, Amar M. Histology of nasal swell body. Otolaryngol Head Neck Surg 2006 Apr;134(4):596–600.

45. Rai S, Rattan V. Traumatic superior orbital fissure syndrome: Review of literature and report of three cases. Natl J Maxillofac Surg 2012 Jul-Dec; 3(2): 222–225.

46. Stammberger HR, Bolger WE. Paranasal sinuses: anatomic terminology and nomenclature. The Anatomic Terminology Group. Ann Otol Rhinol Laryngol Suppl 1995;167:7–16.

47. Van Alyea OE. Ethmoid labyrinth: Anatomic study with consideration of the clinical significance of its structural characteristics. Arch Otolarygol Head Neck Surg 1939;29:881–902.

48. Van Alyea OE. Frontal cells: An anatomic study of these cells with consideration of their clinical significance. Arch Otolaryngol Head Neck Surg 1941;34:11–23

49. Lee WT, Kuhn FA, Citard MJ. 3D computed tomographic analysis of frontal recess anatomy in patients without frontal sinusitis. Otolaryngol Head Neck Surg 2004;131(3):164–73.

50. Daniel DL, Mafee MF, Smith MM, et al. Frontal sinus drainage pathway and related structure. American Journal of Neuroradiology 2003; 24(8):1618–1627.

51. Yanagisawa E, Joe JK. The surgical significance of the agger nasi cell. Ear Nose Throat J 1999 May;78(5):328–30.

52. Bagatella F, Guirado CR. The ethmoid labyrinth. An anatomical and radiological study.

53. Zhang L, Han D, Ge W, et al. Anatomical and computed tomographic analysis of the interaction between the uncinate process and the agger nasi Cell. Acta Otolaryngol 2006;126: 845–852.

54. Boyer: Traité compl. d. Anat. T. IV. Paris 1805

55. Messerklinger W. The ethmoid infundibulum and its inflammatory diseases. Archives of Oto-rhino-Laryngology,1979; 222: 11–22

56. Wormald PJ, Hoseman W, Callejas C, et al. The International Frontal Sinus Anatomy Classification (IFAC) and Classification of the Extent of Endoscopic Frontal Sinus Surgery (EFSS). International Forum of Allergy and Rhinology, 2016; Vol. 6, No. 7: 677–96.

2

Applied Physiology of the Nose and Paranasal Sinuses

DR Nayak, A Krishnamurthy, A Ravindra

The physiologic functions of the nasal cavities have been well established by various studies since last 40 years and not only be considered as the gateway of the respiration, but also other significant functions including conditioning and moistening of the nasal airflow, filtration of inspired air, specific and non-specific anti-infective activities, reflex action, humidification of expired air flow and olfactory function. In contrast, however, the role of paranasal sinuses is poorly understood (Proctor, 1982, Cole 1998).

Functions of the Nasal Cavity

- Nasal respiration
- Protection of the lower respiratory tract
- Filtration
- Airconditioning of inspired air (temperature and humidity regulation)
- Mucociliary function
- Sneeze reflex
- Olfaction
- Vocal resonance
- Outlet to the lacrimal secretions

NASAL RESPIRATION

The contribution of the nose to the airflow in the respiratory tract is of considerable importance. Everyday about 12,000 litres airflow is passing through the adult nose (Cole 1992). 50% of the total resistance is contributed by the nasal cavities. Man is an obligatory nasal breather for the first 6 months of life. 85% of the adults are nose breathers and only resort to an oral or oronasal route under demanding situation such as exercise or in pathological conditions. It has been estimated that an adult inspires up to 10,000 liters of air daily (Kerr, 1997).

Inspiratory air currents pass vertically up through the anterior nares at a rate of 2 to 3 m/s. The flow converges to a laminar pattern at a velocity of 12 to 18 m/s at the narrowest point, i.e. the nasal valve after which the flow becomes horizontal, it splits into three air streams, the largest of which flows above the upper edge of the inferior turbinate in the middle meatus. The second smaller airflow runs along the olfactory corridor localized on the roof of the nasal cavity, and between the septum and medial surface of the superior and middle turbinates. Very minimal flow of air occurs along the floor of the nasal cavity and inferior meatus. Laminar flow is important for cleaning and conditioning of the air. Most of the air conditioning occurs along the middle meatus and the floor of the nose, but eddying occurs in olfactory area (Fig. 2.1a and b).

Expiratory air currents are most turbulent, with air flowing through the nasal cavity, sweeping inspired air out of the olfactory region. The expiratory flow produces eddies in the region of the middle meatus. The sinuses are ventilated only in the expiratory phase by air that has been pre-treated by the respiratory mucosa and are relatively sterile. The uncinate process probably protects the sinuses by diverting the inspired air that is rich in allergens and bacteria (Nayak, *et al.*, 2001). Figure 2.2 shows the inspiratory and

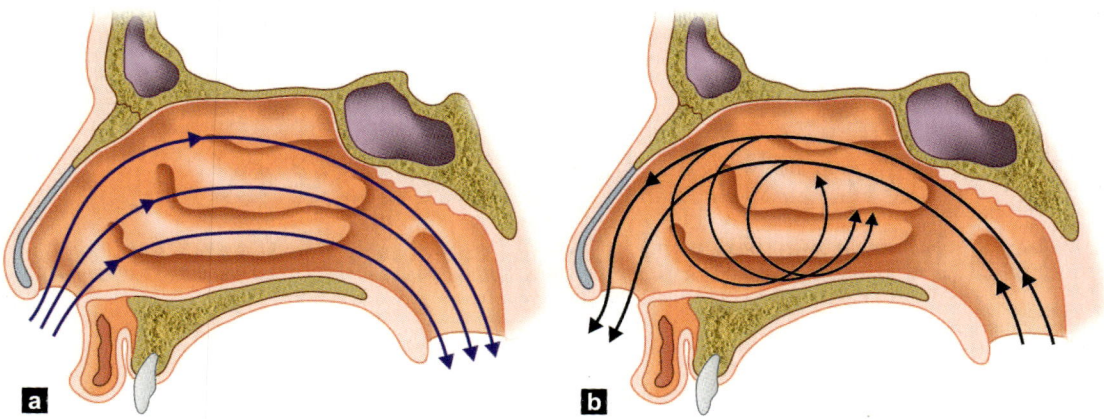

Fig. 2.1: Inspiratory and expiratory phases of nasal airflow

expiratory flow that may get affected by the removal of uncinate process.

Nasal airway resistance: The nasal vestibule is the first component of nasal resistance. The nasal vestibule is composed of compliant walls that are liable to collapse from the negative

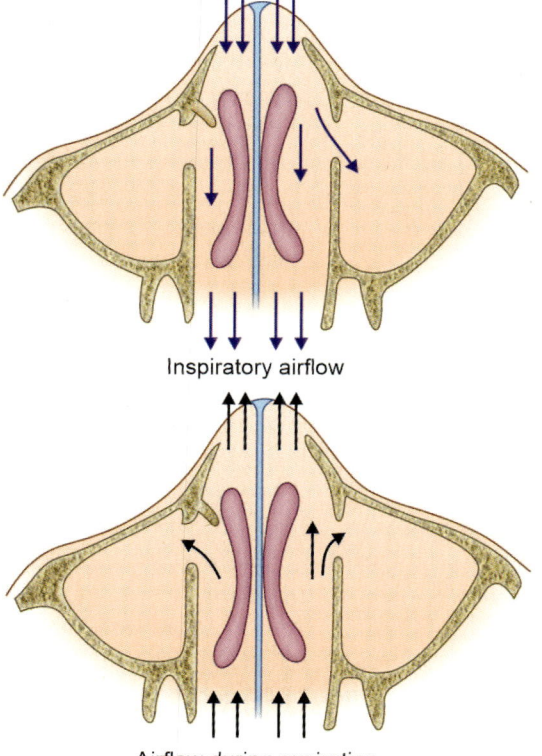

Inspiratory airflow

Airflow during expiration

Fig. 2.2: Ventilatory mechanism of paranasal sinuses with or without uncinate process preservation (Nayak, *et al.*, 2001)

pressures generated during inspi-ration (Kerr, 1997). The vestibule has been termed the external nasal valve. Vestibule contributes to one-third of the nasal airway resistance. The valve region is formed slightly posterior to the posterior edge of the lower lateral cartilage and the nasal septum contri-butes most of the remaining two-thirds of the resistance. The **internal nasal valve** is the narrowest part of the nasal cavity responsible for controlling the nasal airway resistance and is situated between the cartilaginous nasal septum and lower border of upper lateral cartilage (ULC) + anterior end of inferior turbinate. The term of nasal valve has been coined by Mink in 1903 and was subsequently characterized in more detail by Bridger (1970).

Inferior and middle turbinate and corres-ponding part of the septum (septal swell bodies) contain erectile tissue (Wustrow 1951); the anterior end of inferior turbinate has a major effect on nasal resistance and it functions as a physiological internal nasal valve (Fig. 2.3). The nasal valve area is a complex three-dimensional unit that consists of the mobile lateral nasal wall, the anterior septum with the swell body, the head of the inferior turbinate and the osseous pyriform aperture. From the physiologic point of view, it is the place of maximum nasal flow resistance (flow limiting segment). Therefore, according to Poiseuille's law, even minor constrictions of this area result in a clinically relevant impairment of nasal breathing for the patient. This narrow passage,

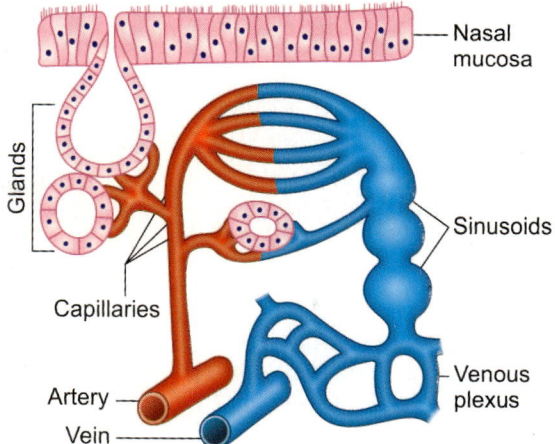

Fig. 2.3: Subepithelial erectile tissue of nasal cavity

also called "ostium internum nasi", is formed by the mobile lateral nasal wall, the anterior septum with the swell body, the head of the inferior turbinate and the osseous pyriform aperture (Bloching 2007).

The nasal valve can be assessed subjectively using the Cottle's test to know about nasal patency while rhinomanometry is the best way to assess objectively (Cole 2000, Clemant 1984).

Changes in the nasal resistance are primarily the result of a vascular response of erectile tissue controlled by autonomic nervous system, mainly the sympathetic system. This determines the state of engorgement of the erectile tissue. Sympathetic activity causes vasoconstriction, leading to decrease in nasal resistance, whereas parasympathetic activity causes vasodilatation leading to increase in nasal resistance.

Factors Affecting the Nasal Resistance

About 10,000 literes of air is passed through the nasal cavity on inspiration per day. Nasal airway resistance plays an important role with respect to various factors that can affect them as described below (Kerr 1997 & Maran & Lund 1990).

a. *Age:* Maximum resistance is found in infancy and it reduces as the age advances.
b. *Nasal cycle:* A physiological cycle of spontaneous reciprocating nasal congestion and decongestion alternating between the two

nasal cavities. This was first described by Kayser in 1895 and is probably controlled by respiratory areas in the brainstem closely associated with respiratory activity. The duration of the cycle varies from 2 to 7 hrs. It is absent in laryngectomies and tracheostomized patients. White, et al (2015) suggested the contrasting role of nasal cycle in eliminating contaminants while facilitating air-conditioning through fluctuating airflow in each nostril.

c. *Exercise:* With increase in exercise, the nasal resistance decreases probably due to increase in the sympathetic action on the erectile tissue (Eccles 2000).

d. *Respiration:* Resistance is slightly lower during inspiration compared to that during expiration. Hyperventilation results in vasodilatation and a rise in resistance.

e. *Posture:* Change of posture leads to change in nasal resistance due to alteration in jugular venous pressure.

f. *Nasal reflexes:* Sneezing can influence the nasal resistance. Sneezing results from a number of mild mechanical and chemical stimuli to the nasal mucosa and is associated with increased secretion and congestion. The trigeminal nerve, respiratory muscles and the autonomic nervous system usually mediate this.

g. *Skin and air temperature:* Atmospheric air can affect the skin temperature, which reflexly alters the nasal mucosal blood flow as part of the thermoregulatory mechanism. Cool inspired air can cause congestion and increased resistance.

h. *Emotional and psychological response:* This causes autonomic imbalance and alteration in the nasal resistance by regulating the erectile tissue.

Protection of the Lower Respiratory Tract

Filtration

Vibrissae in the nasal vestibule prevent the large particles in the inspired air to pass through the nasal cavity depending on the size of the particulate matter (Muir 1972). Deposited particles, between 10 and 1 μm in diameter, are removed from the nasal mucosa within 6–15 min depending on the efficacy of the mucociliary system (Tomenzoli 2005). The nasal airway filters 95% of particles of more than 15 μm diameter from the inspired air (Cole 1992). Zhou, et al, 2007 found inhaled aerosol dose deposited in the alveolus is reduced considerably while inhaling through nose than through mouth.

Air-conditioning of the Inspired Air (Fig. 2.4)

The temperature and humidity of the inspired air is regulated by the nasal mucosa. The blood flow of the nasal cavity is from the posterior to anterior direction as shown in Fig. 2.4, which is opposite to the flow of inspired air.

This mechanism is applied in refrigeration industry and is called countercurrent mechanism. This allows the inspired air to be humidified as it comes in contact with the mucous blanket, which also traps the dust particles. The humidification of the inspired air occurs from the evaporation of mucous blanket. The countercurrent effect also allows heating of the inspired air that gets pretreated in the nasal chamber. This air-conditioning function is controlled by the autonomic nervous system. Cauna 1970 reported the total absence of the internal elastic membrane in the arterioles, so that the endothelial basement

membrane is continuous with the basement membrane of the smooth muscle cells besides having porosity in the membrane. It along with the venules has interposed cavernous and sinusoidal system deep to the lamina-propria that can regulate the blood flow and facilitate heating and humidification of the inspired air.

Mucociliary Function

The respiratory area of the nasal cavity is covered by 120 cm² of pseudostratified columnar ciliated epithelium and has a thickness of 0.3 to 0.5 mm which are attached to the basal cell layer of the basement membrane. The columnar cells with 300–400 microvilli per cell represent up to 70% of the epithelium and facilitates in increasing the surface area (Mygind 1982). The ciliated cells with approximately 200–300 cilia on each cell consist of about 20–50% of the epithelium and are responsible for mucociliary clearance. Mucociliary clearance is one of the major functions of the nasal epithelium. Respiratory mucosa is coated by a 10–15 μm thick layer of mucous secretions called mucous blanket, which helps in cleaning the fine particulate matters that are trapped in it during the inspiratory phase and also helps the cilia to function smoothly to facilitate proper

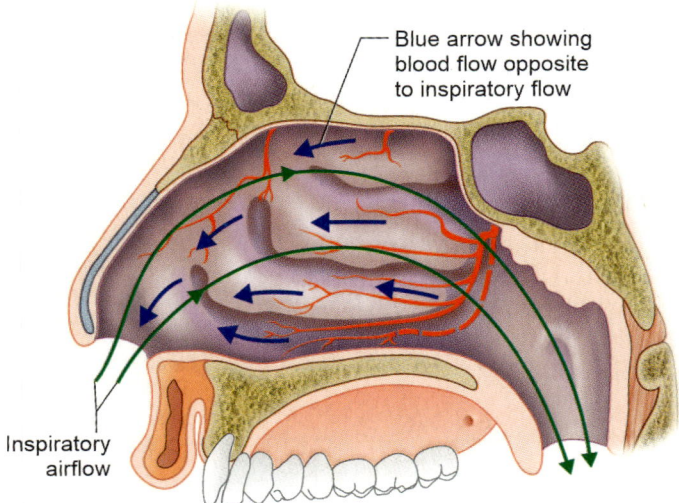

Blue arrow showing blood flow opposite to inspiratory flow

Inspiratory airflow

Fig. 2.4: The countercurrent mechanism of the air-conditioning function of the nose. Blue arrows show the direction of the blood supply and green arrows showing the direction of the inspiratory airflow

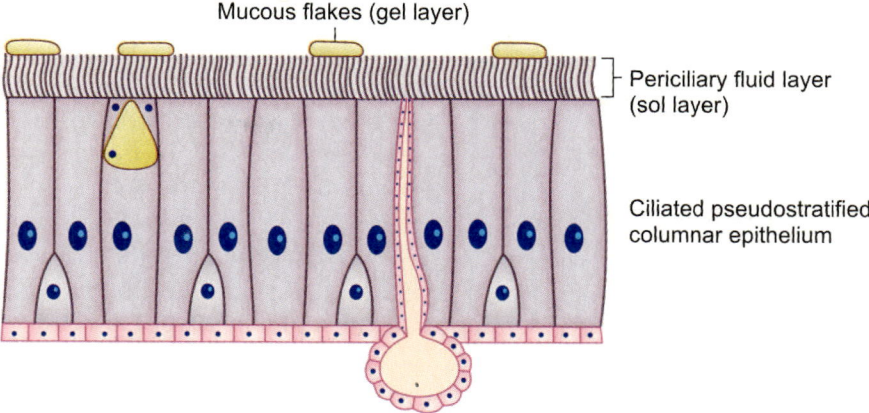

Fig. 2.5: Mucous blanket function

mucociliary clearance. It consists of superficial thick mucous layer (gel) and deep thin periciliary layer (sol) (Fig. 2.5). Mucociliary transport occurs in an unidirectional manner because of the unique characteristics of cilia. Ciliary beating produces a current in the superficial layer of the periciliary fluid in the direction of the effective stroke. Studies on healthy adult subjects by the tagged particle or saccharin method have consistently shown that 80% exhibit clearance rates of 3 to 25 mm/minute (average, 6 mm/min), with slower rates in the remaining 20% (Proctor 1982).

The mucous secreting glands and goblet cells of the nasal and sinus mucosa secrete the mucous. The mucous is rich in lysozymes, an important enzyme that initiates bacterial destruction. In addition, it contains secretory IgA, which neutralizes allergens and bacterial toxins (Fig. 2.6).

The cilia of the respiratory epithelium beat in a specific manner and direction and propel the mucous blanket towards the pharynx, where it is swallowed. The beat of a single cilium consists of a rapid forward beat and a slow return beat with a time ratio of 1:3 (Cole, 1998). The cilia are composed of multistructural axonema which are composed of nine doublets of peripheral microtubules and two single central microtubules (9+2 pattern). Among the paired microtubules, one (A) contains two dynein arm (outer and inner) extending towards the other microtubules (B) the dynein arm contains ATPase responsible

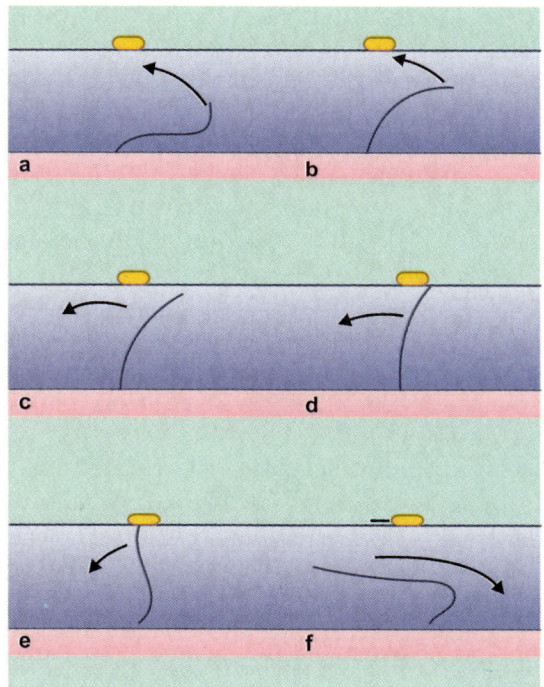

Fig. 2.6: Ciliary beat in stages: a. Initiation of beat of cilia. b to e. Propelling of cilia making the mucous blanket to move. f. Recovery stage

for ciliary motility (movement) (Fig. 2.7) also called sliding fillament mechanism (Widdicombe, 1997).

Nasal Reflex Function and Protection

Clinical observation suggests the existence of poorly characterized reflex pathway between upper and its interaction with contiguous

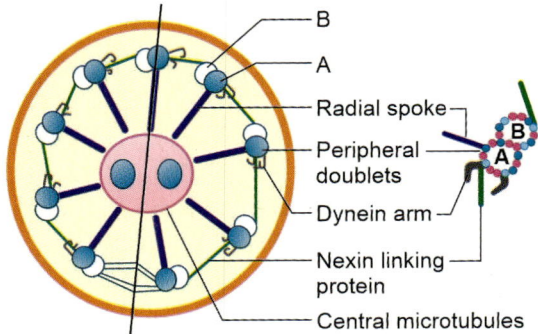

Fig. 2.7: The structure of cilia

structures (eye, ear, sinuses) and lower respiratory pathway (Baroody, 2010). Nasal mucosa receives nerve supply from the somatic (trigeminal nerve) and autonomic systems (vidian nerve). The response of the nasal mucosa to irritants and harmful stimuli results in sneezing, watery rhinorrhea and changes in blood flow (Allison and Powel, 1971). Sneezing is also a protective function in response to irritants and harmful stimuli. Animal and *in vitro* studies indicate that the chemosensitive neurons and airway epithelium may be critical targets for irritants that participate in the induction of inflammation (Bascon, 1991).

Nasolacrimal reflex is another reflex mechanism that can occur due to chemical or mechanical stimulation of the ciliated nasal epithelium, resulting in increased lacrimal secretion. Afferent, C-fibres run along with the trigeminal nerve to the superior salivary nucleus via geniculate ganglion and greater superficial petrosal nerve and through the vidian nerve to the sphenopalatine ganglion. Cholinergic fibres reach together with the maxillary nerve to the lacrimal gland (Baraniuk and Kim, 2007)

Vocal Resonance

The nasal cavities and the sinuses add nasal tone to the articulated voice by acting as resonators. Nasal speech (rhinolalia) results due to nasal or nasopharyngeal obstruction (rhinolalia clausa) or due to abnormal communication between the oral and nasal cavities as in cleft palate and palatal paralysis (rhinolalia aperta).

Olfaction

It is defined as a mechanism by which the smell is perceived. The olfactory area of the nasal cavity as described earlier is responsible for this function of the nasal cavity. The main functions of olfaction are:

- Regulation of the food intake and perception of flavor and palatability
- Regulation of reproductive behavior (more developed in lower animals)
- Protective function: Detection of the noxious and toxic substances.

Mechanism of Olfaction

The mechanisms by which mammals discriminate a vast array of diverse odors are poorly understood. Olfactory receptors situated in the upper part of the nasal cavity above the level of the superior turbinate sense the odorant particles in the inspired air. Each olfactory receptor neuron has 8–20 cilia that are whip-like extensions 30–200 microns in length. The olfactory cilia are the sites where molecular reception with the odorant occurs and sensory transduction (i.e. transmission) starts. The amount of inspired air reaching this area depends on the nasal anatomy and pathological abnormalities. Sniffing increases the availability of inspired air into the olfactory area. The regulation of the olfactory system is mainly achieved by the olfactory mechanism, which consists of the olfactory epithelium and its central connections and to some extent by the non-olfactory receptors of the V, VII, IX and X cranial nerves. The Vth cranial nerve perceives odor up to 30%.

OLFACTORY PATHWAY (Figs 2.8, 2.9 and Flowchart 2.1)

Mechanism of Odour Perception

Olfactory epithelium situated over the olfactory area is a highly specialized sensory epithelium. Bowman glands of olfactory mucosa secrete serous fluid rich in glycoprotein, which warms, moistens, and traps air, helping dissolve gaseous odourant particles. The odour perception from these particles is mediated by olfactory receptors. The olfactory

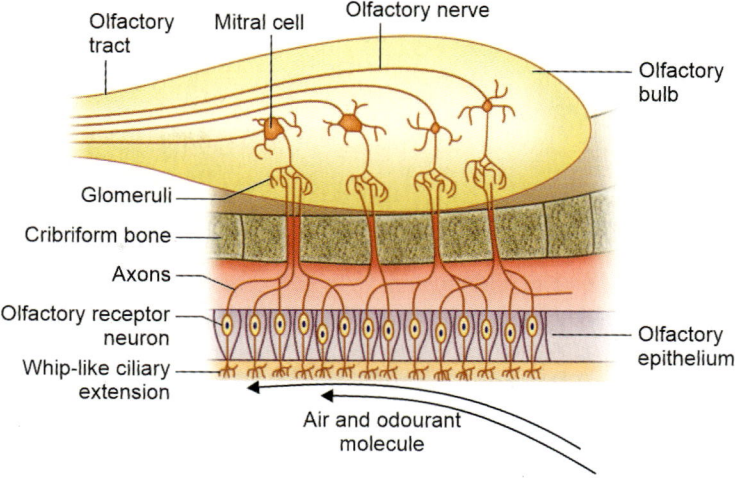

Fig. 2.8: Olfactory mechanism

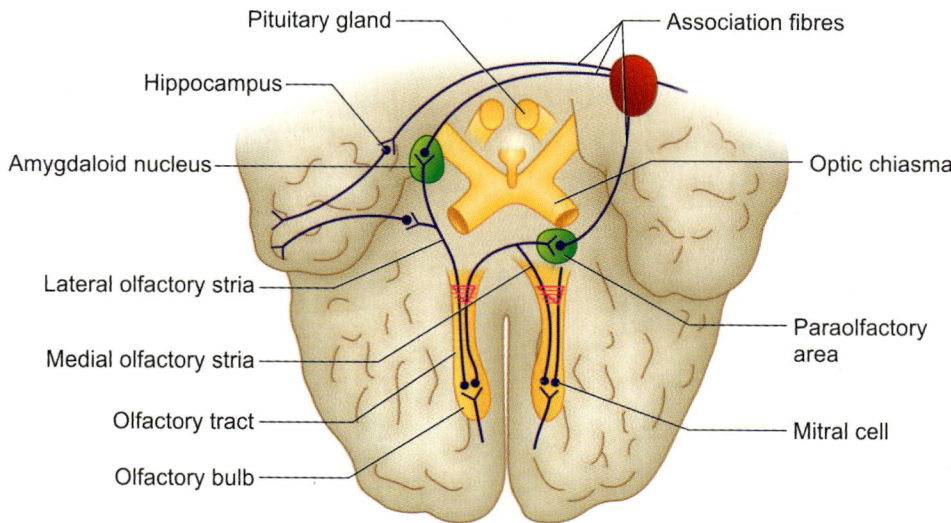

Fig. 2.9a: Olfactory structures related to anterior part of base of the brain

signals are further transmitted to olfactory bulb. Through the olfactory glomeruli and olfactory nerve, it reaches the olfactory nuclei which transfer olfactory memory from one side to the other. Olfactory discrimination occurs at the pyriform cortex. Amygdala gives emotional response to olfactory stimuli. The olfactory memories are stored in the entorhinal cortex, that receives input from pyriform cortex and olfactory bulb (Pavelka & Roth 2010). Many theories exist to explain the mechanism of odour perception. Among them,

the Lock and Key concept of chemical recognition is widely held. Perception depends on the interaction of the odourant molecules with highly specialized and highly specific olfactory receptor sites in the olfactory cell membrane. The electrical impulse thus generated is transmitted to the higher centers. The odour particles have to cross the mucus to reach the receptor cells, which necessitates it to be water soluble to some extent, but lipid solubility will enhance interaction with the plasma membrane. Because of the pigments

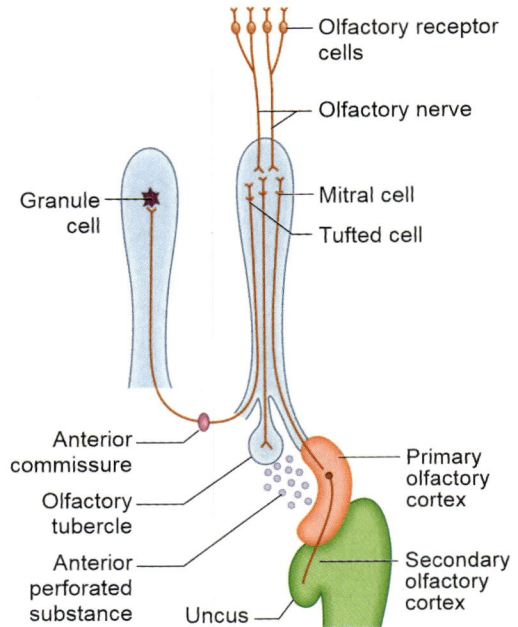

Fig. 2.9b: Olfactory pathway from olfactory area to secondary olfactory cortex

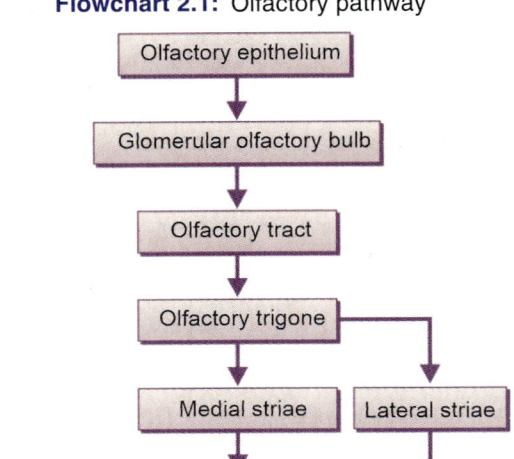

Flowchart 2.1: Olfactory pathway

like carotenoids which are found in the Bowman's glands, a role similar to that of retina has been proposed. Triller, et al (2008) said 'lock and key' models of olfaction based on a concept of odor-quality-tuned receptors are inadequate, irrespective of the nature of the lock-key interaction.

Olfaction is the dominant sensory modality for most animals and chemosensory communication is particularly well developed in many mammals. Our understanding of this form of communication has grown rapidly over the last 10 years since the identification of the first olfactory receptor genes. The subsequent cloning of genes for rodent vomeronasal receptors, which are important in pheromone detection, has revealed an unexpected diversity of around 250 receptors belonging to two structurally different classes. Recent studies using genetically modified mice and electrophysiological recordings have highlighted the complexities of chemosensory communication via the vomeronasal system and the role of this system in handling information about sex and genetic identity. Although the vomeronasal organ is often regarded as only a pheromone detector,

evidence is emerging that suggests it might respond to a much broader variety of chemo signals (Brennan & Keverne, 2004).

Outlet for Lacrimation Secretion

The nasolacrimal duct drains into the inferior meatus. Blockage of this duct can lead to epiphora. Inflammatory conditions of the nose and sinuses like sinusitis and rhinitis, malignancy of the nose and paranasal sinuses can cause obstruction to the lacrimal apparatus and epiphora.

The lacrimal drainage system consists of upper and lower puncta which are situated in the medial aspect of respective eyelids. The puncta lead to the respective vertical and then to horizontal canaliculus. The upper and lower canaliculi join to form a common canaliculus. The common canaliculus enters the lacrimal sac through the valve of Rosenmuller. This valve of mucosal flap prevents reflux obstruction of common canaliculus that can cause epiphora. The lacrimal sac funnels to form the nasolacrimal duct which opens into the inferior meatus (Fig. 2.10).

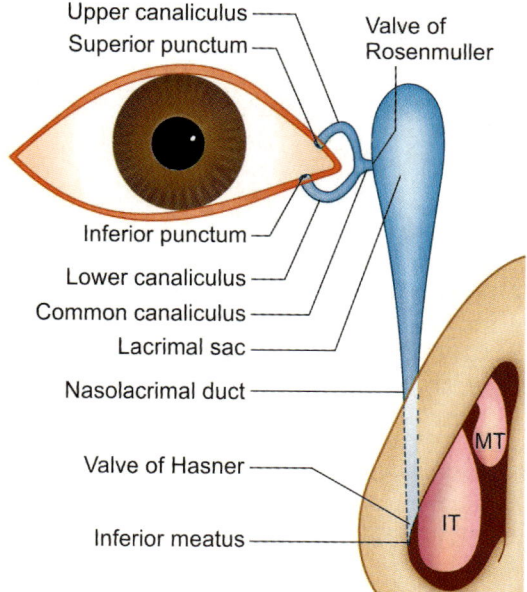

Fig. 2.10: The drainage of lacrimal secretions to inferior meatus (IT–inferior turbinate, MT–middle turbinate)

About 70% of lacrimal secretions drain through the lower punctum, while 30% drain through the upper punctum to the lacrimal sac. The main function of the lacrimal apparatus is to moisturize the cornea and conjunctiva. It also provides the correct balance between inflow and outflow of tears to the lacrimal sac (Maliborsky and Rozyki, 2014). The lacrimal canaliculi pump the excess secretion to the lacrimal sac. The lacrimal sac dilates due to Horner's muscle contraction following eye closure, thus allowing the the secretions to get collected that finally drains into the nasal cavity through inferior meatus (Dei Cas, 2002). Chronic rhinitis and sinusitis can cause inflammatory disease of lacrimal apparatus leading to obstruction of naso-lacrimal duct.

Endoscopic dacryocystorhinostomy is an effective surgical approach to treat this problem.

Functions of the Paranasal Sinuses

The functions of paranasal sinuses are not very clear and no clear cut opinion have been expressed in the past. Flottes, Guillerm and

Riu (1960) focused on sinus ventilation and conclude that "The human sinuses are diverticula of the nasal cavities, with which they communicate via narrow passages, and undergo minimal ventilation and drainage". Various hypotheses have been proposed in this regard as follows (Gluck 1991):

1. They lighten the bones of the skull.
2. Improve the resonance of voice.
3. Humidify and warm the inspired air.
4. Increase the area of olfactory membrane.
5. Serve as shock absorbers in mechanical impacts.
6. Act as thermal insulators of the brain.
7. Promote facial growth and architecture.
8. Persist as evolutionary relics or faults.

Scrutiny of these hypotheses shows that none has a scientific basis (Gluck 1991). The most important function probably is the mucociliary clearance.

Mucociliary clearance: The sinuses act as a constant source of sterile mucous blanket, which is essential to replace the contaminated secretions in the nasal cavity. Secretory mucosa and unobstructed mucociliary transport are absolutely essential for the normal respiratory and olfactory function of the nose and sinuses. Development in nasal endoscopy has revealed more information about the sinus mucociliary clearance activity and in the pathogenesis of sinusitis. Anatomical abnormalities in the nasal cavity especially in the middle meatus can obstruct the outlet of the paranasal sinuses causing persistent inflammatory disease in the sinuses. Mucociliary clearance is described in detail in Chapter 3. The discovery within the paranasal sinuses of the production of nitric oxide (NO) has altered the traditional explanations of sinus physiology and has major implication on respiratory physiology and clinical implication (Marquez 2008). Nitric oxide may be regarded as an "aerocrine" hormone that is produced in the nose and sinuses and the role of NO in the sinuses is likely to enhance local host defense mechanisms via direct inhibition of pathogen growth and stimulation of mucociliary activity (Lundberg 2008).

Studies have demonstrated that paranasal sinuses may facilitate in the production of nitric oxide (NO) and in aiding the immune defences of the nasal cavity (Keir 2008). The paranasal sinuses seem to develop after regression of the erythropoietic marrow in the maxillary, frontal and sphenoid bones and its replacement by cavities filled with gas, which escapes into the nasal fossae through the ostium. The sinus epithelium synthesizes NO continuously. The paranasal sinuses provide a compartmentalized reservoir of NO, that are released discontinuously in the form of boli, when the ostium opens. The NO also plays the role of an "aerocrine" messenger between the upper and lower respiratory tracts, reducing pulmonary vascular resistance (Jankowski 2016).

BIBLIOGRAPHY

1. Allison DJ, Powis DA. Adrenal catecholamine secretion during stimulation of the nasal mucous membrane in the rabbit. J Physiol (Lond) 1971;217:327–339.

2. Ballengar JJ. Diseases of Ear Nose Throat, 13th edition, Philadephia, Lea Feiger 1985.

3. Baraniuk JN, Kim D. Nasonasal reflexes, the nasal cycle, and sneeze. Curr Allergy Asthma Rep 2007; 7: 105-111. DOI: 10.1007/s11882-007-0007-1

4. Baroody FM. How nasal function influences the eyes, ears, sinuses, and lungs. Proc Am Thorac Soc, Vol 8. pp 53–61, 2011. DOI: 10.1513/pats.201007-049RN

5. Beauchamp GK, Yamazaki K. Chemical signalling in mice. Biochem Soc Trans 2003; 31:147–151.

6. Boscom R. The upper respiratory tract: mucous membrane irritation. Environ Health Perspect 1991 Nov;95:39–44.

7. Brennan PA, KeverneEB. On mammalian pheromones, Neurobiology (Current Biology 2004, 14:R81).

8. Cauna N. Electron microscopy of the nasal vascular bed and its nerve supply. Ann Otol 1970,79:443–45.

9. Clement PAR. Committee Report on Standardization of Rhinomanometry. Rhinology 1984;22: 151–55.

10. Cole P. Biophysics of nasal airflow: A review. Am J Rhinol 2000;14(4):245–49.

11. Cole P. Nasal and oral airflow resistors: Site, function, and assessment. Arch Otolaryngol Head Neck Surg 1992; 118: 790–93.

12. Dei Cas RE. Evaluation of tearing in children. In: Katowitz JA (ed). Pediatric Oculoplastic Surgery. Springer Verlag; 2002. pp. 301–56.

13. Doty RL. Mammalian pheromones: Fact or fantasy? In: Doty RL (ed). Handbook of Olfaction and Gustation. Marcel Dekker Inc, 2003.

14. Eccles R. Nasal airflow in health and disease. Acta Otolaryngol 2000; 120(5):580–95.

15. Gluck U. The physiological significance of paranasal sinuses in man: Speculations for 1800 years. Schweiz Med Wochenschr 1991 Jun 22;121(25):925–31.

16. Jankowski R, Nguyen DT, Poussel M, et al. Sinusology; European Annals of Otorhinolaryngology, Head and Neck Diseases 2016;133: 263–268

17. John Grooves, Roger Gray. Synopsis of otolaryngology, John Wright and Sons Ltd. 4th and 5th edition.

18. Kayser R. Die exakteMessung der Luftdurchgängigkeit der Nase. Arch Laryngol Rhinol 1895; 3: 101–120.

19. Keir J. Why do we have paranasal sinuses? The Journal of Laryngology and Otology (2008) 123(1):4-8; DOI: 10.1017/S0022215108003976

20. Kerr A, ed. Rhinology. In: Scott-Brown's Otolaryngology. 6th ed. Oxford: Butterworth-Heinemann;1997.

21. Kerr P, Millar T, Buckle P, Kryger M. The importance of nasal resistance in obstructive sleep apnea syndrome. J Otolaryngol 1992;21: 189–195.

22. L Flottes, P Clerc, R Riu, F Devilla (Eds.). La physiologie des sinus, Librairie Arnette, Paris (1960).

23. Logan Turners' Diseases of Nose, Throat, Ear by Aruthur Logan Turner and AGD Maraer, Bristol:Wright 1988.

24. Lundberg JO, Nitrous oxide and paranasal sinuses. Anat Rec (Hoboken) 2008 Nov;291(11): 1479–84.

25. Maliborsky A, Rozyki R. Diagnostic imaging of the nasolacrimal drainage system. Part I. Radiological anatomy of lacrimal pathways. Physiology of tear secretion and tear outflow. Med Sci Monit 2014;20:628–638.

26. Maran A, Lund V. A basic science investigation test. Clinical Rhinology, Maran A and Lund V (editors), Goerge Thiemes (StuGgart, New York): 1990;51–58.

27. Marquez S. The Paranasal Sinuses: The Last Frontier in Craniofacial Biology. The Anatomical Record 2008;261:1350–1361.

28. Muir DCF. Clinical aspects of inhaled particles. Heinemann, London 1972.

29. Muir DCF. Deposition and clearance of inhaled particles. (Chapt. 1) In: Muir DCF (ed). Clinical aspects of inhaled particles. William Heinemann Medical Books, Ltd, London; 1972

30. Mygind N, Pedersen M, Nielsen M. Morphology of the upper airway epithelium. In: Proctor D, Andersen I (eds). The Nose. Amsterdam: Elsevier; 1982.

31. Nayak DR, Balakrishna R, Murthy KD, "Endoscopic Physiologic Approach to Allergy associated chronic rhinosinusitis a preliminary study ENT Journal 2001;80(6):392–403.

32. Nayak DR, Balakrishnan R, Murthy KD. "Functional Anatomy of the uncinate process and its role in endoscopic sinus surgery". Indian Journal of Otolaryngology And Head and Neck Surgery 2001:53(1):27–31.

33. Proctor DF. The mucociliary system. In: Proctor DF, Andersen IB (eds). The Nose: Upper Airway Physiology and the Atmospheric Environment. Amsterdam: Elsevier Biomedical Press; 1982.

34. Rui L. Contribution a lëtude du role des sinus paranasaux. Revue de Laryngologie et Oto-Rhinologie 1960;81:796–839

35. Sir Victor Negus. Functions of paranasal sinuses; AMA Arch Otolaryngol 1957;66(4): 430-442. doi:10.1001/archotol.1957.038302800 60007.

36. Stammberger H. Endoscopic endonasal surgery. Concepts in treatment of recurring rhinosinusitis. PartI. Anatomic and pathophysiologic considerations. Otolaryngol—Head and Neck Surgery 94:143–155.

37. Tomenzoli D. Physiology of Nose and PNS in Imaging in Treatment Planning for Sinonasal Diseases, edited by Maroldi R and Nicoli P; ISBN 3-540-42383-4 Springer Berlin Heidelberg New York.

38. White DE, Bartley J, Nates RJ. Model demonstrates functional purpose of the nasal cycle. Biomed Eng Online 2015;24;14:38.

39. Widdicombe JH, Bastacky SJ, Wu DX, Lee CY. Regulation of depth and composition of airway surface liquid. EurRespir J. 1997;10:2892–2897. DOI:10.1183/09031936.97.10122892

40. Wustrow F. Septal turbinate. Zeitschrift Anatomic Entwicklungsgeschichte 1951;116: 139–142.

41. Zhou Y, Benson JM, Irvin R, et al. Particle size distribution and inhalation dose of shower water under selected operating conditions. Inhalation Toxicology; May 2007;19(4):333–42. doi:10.1080/08958370601144241.

42. Triller A, Boulden EA, Churchill A, et al. Odorant-receptor interactions and odor percept: a chemical perspective. Chem Biodivers 2008 Jun; 5(6):862–86.

43. Brennan PA, Keverne EB. Something in the air? New insights into mammalian pheromones. Curr Biol 2004 Jan 20;14(2):R81–89.

Anatomical Abnormalities, Pathophysiology and Etiopathogenesis of Chronic Sinusitis

DR Nayak, S Nayak, R Balakrishnan, LC Prasanna

Definition of Sinusitis

Inflammation of the mucosa of one or more paranasal sinuses where the mucociliary clearance function is affected as a result of anatomical or pathological abnormalities can lead to blockage of the sinus ostia.

Acute rhinosinusitis (ARS): Acute inflammation of mucosal lining of nasal cavity and paranasal sinuses that starts with and attack of viral infection followed by seconadary bacterial infection where the symptoms last for less than 12 weeks. When complete remission of symptoms and signs occurs between the episodes of acute rhinosinusitis, the term "**acute recurrent rhinosinusitis**" is used (Foreman, et al. 2009). When the symptoms persists for more than 12 weeks with or without treatment, the term "**chronic rhinosinusitis**" is used (Foken, et al 2012).

Depending on the site of involvement, it can be described as:

- Frontal sinusitis
- Maxillary sinusitis
- Ethmoidal sinusitis
- Sphenoidal sinusitis
- *Pansinusitis:* All sinuses are involved which could be unilateral or bilateral.

In the past, sinusitis was addressed individually with respect to site. The etiopathogenesis, clinical features, investigations and treatment were individualistic. More emphasis was given to maxillary sinus as the most common site of infection.

With clear understanding of ostiomeatal complex anatomy and its role in the pathogenesis of chronic sinusitis and with the availability of nasal endoscope and CT imaging for study of sinus pathology, the concept of sinus pathology and its treatment has changed rapidly. The intimate relation-ship of the sinus system to the nasal cavity and also that of upper and lower respiratory tracts, the role of ostiomeatal complex and middle meatus in the etiopathology of chronic infection of the major sinuses has been better understood and has changed the treatment policy. Conventional procedures like intranasal antrostomy, Caldwell-Luc operation, etc. have become almost obsolete and are reserved only for irreversible disease. Present treatment is directed at the disease causation than the result. The ostiomeatal disease is endoscopically dealt by functional endoscopic sinus surgery and the physiological sinusotomies are created for better drainage of major sinuses, e.g. middle meatal antrostomy for treatment of maxillary sinusitis, frontal recess clearance for frontal sinusitis, etc. (Fig. 3.1).

Pathophysiology

Mucociliary clearance of the nasal cavity and paranasal sinuses is a primary defence mechanism that clears the mucus secreted into the upper airways by the secreting cells. This secretion traps inhaled particulate matter, allergens, and pathogens by the mucus flakes (gel layer of mucus blanket) and transport them to the pharynx (Cohen 2006). Normal mucociliary function of nose and sinuses provides a first line defense to the health of the

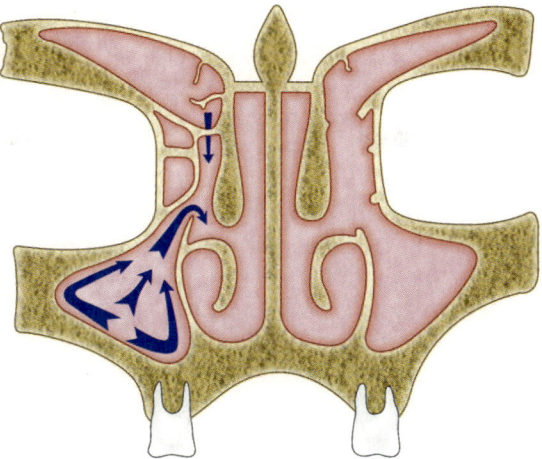

Fig. 3.1: Mucociliary clearance before and after endoscopic sinus surgery (after Stammberger)

respiratory tract. Failure of normal mucus transport and decreased sinus ventilation are the major factors contributing to the development of sinusitis. Mucosal edema and the anatomic abnormality can interfere with drainage of the sinuses as a result of obstruction of the sinus ostium. Figures 3.2a and b show normal mucociliary clearance and mucociliary clearance of the maxillary sinus is affected by Haller cell and by uncinate bulla

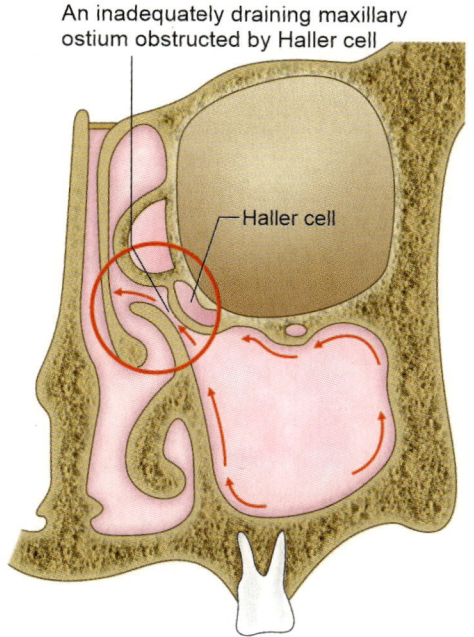

Fig. 3.2b: Normal mucociliary clearance of the maxillary sinus is affected by Haller cell

(Fig. 3.2c). Better understanding of the mucociliary activity of the paranasal sinuses and the nasal cavity has made the modern rhinologists aspire for a more physiological and hence a functional surgical modality of treatment for chronic and recurring sinusitis. Details of the mucociliary activity are described below to facilitate better understanding of the pathogenesis of chronic sinusitis.

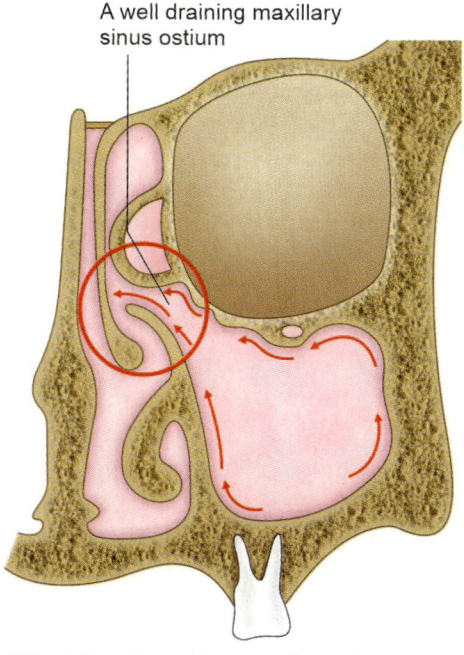

Fig. 3.2a: Normal mucociliary clearance

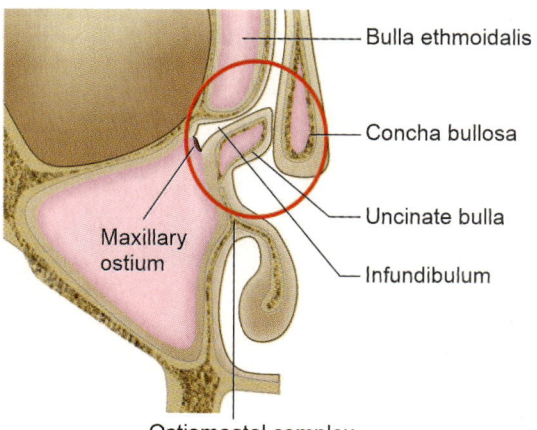

Fig. 3.2c: Obstruction of infundibulum and middle meatus due to pneumatized uncinate process (uncinate bulla) and concha bullosa

Mucociliary Activity of Maxillary Sinus (Fig. 3.3)

The mucociliary activity occurs due to ciliary beating facilitated by the periciliary layer of the double layered mucus blanket and depends on the number, structure and coordinated stroke of the cilia in the ciliated columnar epithelium. The mucociliary clearance refers to the clearance of sterile and contaminated secretions from the upper and lower respiratory tracts due to ciliary beating

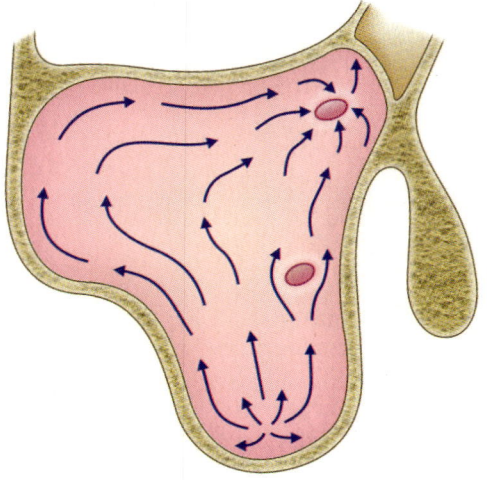

Fig. 3.3a: Mucociliary activity of maxillary sinus. Note how the mucous stream is bypassing the accessory ostium and moves towards the natural ostium (after Stammberger)

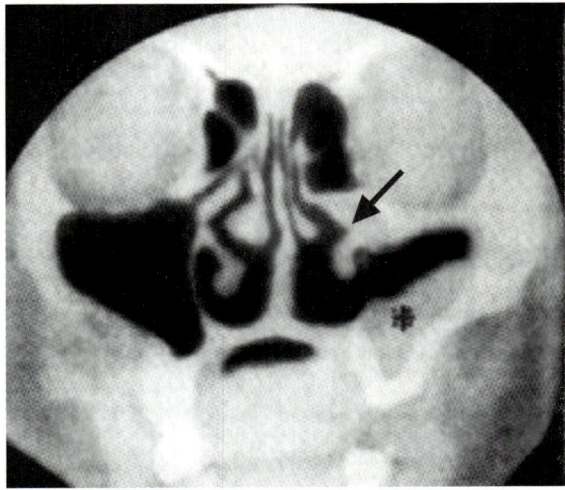

Fig. 3.3b: A case of inferior meatal antrostomy (IMA). Note collection of discharge in the floor of the left maxillary sinus (*) inspite of IMA and drainage is toward the sinus ostium (black arrow)

depending upon the cordinat. The cilia beat synchronously within the nasal cavity from anterior aspects towards the nasopharynx. Within the paranasal sinuses, they beat towards the natural ostium to drive the secretions out into the nasal cavity. Several investigations demonstrate a sharp decrease in mucociliary clearance among patient with chronic rhinosinusitis (Cohen 2006). The nasal mucus is slightly acidic in pH which varies from 5.5 to 6.5 (Quraishi, et al 1998). The optimal mucociliary clearance occurs at 37°C and 100% humidity (Williams, et al 1996).

The secretions from the maxillary sinus start in a star-like shape from the floor of the sinus along its walls to reach the inner maxillary ostium at the uppermost and posterior corner of the sinus in the lateral nasal wall. Messerklinger (1978) observed the light reflex movement of the cilliary beat by using Bismuth subgallium powder under antroscopy. Stammberger and Hawke (1993) observed alternating localized areas of slow and fast (express) mucociliary clearance pathways that can be detected in normal and chronic rhinosinusitis patients.

From the ostium, the secretions is actively transported through the ethmoid infundibulum over the rear margin of uncinate process onto the medial surface of inferior turbinate and then towards the nasopharynx.

The mucous moves along the margin of the ostium towards the natural ostium, when an accessory ostium is present probably guided by gravity. Similarly, a surgically made inferior meatal window fails to actively drain the sinus, but does drain to some extent guided by gravity.

Mucociliary Activity of the Frontal Sinus (Fig. 3.4a)

Messerklinger demonstrated an inward transport along the interfrontal septum, along the roof and walls of the sinus laterally, returning to the floor of the sinus and leaving the inner ostium laterally.

Not all the secretions leave the sinus at once. The ethmoidal prechamber to frontal sinus, a certain amount of secretion again joins

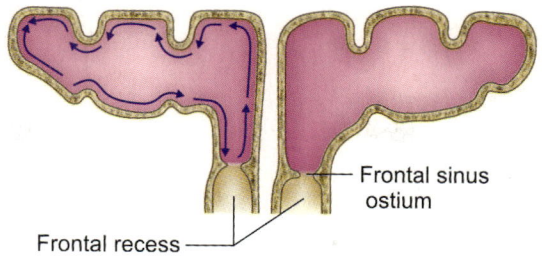

Frontal sinus ostium

Frontal recess

Fig. 3.4a: Mucociliary activity of the frontal sinus

the inwardly directed pathway and thus enters the sinus again. This retrograde pathway into the sinus helps in spread of infection from the ethmoids to the frontal sinus.

Ethmoidal infundibulum is considered as ethmoid prechamber of maxillary sinus and probably similar retrograde flow exists here also. The frontal sinus drains into the infundibulum or middle meatus through the frontal recess (a space to which frontal sinus drain) depending on the anatomical variation of the attachment of uncinate process. If the uncinate process is attached to the skull base superiorly and it drains directly into the middle meatus and if the attachment is to the lamina papyracea, it drains into the infundibulum (Figs 3.4b and 3.4c).

From the frontal recess, the secretion passes to the ethmoid infundibulum, joins the secretion from maxillary sinus and then it is

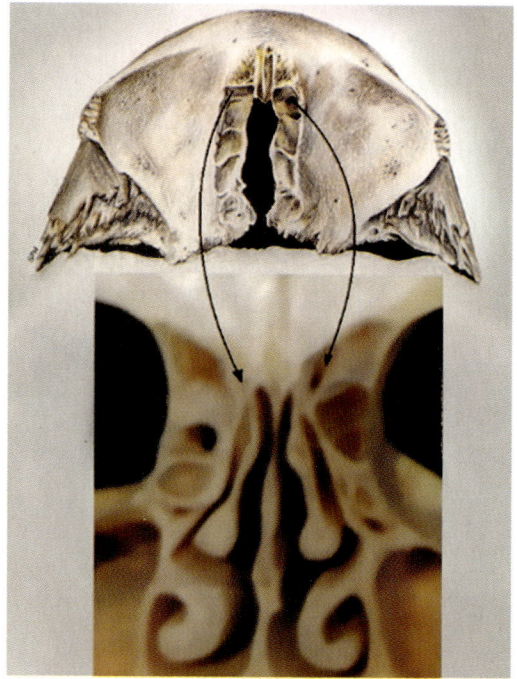

Fig. 3.4b: Drainage of the frontal sinus into ethmoidal prechamber

transported towards the nasopharynx. Drainage of frontal sinus can be affected by obstruction to the frontal recess (Fig. 3.4b) due to anatomical variation in the agger nasi, supra-agger cell or supra-agger frontal cell and suprabullar frontal cell (Wormald, et al 2016).

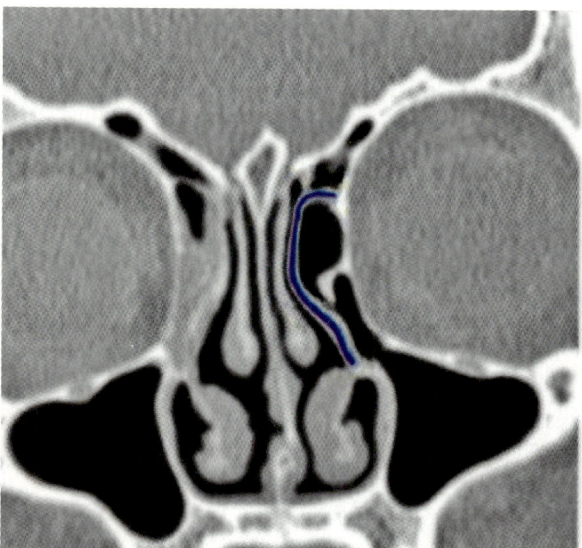
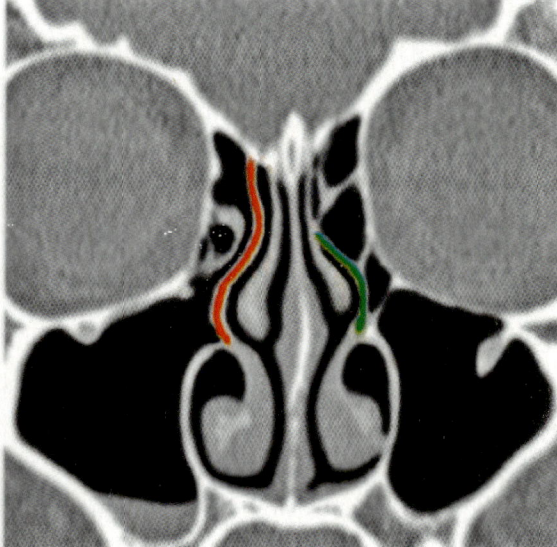

Fig. 3.4c: Mucociliary drainage of frontal recess and maxillary sinus is affected by septoturbinal compression

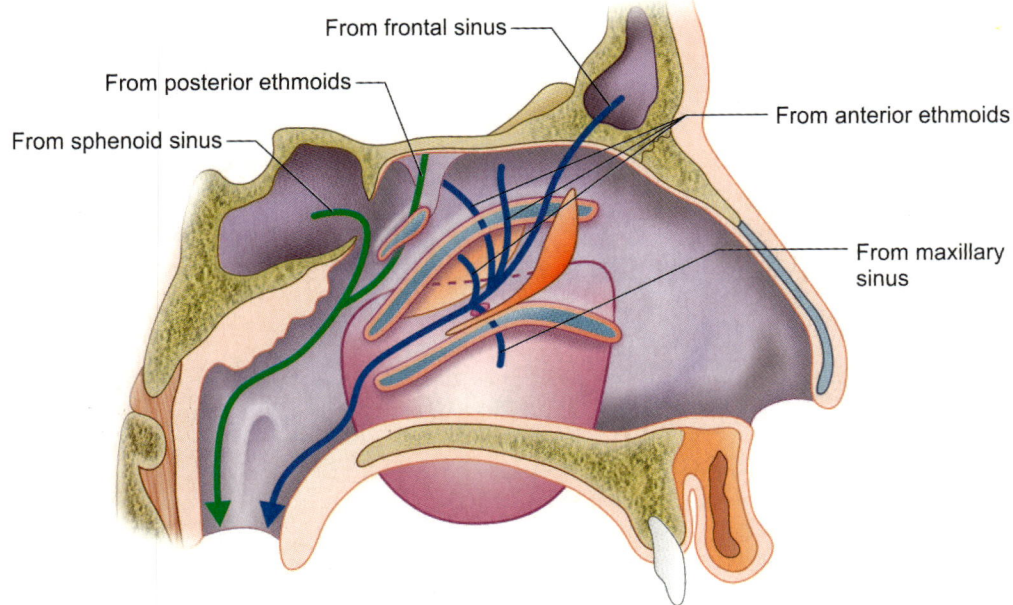

Fig. 3.5: Mucociliary activity of lateral wall of nasal cavity (Messerklinger 1969)

The mucociliary drainage of the sphenoid sinus depends on the site of the ostium and usually it has a spiral transportation. The ethmoidal cells may have a direct or a spiral drainage pathway depending on the site of the ostium into their respective meatuses (Stammberger & Hawke 1993).

Mucociliary Activity of Lateral Wall of Nasal Cavity (Fig. 3.5)

Two streams of mucous pass on the lateral wall nasal cavity. The first from the anterior group sinuses onto the medial surface of inferior turbinate via infundibulum and then anterior and inferior to the tubal orifice in the nasopharynx. The second stream from the posterior group of sinuses passes above the middle turbinate and then posterior and superior to the tubal orifice. Thus in relation to the tubal orifice, two streams are supratubal and infratubal streams of mucous from posterior and anterior groups of sinuses, respectively (Fig. 3.5).

Acute or chronic nasal and sinus inflammation causes alteration in the normal and well-defined pathway. As illustrated the following may occur (Fig. 3.6).

- The routes can join before reaching the tubal orifice (Fig. 3.6).
- One or both routes may form whorls around or even in the orifice itself (Fig. 3.6).
- Abnormal secretions may thus move directly over the orifice (Fig. 3.6).

Any factor that impedes the physiologic mucociliary clearance and ventilation of the sinuses cause chronic sinusitis.

Unfortunately the sinuses drain into the nasal cavity through a complex micro-architectural pathway through the anterior ethmoid and the middle meatus. This system of fissures and clefts within the anterior ethmoid draining the maxillary and frontal sinuses is called ostiomeatal complex and comprises ethmoid infundibulum, frontal recess and maxillary sinus ostium.

These microchannels can be obstructed by various anatomical and pathological variations, however, trivial they may be. Also, the ethmoid sinus because of its topographical situation, is the primary site of deposition of bacterial and allergic particles and thus a primary site of inflammatory disease.

Procter in 1966 said, *"The ethmoid sinuses are usually the key to any problem involving*

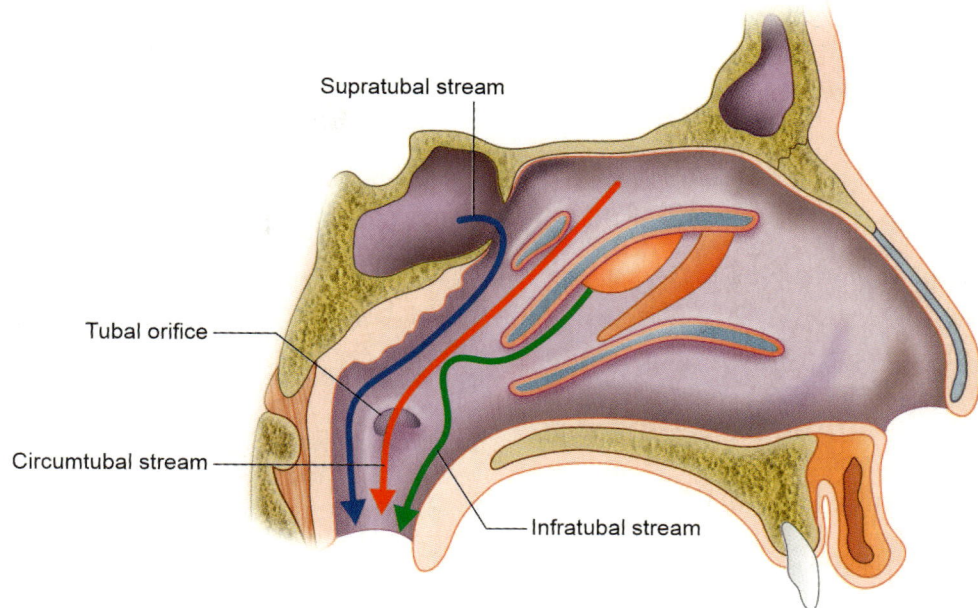

Fig. 3.6: Alteration in normal mucociliary pathway associated with sinus inflammation (Messerklinger 1969)

the infectious sinusitis. Infection begins there and persistent infection there is usually the reason for failure of therapy directed at any of the other paranasal sinuses".

Thus the ethmoid sinuses and the ostio-meatal complex play a crucial role in pathogenesis by:

1. Obstruction to the drainage pathway can occur due to anatomical variations that are very common in anterior ethmoid and as it is the primary site of inflammatory disease, pathological variations are also very common.
2. Acting as the reservoir of infection.
3. Reinfects the dependent sinuses by means of retrograde flow.

Most infections of the PNS are rhinogenic. Other sources of primary infection are dental, blood-borne or traumatic. Whatever the source of infection is, in chronic sinusitis, even though the primary source of infection is cured, the ethmoid sinus continues to harbour infection.

Rhinogenic cause of infection is either due to:
• Primary infection of the nasal and sinus mucosa by bacteria, viruses, etc.

• Secondary to chronic rhinitis due to allergy, vasomotor response or obstructive pathologies of nasal cavity like DNS, polyps, tumour, synechiae, foreign bodies, etc.

Thus, in most of the cases, chronic sinusitis is actually a chronic rhinosinusitis. (CRS). CRS with nasal polyposis has been found to be associated with defective epithelial barrier along with a decreased expression of TJ proteins. The disruption of epithelial integrity by IFN-γ and IL-4 *in vitro* indicates a possible role for these proinflammatory cytokines in the pathogenesis of patients with CRS (Soyka, et al 2012). Thus the treatment of this condition should also eliminate the rhinogenicity. Giacchi, et al (2001) have demonstrated changes in the extracellular matrix, such as bone resorption and neo-osteogenesis on polarized light microscopy. Their findings suggest that CRS may be associated with osteitis of the underlying ethmoid bone. These osteitic bones can obstruct the drainage pathway associated with chronic or reccurent sinusitis.

The ostiomeatal obstruction can occur either due to anatomical variations or pathological variations like infections and oedema in the ostiomeatal complex.

ANATOMICAL VARIATIONS

Anatomical variations in the paranasal sinuses, especially in the middle meatus, lead to increase in susceptibility for recurrent sinusitis (Bolger, et al 1991). The following variations can be observe commonly in the middle meatus.

Variations of Uncinate Process

Medially Turned Uncinate Process

The free posterior margin may be deflected medially, narrowing the middle meatus, thus obstructing the drainage pathway. This may also contact the middle concha.

Laterally Turned Uncinate Process

This narrows the ethmoid infundibulum and if occurs anteriorly, blocks the frontal recess.

Anteriorly Bent Uncinate Process

This may contact the middle turbinate. It narrows the middle meatus and may appear as an additional turbinate. Such a situation is referred to as double middle turbinate.

Fracture of the Uncinate Process

This could be either traumatic or iatrogenic, due to infracture of the inferior turbinate as in procedures like INA, Caldwell-Luc, etc. This infracture produces lateral movement of uncinate process, thus obstructing the ethmoid infundibulum.

Uncinate Bulla (Fig.3.2c)

It refers to pneumatization of uncinate process (Fig. 3.7) which may get aerated from the agger nasi cell and can significantly alter the ventilation and drainage of frontal sinus and ethmoidal infundibulum (Gungor, et al 2008). Term uncinate bulla was coined by Gumusburun et al. (1996) to a well-pneumatized uncinate process. The pneumatization varies between 1 and 9% of cases. The uncinate process can also be hypertrophied besides being laterally or medially bent (Fadda, et al 2012).

Variations of Middle Turbinate

Paradoxically Turned Middle Turbinate

It has its convexity towards lateral nasal wall thus narrowing the middle meatus. This is often found bilaterally and in the anterior aspect of middle meatus. In severe cases, it may compress all the delicate structures in the lateral middle meatal wall.

Concha Bullosa

Concha bullosa (pneumatized middle turbinate), the term was coined by Zuckerlandl in 1862 to define a pneumatized middle turbinate the incidence of which varies between 9 and 12% and can be unilateral or bilateral (Fadda, et al. 2012).

The pneumatization makes the middle turbinate bulky, narrowing the airway, middle meatus, frontal recess, ethmoid infundibulum and hiatus semilunaris. Also, the cell may get infected aggravating its pathogenicity.

Three patterns of pneumatization have been described with respect to their position in the MT (Bolger, et al 1991):

1. In the inferior or bulbous segment (31.2%)
2. In the superior or lamellar segment (46.2%)
3. Extensive pneumatization of both (15.7%)

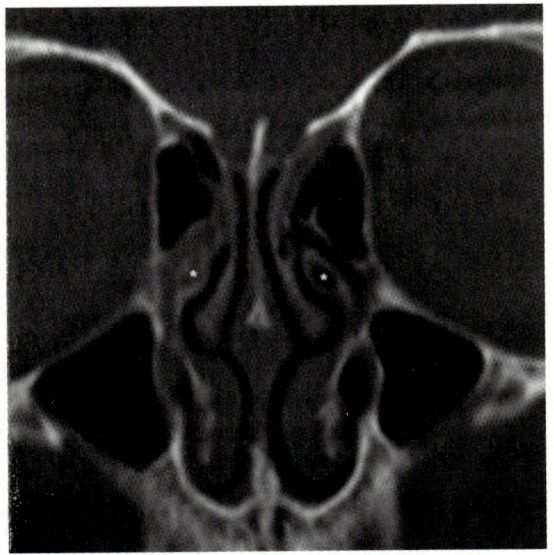

Fig. 3.7: Pneumatized uncinate process(*)

The types 1 and 3 are said to be more significant. The other infrequently found abnormalities of the middle turbinates are: hypoplasia of middle turbinate, accessory middle turbinate, secondary middle turbinate, bifurcate or trifurcate middle turbinate (El-Anwar, et al 2020).

Overpneumatized Bulla

This makes bulla more bulky, and may compress the uncinate process associated with narrowing of the infundibulum, frontal recess, obstructing the hiatus semilunaris. It may also fill in the middle meatus, touching the middle turbinate and thus narrowing the middle meatus. Infected bullar cells aggravate the situation by producing mucosal thickening on the surface of the bulla.

Sinus lateralis: The space above (suprabullar recess) and posterior (retrobullar recess) to the bulla is called sinus lateralis. This is another narrow, hidden space. Disease from bulla may reach posterior ethmoid through this space.

Haller's Cells

These are anterior ethmoid cells, pneumatizing the floor of the orbit, precisely in the region above and lateral to the maxillary sinus ostium and infundibulum. This can narrow the ostium or the infundibulum mechanically by virtue of either dimension of the cell or due to disease within it. These cells are implicated as possible etiologic factor in recurrent maxillary sinusitis (Fig. 3.2b).

Overpneumatized Agger Nasi Cells

Agger cells which are the anterior most cells of anterior ethmoids are situated anterior and superior to the insertion of the middle turbinate to lateral nasal wall (Fig. 6.7, Chapter 6).

This may be over pneumatized usually bilaterally and usually starting from the frontal recess area.

This may narrow the frontal recess and also the middle meatus at the insertion of middle turbinate, leaving only a tiny fissure. When diseased, it may completely block the above.

Nasal Septal Abnormalities

Nasal septal spur: Bony spur of nasal septum can occupy and obstruct the middle meatus.

Pneumatization of nasal septum and interfrontal septum: Some times pneumatization can occur in the perpendicular plate of the nasal septum and interfrontal sinus septum. The pneumatized perpendicular plate of ethmoid can cause obstruction of the olfactory recess causing hyposmia and also can get infected and cause septal mucocele (Lei, et al. 2004). The interfrontal septal pneumatization (cell) can obstruct the frontal recess causing sinusitis and even frontal sinus mucocele. This cell, if not addressed during endoscopic sinus surgery, can result in failure with closure of frontal sinusotomy and recurrence of frontal sinus disease (Som & Lawson 2008).

Pathological Changes in the Middle Meatus

Polypoidal changes are seen frequently invoving the middle turbinate and can be associated with polyposis of paranasal sinuses. While changes in the middle turbinate is atributed to allergic rhinitis, polyps are associated with chronic rhinosinusitis which can significantly affect the quality of life (Brunner 2017). Pathological variations like mucosal oedema or hyperplasia, polypi, etc. could be due to persistent infection or allergy. They commonly occur in the anterior ethmoids as they are the primary sites of inflammation. In addition, the anatomical variations which are very common in anterior ethmoids predispose to the formation of polypi by creating narrow pathways for passage of air (Bernoulli's phenomenon). Also, contact areas may cause polyp growth by the local liberation of neuropeptides such as substance P, which is also a factor in mediating pain can be responsible in pathogenesis of some forms of polyp (Beatrice 1994). Thus small polypi are frequently found within the hiatus, infundibulum, frontal recess and for that matter in any area of mucosal contact like between over pneumatized bulla and middle turbinate.

Flowchart 3.1: Pathogenesis of chronic rhinosinusitis with/without polyposis

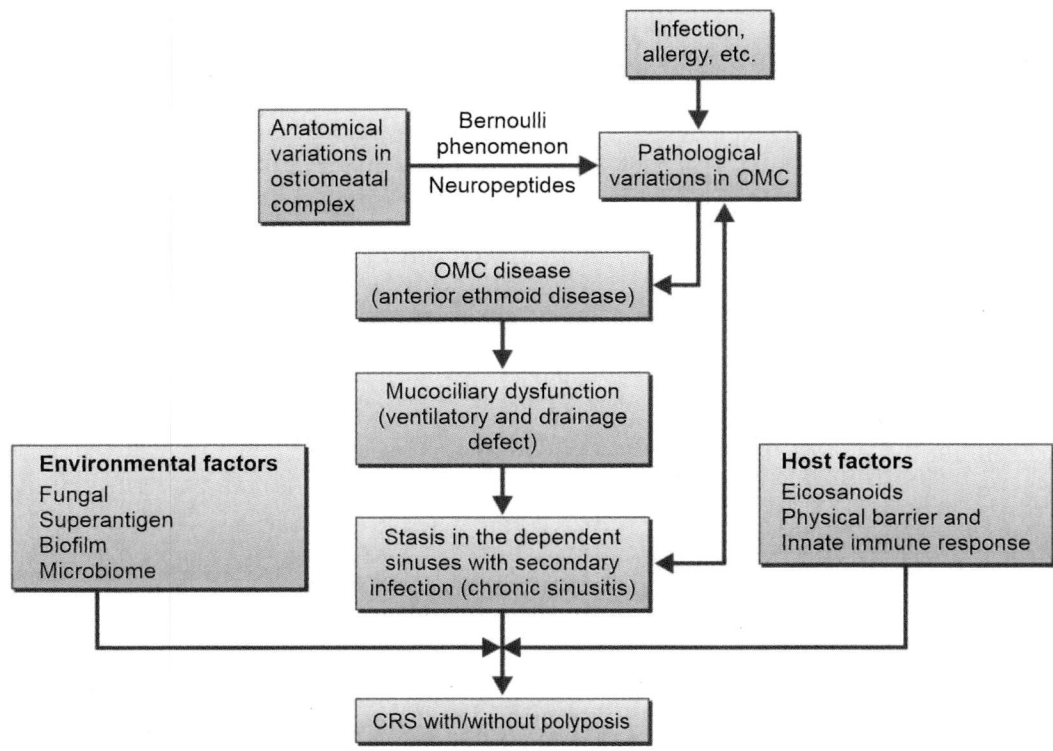

The infundibular diseases are reflected on the medial surface of uncinate process as congested, thickened mucosa, with or without polypi and perforations in uncinate process discharging mucopus. The disease in the bullar cells is reflected on the surface of bulla with similar findings. In diseased frontal recess, in addition to the anatomical variations like prominent agger nasi, congestion and mucopus discharge may be found in this area endoscopically.

Synechiae formed in the middle meatus either due to previous surgery or trauma from nasal packing, nasotracheal or nasogastric intubation, etc. can cause OMC disease.

Thick viscid mucous can plug the intricate passages of anterior ethmoid. Ciliary motility disorders like Kartagener's syndrome, muco-viscidosis, polycystic disease, bronchiectasis, cystic fibrosis, etc. can impair mucociliary activity causing chronic sinusitis.

Thus a functional endoscopic sinus surgery should aim at:

1. Elimination of the ethmoid reservoir of infection by anterior ethmoidectomy.
2. Creation of physiological sinusotomies for mucociliary guided drainage.

By achieving the above (as in Fig. 3.1), it has been shown that even the mucosal disease in the major sinuses, which was considered irreversible, reverts to normal.

The pathogenesis of chronic rhinosinusitis (CRS) is summarized in Flowchart 3.1. Although CRS is traditionally believed as an inadequately treated or unresolved acute bacterial infection and CRS with nasal polyp results from atopy, the entire pathogenesis is quite complex (Fokkens, et al. 2020). Various hypotheses have been implicated based on environmental and host factors. The environmental factors include fungal, staphylococcal superantigen, biofilm and the microbiome. The fungus like alternaria causes a cytokine response on exposure to fungal protein associated with aberrant host defense response although they are not considered as primary cause for CRS (Lam, et al 2015).

Staphylococcal super antigenic exotoxins can enhance eosinophilic response and have been implicated in CRS with nasal polyps (Bernstein, et al. & Zele, et al 2011). Biofilms have been considered as important factor that inactivate the host defense response and effectiveness of antibiotic against infection associated with CRS (Lam, et al 2015). Microbiome of nasal flora plays an important role in preventing pathogenic bacterial growth that can be altered in CRS. The host factor hypothesis includes the eicosanoids pathways and the immune barrier mechanism. The eicosanoid pathways have been involved in aspirin intolerance and is implicated for CRS with nasal polyps (Van et al 2011). The other being physical barrier and the innate immune response may be affected genetically as seen in cystic fibrosis and Kartagener's syndrome (Fokkens, et al 2015).

BIBLIOGRAPHY

1. Beatrice F, Allufi P. Bottomicca F. Nasal polyps and substance P: A preliminary report. Acta Otorhinolaryngol Ital 1994;14 Suppl 41:35–9.

2. Bolger, et al. Paranasal sinus surgery. Anatomic variations and mucosal abnormalities. CT analysis for endoscopic sinus surgery. Laryngoscope 101, Jan. 1991;56–64.

3. Brunnej, et al. Polypoid change of the middle turbinate and paranasal sinus polyposis are distinct entities. Otolaryngol Head Neck Surg 2017;157 (3):519–23.

4. El-Anwar MW, et al. Radiological middle turbinate variations and their relation to nasal septum deviation in asymptomatic adult. Egyptian Journal of Radiology and Nuclear Medicine 2020; 51:104.

5. Fadda G, et al. Multiparametric statistic al correlation between paranasal sinus anatomic variations and chronic rhinosinusitis; Acta Otorhinolaryngol Ital 2012;32:244-251 tween_paranasal_sinus_anatomic_variations_ and_chronic_rhinosinusitis [accessed Feb 24 2020].

6. Gumusburun E, et al. The uncinate bulla. Okajimas Folia Anat Jpn 1996 Aug;73(2-3):101–3.

7. Gungor G, Okur N, Okur E. Uncinate process variations and their relationship with ostiomeatal complex: A pictorial essay of multi-dedector computed tomography (MDCT)

findings. Pol J Radiol 2016;81:173–180. 1994;14 Suppl 41:35–9.

8. Howard L Levine. Functional endoscopic sinus surgery. Evaluation, surgery and follow up of 250 patients. Laryngoscope 100, Jan. 1990;79–84.

9. Kennedy, et al. Endoscopic middle meatal antrostomy. Theory, technique and patency. Laryngoscope 1987; Vol. 97, Supp., pp 143.

10. Kennedy, et al. Functional endoscopic sinus surgery. Part 1. Theory and diagnostic evaluation. Arch otolaryngol Vol. III. Sept. 1985; 576–582. Part II. Surgical technique. Arch otolaryngol Vol. Ill, Oct. 1985;643–649.

11. Kerr A (ed). Rhinology. In: Scott-Brown's Otolaryngology. 6th ed. Oxford: Butterworth-Heinemann; 1997.

12. Lei L, Wang R, Han D. The frontal intersinus septal air cell. Acta Otolaryngol 2004 Mar; 124(2):221–22.

13. Cohen NA. "Sinonasal mucociliary clearance in health and disease". The Annals of Otology, Rhinology and Laryngology. Supplement, 2006; vol. 196:pp. 20–26.

14. Nayak, et al. Endoscopic physiological approach to nasosinus allergy. Ear Nose Throat Journal, Jan (2001).

15. Proctor DF. The nose, paranasal sinus and pharynx. In: Walters W (ed). Lewis Walters, Practice of Surgery, Hagerstown, Maryland, WF Prior, 1966; Vol 4: pp 1–37.

16. Quraishi MS, Jones NS, Mason J. The rheology of nasal mucus: A review. Clin Otolaryngol Allied Sci. 1998;23:403–413. DOI: 10.1046/j.1365-2273.1998.00172.x

17. R Williams, N Rankin, T Smith, et al. Ralationship between humidity and temperature of inspired gas and the function of the airway mucosa. In: Crit Care Med, 1996, Vol. 24, no11: 1920–1929, ISBN 0090-3493.

18. Som PM, Lawson. Interfrontal sinus septal cell: Acause for obstructing inflammation and mucocele. American Journal of Neuroradiology August 2008;29(7):1369–1371.

19. Stammberger H, Wolf. Headaches and sinus disease: The endoscopic approach. Ann: Otol. Rhinol. Laryngol 1988. Supp. 134, 3–23.

20. Stammberger H, Hawke M. Essentials of endoscopic sinus surgery. St. Louis: Mosby 1993.

21. Stammberger H. An endoscopic study of tubal function and the diseased ethmoid sinus. Arch. Otorhinol. Laryngol 1986; 243:254–59.

22. Stammberger H. Endoscopic endonasal surgery. Concepts in treatment of recurring rhinosinusitis. Part I. Anatomic and patho-physiologic considerations. Otolaryngol-Head and Neck Surgery 94:143–155.

23. Stammberger H. Endoscopic surgery for myeotic and chronic recurring sinusitis. Ann. Otol. Rhinol. Laryngol 1985; Supp. 94:101–119.

24. Stammberger H. Nasal and paranasal sinus endoscopy. A diagnostic and surgical approach to recurrent sinusitis. Endoscopy 1986 Nov; 18(6): 213–18.

25. Zinreich, et al. Paranasal sinus, CT imaging requirements of endoscopic surgery. Radiology 163. 1987; 769–775.

26. Messerklinger W. The normal secretion pathways in the human nose. Arch Clin exp Ear, Nose u. Kehlk.-Heilk. 1969;195:138–151.

27. Wormald PJ, Hoseman W, Callejas C, et al. The International Frontal Sinus Anatomy Classification (IFAC) and Classification of the Extent of Endoscopic Frontal Sinus Surgery (EFSS). International Forum of Allergy & Rhinology, 2016; Vol. 6, No. 7: 677–696.

28. Fokkens WJ, Lund VJ, Hopkins C, et al. European Position Paper on Rhinosinusitis and Nasal Polyps 2020. Rhinology. 2020 Feb 20; 58(Suppl S29):1–464.

29. Lam K, et al. The Etiology and Pathogenesis of Chronic Rhinosinusitis: a Review of Current Hypotheses. Curr Allergy Asthma Rep 2015 Jul; 15(7): 41.

30. Van Crombruggen K, Zhang N, Gevaert P, et al. Pathogenesis of chronic rhinosinusitis: inflammation. J Allergy Clin Immunol 2011; 128:728–31

31. Foreman A, Psaltis AJ, Tan LW, Wormald PJ. Characterization of bacterial and fungal biofilms in chronic rhinosinusitis. Am J Rhinol Allergy 2009;23:556–61.

32. Fokkens WJ, Lund VJ, Hopkins C, et al. European Position Paper on Rhinosinusitis and Nasal Polyps 2020. Rhinology 2020 Feb 20;58 (Suppl S29):1–464.

33. Zele VT, Gavaert P, Watelet JM, et al. Staphylococcus aureus colonization and IgE antibody formation to enterotoxins is increased in nasal polyposis. J Allergy Clin Immunol 2010; 126:962–8, 68 e1-6. 37

34. Fokkens WJ, Lund VJ, Mullol J, et al. EPOS 2012: European position paper on rhinosinusitis and nasal polyps 2012. A summary for otorhino-laryngologists. Rhinology 2012; 50:1–12.

4

Diagnostic Nasal Endoscopy

DR Nayak, PSN Murthy, S Behera, RN Biswal

Diagnostic nasal endoscopy is a minimal invasive procedure to examine the interior of nasal cavity for diagnostic evaluation and therapeutic decision making by using an angled nasal endoscope preferably with 30°. Nasal endoscopy was first introduced by Hirshman in 1901, used a modified cystoscope to examine the sinonasal cavity whereas Maltz (1925) used it for diagnostic evaluation and called it sinuscopy (Tajudin and Kennedy, 2017). Messerklinger (1978) described the necessity of diagnostic evaluation of middle meatus and its therapeutic implication. Harold H Hopkins deveoped the rod optic nasal endoscope what we are using today and is still evolving with its excellent optical quality and detailing (Tajudin & Kennedy, 2017). Diagnostic nasal endoscopy and functional endoscopic sinus surgery are relatively new techniques that have expanded our under-standing of sinus physiology and the etio-logies of sinus pathology. Diagnosis at an early stage of chronic sinus disease demonstrates that pathological changes are often limited to the ostiomeatal complex and the anterior sinus group. Early disease refractory to aggressive medical management usually responds to surgical treatment (Levine 1991).

One of the most revolutionary changes seen in rhinology in the recent past is the use of telescope to visualise the lateral nasal wall pathologies as a cause of recurrent sinusitis and to treat these effectively. Antroscopy and nasal endoscopy help to peep inside maxillary sinus and nose, and provide information which is superior to that obtained by other investigations. Both these can be conveniently performed as an outpatient procedure under local anaesthesia.

Narrow, stenotic areas in the anterior ethmoid especially in the vicinity of infundibulum where the frontal and maxillary sinuses drain, are the key areas for detection and cure of infection of the anterior group of paranasal sinuses which is made possible by the use of nasal endoscopy. Nasal cavity findings obtained by nasal endoscopy were more conclusive in the elucidation of diagnosis than those obtained by computer tomography of the paranasal sinus (Duarte, et al. 2005).

Technology

Major technical advances in optics and lighting have produced rigid endoscopes suitable for use in nasal and sinus endoscopies.

Hopkins optical rod lens system has improved upon traditional endoscopes by producing bright and sharp images with a larger viewing angle. Hopkins rod lens system was introduced in 1960. Traditional telescopes employed a group of lenses constituting an objective followed by a succession of relay systems.

In rod lens system, the image is relayed by a succession of rod lens. The traditional systems consisted of a tube of air with thin lens of glass. By contrast, the new system may be regarded as a tube of glasses with thin lenses of air (Hopkins—Modern urological endoscope).

Advantages of using rod lenses are:

1. The total light transmitted is increased by factor n^2, where n is the refractive index of glass used for lenses.

2. Mechanically the outer case and precision of mounting of rod lenses permit a greater diameter to be used for lenses for a given outer diameter of telescopes.

3. The use of efficient, multilayer, anti-reflection coatings on the surface of lenses contribute notably to the brightness.

The function of endoscopy itself is to render the interior of body cavity observable to the endoscopist exactly, as if it were being viewed by him directly.

The nasal endoscope is an optical instrument for examining the nasal cavity. This examination is known as diagnostic nasal endoscopy. As the endoscope is between 2.7, 3 and 4.0 mm in diameter, it can be passed easily through the nostril to examine the nasal passages and the sinuses. In 0° nasal endoscopes, the view is straight ahead from the tip of the instrument, whereas in other endoscopes, the view is at an angle from the tip of the endoscope. These angled endoscopes can be used to visualise the remote areas of the nasal cavity and paranasal sinuses. The Hopkins rod-lens system has brought about a revolutionary change in technology of endoscopy (Fig. 4.1).

In the performance of comprehensive diagnostic nasal endoscopy, the most commonly employed telescopes are the 0° and 30° endoscopes. The instruments are 18 cm long glass rod lenses, with an outside diameter of 4 mm. For special indications like children

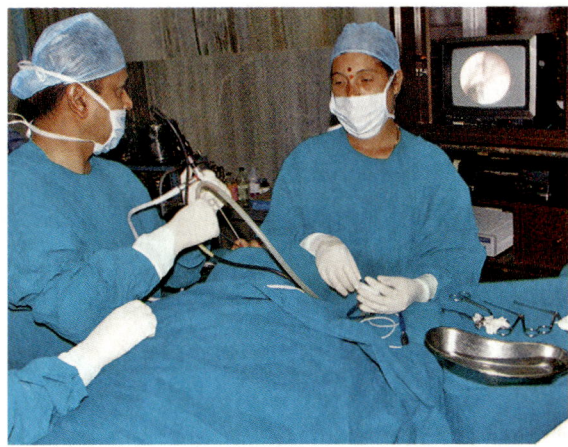

Fig. 4.2: Video nasal endoscopic assessment before starting functional endoscopic sinus surgery

or in patients with stenotic meati, the 0° and 30° lenses with 2.7 mm outer diameter scopes are used. The telescope with a deflection angle of 70° is helpful in visualising frontal recess.

For routine examination, illumination is provided by Karl Storz 481-C miniature light source, whereas for photo documentation a Karl Storz 610 Xenon light source with built in flash generator is employed.

The video equipment includes a television camera, beam splitter, colour monitor and recorder (Fig. 4.2).

Indications for Diagnostic Nasal Endoscopy

Diagnostic nasal endoscopy is an essential investigative modality in the following situations:

1. Patients with gross sinusitis diagnosed clinically to reach a pathological diagnosis (ostiomeatal complex disease).

2. In patients with symptoms attributable to sinusitis to confirm diagnosis including sinus barotrauma.

3. In patients whose problems are not clear and in whom there seems to be no overt indication of sinus disease, this group of patients present rewarding challenge for the nasal endoscope (Stammberger 1988).

4. In patients with headaches to rule out occult sinus infections and contact headaches.

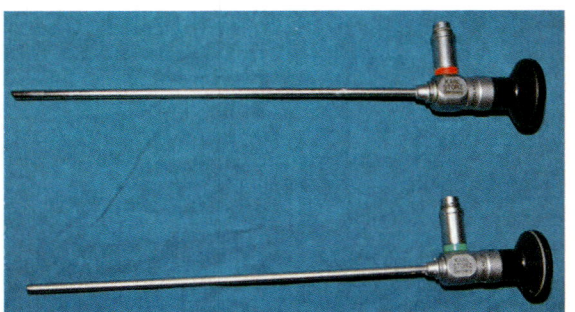

Fig. 4.1: Karl Storz 0° and 30° nasal endoscopes

5. In allergic rhinosinusitis for early detection of nasal polyps.
6. In patients with chronic dacryocystitis to visualize the nasolacrimal duct and to rule out any nasal causes.
7. In cases of rhinosinusitis and sinus abnormality on CT evaluation to decide, if surgery will be the effective therapy.
8. For postoperative objective evaluation after sinus surgery.
9. For taking nasal swabs for cultures under endoscopic control (Kennedy, 1985).
10. In tubotympanic disease to detect occult sinusitis.
11. In patients with epistaxis to localise bleeding points.
12. To detect small foreign bodies in the nose.
13. To establish if a deflected nasal septum is significant enough to cause the symptoms.
14. To diagnose adenoids and other naso-pharyngeal masses. It has replaced Yanker's nasopharyngeal speculum to examine nasopharynx.
15. To evaluate eustachian tube orifice.
16. To diagnose chronic nasal diseases like rhinosporidiosis, mycosis, rhinolith, etc.
17. For post maxillectomy evaluation.
18. In pain therapy by blocking the spheno-palatine ganglion.
19. To evaluate anosmia and hyposmia.
20. Oroantral fistula. Rhinorrhea suggestive of CSF leak.

Selection of Patients

Diagnostic nasal endoscopy has to be done in a quiescent stage of sinusitis. Patients encountered with acute exacerbation of chronic sinusitis may be put on medical treatment for 7–10 days before embarking on diagnostic nasal endoscopy.

Diagnostic endoscopy can be performed in any age or sex. Nasal endoscopy is a safe, objective and useful means of identifying potentially significant abnormalities in children with nasal obstruction (Kubba and Bingham 2001).

Before doing a nasal endoscopy checking lignocaine sensitivity is a must to avoid catastrophies. Blood pressure estimation will detect hypertensive patients in whom adrenaline should not be used for nasal decongestion.

Other systemic diseases like diabetes mellitus, tuberculosis, bronchial asthma and bleeding diathesis pose no contraindication to nasal endoscopy. As for apprehensive patients, a gentle reassurance will allay anxiety. Patients with HIV, hepatitis B and rhinosporidiosis can be done at the end of the day. In the COVID-19 pandemic, personal protectives are equally important espacially face shield, N95 masks, protective gown and surgical cap. Prior RT PCR testing is preferable. Nasal irrigation with dilute povidone-iodine solution (1.25%) can inactivate SARS COV2 before nasal endoscopic procedure or surgery and is safe to use (Frank, et al. 2020).

1. Equipment

- **Nasal endoscopes:** Hopkins rod optical system with cold light source and fiber-optic light delivery system provides excellent illumination and optical quality. Endoscopes are available with 0°, 30°, 70°, 90°, 120° angles of view and 2.7 and 4 mm diameter (Fig. 4.1).
- Topical decongestant and anaesthetic agent and applicators. 4% xylocaine with 1:100,000 adrenaline.
- Antifog solution
- Suction apparatus and suction cannula

2. Position

Supine with head slightly turned towards the examiner who is seated on the right side of the patient (Fig. 4.3).

Gustafson, et al. (1989) describe the patient in sitting position, with the examiner sitting opposite, facing him.

Anaesthesia

Topical decongestant anaesthetic spray (4% lignocaine + 1:100,000 adrenaline) followed by application of the same solution

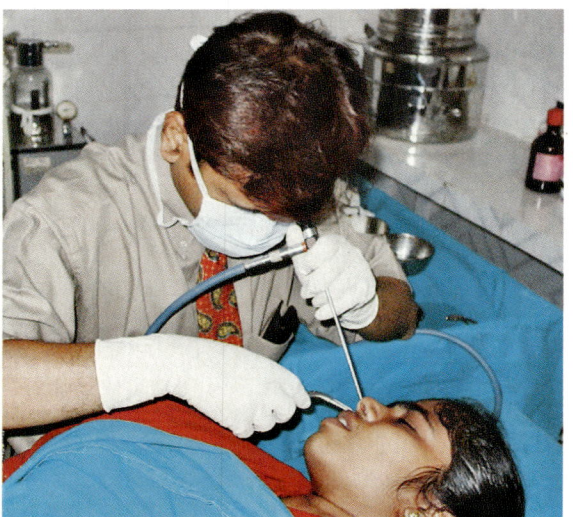

Fig. 4.3: Outpatient diagnostic nasal endoscopy in progress. In the present scenario of COVID-19 outbreak, the endoscopist should wear proper personal protective equipment for self protection.

using applicator like cottonoid strips on the floor of nasal cavity, over the inferior turbinates, sphenopalatine foramen area, middle meatus and the anterior aspect of the roof, to block anterior ethmoidal nerve. Applicator is left in position for 10 minutes.

Gustafson, et al. (1989) used phenylephrine hydrochloride as decongestant. Huerter (1992) used mixture of oxymetazoline in 4% lignocaine in 1:1 ratio. Kennedy used 5% cocaine on a nasal applicator to the inferolateral surface of the middle turbinate and to other sites, where passage of endoscope may exert slight pressure. In case where significant septal deviation is present, topical cocaine is also applied to the posterior nasal mucosa on the side of convexity.

3. Antifog Solution

The scope may be get fogged due to deposition of moisture. Huerter (1992) used antifog solution FRED to prevent fogging. Kennedy says that if telescope lens is touched against clean mucous membrane such as anterior end of inferior turbinate, is all that is needed to prevent fogging.

In our set-up, we use savlon solution, and also ask the patient to breath through the mouth to prevent fogging.

4. Endoscopy

The endoscope is gently held using both hands. The left hand rests on the patients face and holds the endoscope using thumb and index finger. Right hand holds the eyepiece. Movements are made gently avoiding trauma. It is essential that the instrument is gripped lightly so that the examiner readily detects undue pressure and avoids discomfort. In adult, 4 mm 30° telescope is selected first. This provides an excellent overall view of nose and nasopharynx (Kennedy 1985).

Huerter (1992) used 2.7 mm 30° endoscope as it allows good visualization of even narrow noses. Gustafson (1989) used 4 mm, 0°–30° and 70° for routine examination.

Ist Pass

In this pass, the endoscope is passed along the floor of nasal cavity towards nasopharynx, look for:
a. Status of inferior meatus and turbinate should be noted. Hypertrophic turbinates are usually associated with DNS and chronic rhinitis. Turbinates may be atrophied in atrophic rhinitis (Fig. 4.4b).
b. Patency of nasolacrimal duct orifice.
c. Status of INA window, if present and status of antral mucosa, if visualised.
d. Septal spur (Fig. 4.5)
e. Eustachian tube orifice and nasopharyngeal mucosa. Look for stream of mucus, which could be supratubal, infratubal circumtubal or over the orifice (Fig. 4.4a).
f. Dynamic action of tubal orifice may be visualised. Fossa of Rosenmuller is examined for any lesion (Fig. 4.4c).

IInd Pass

After completing examination in the Ist pass, the scope is withdrawn and slide over the medial surface of the middle turbinate floor of the posterior choana. The scope is further advanced between the middle turbinate and the septum to reach the sphenoethmoidal recess. Any discharge, if present, should be noted (Figs 4.4a and 4.4d). Further advancing the scope upwardly in the region will allow the visibility of the sphenoid sinus ostium. Decongestion of this area between the septum

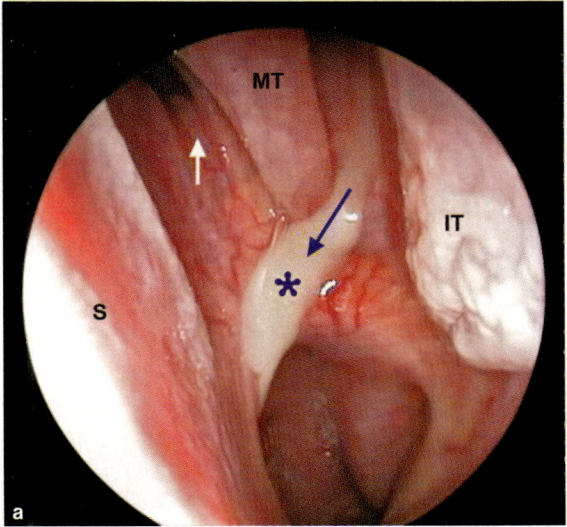

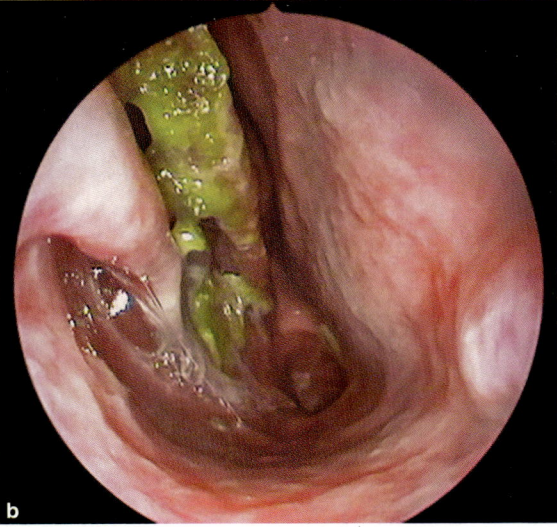

Fig. 4.4: a. Thick purulent discharge from left middle meatus seen above the eustachian tube orifice. White arrow shows sphenoethmoidal recess leading to sphenoid sinus ostium. **b.** Greenish yellow crusts seen in the posterior part of nasal cavity associated with atrophy of the turbinates

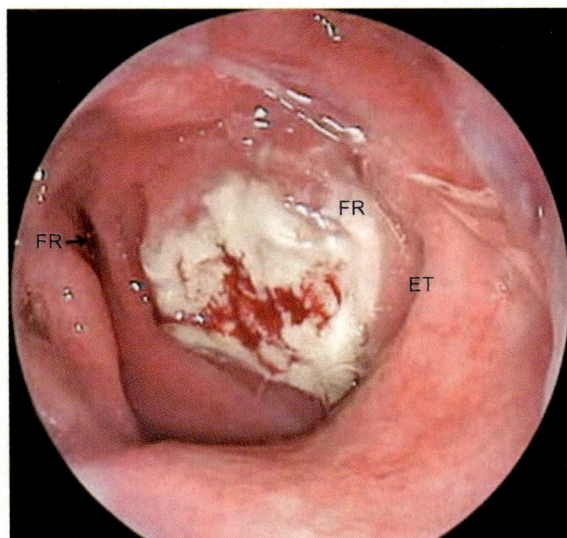

Fig. 4.4c: Ulcerative lesion in the left **fossa of Rosenmüller** (FR) extending to the roof of nasopharynx and left eustachian tube (ET) in a case of nasopharyngeal cancer

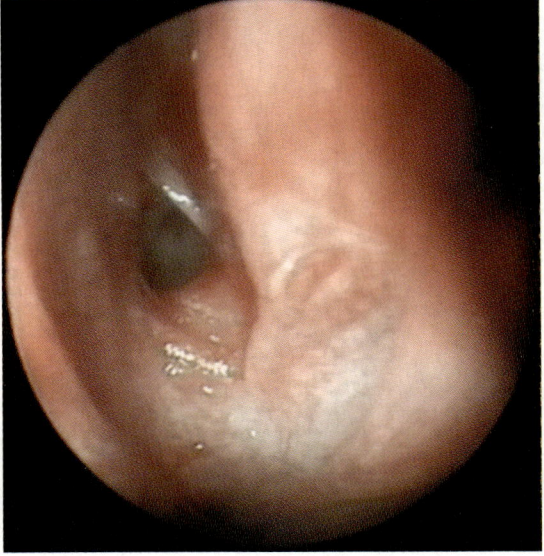

Fig. 4.4d: Sphenoidal ostium in the sphenoethmoidal recess after balloon dilatation

and the middle turbinate is very essential for good visualization.

IIIrd Pass

This is the most important pass of the three that evaluates the middle turbinate and the middle meatus and it's contents. The agger nasi is

evaluated at the anterior attachment. Middle meatus is rarely wide enough to admit the telescope anteriorly. It can be frequently inserted into the posterior aspect of middle meatus to inspect bulla, hiatus semilunaris, infundibulum, etc. Look for any anatomical variations in the OMC like concha bullosa (Fig. 4.5) medially turned uncinate process

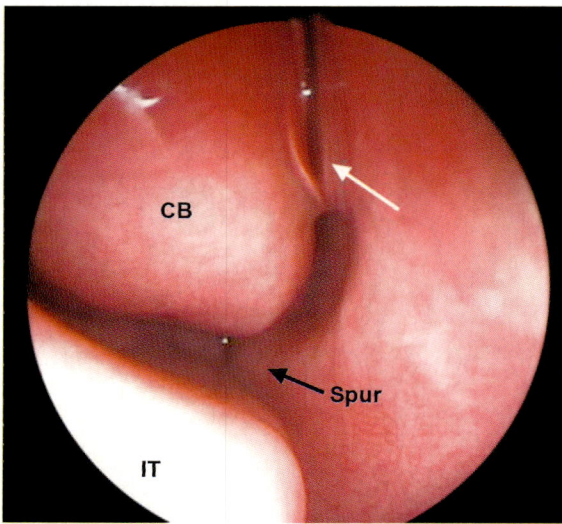

Fig. 4.5: Endoscopic picture of left concha bullosa (CB) and septal spur touching inferior turbinate (IT). Also note mucoid discharge between septum and middle turbinate seen in a case of allergic rhinosinusitis, from posterior ethmoids (white arrow)

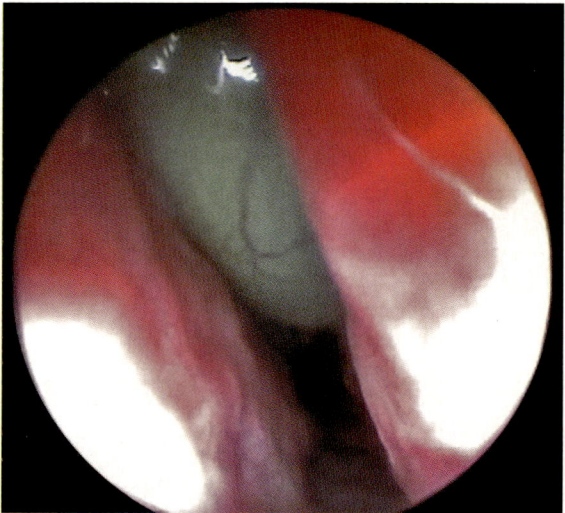

Fig. 4.7: Intranasal meningocele in the nasal cavity presenting as nasal polyp

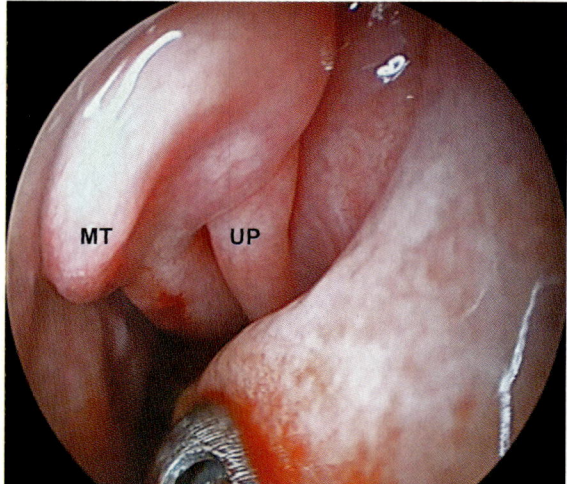

Fig. 4.6: Endoscopic picture of a medially turned uncinate process (UP), upper part is obscured by middle turbinate (MT).

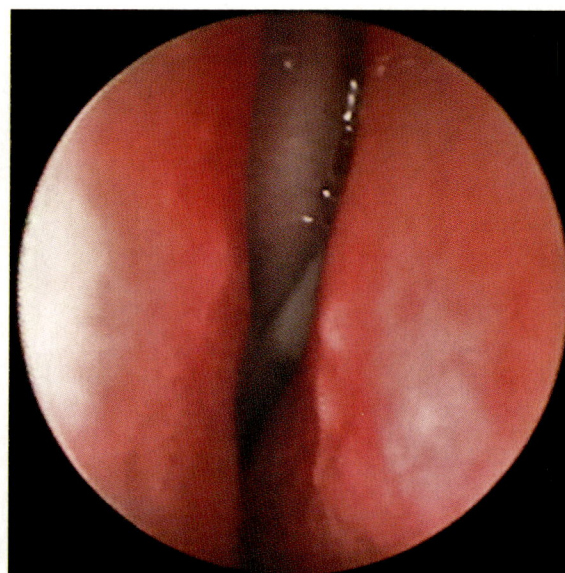

Fig. 4.8: Endoscopic picture showing mucoidal discharge in the middle meatus

(Fig. 4.6), etc. The pathological variations in the OMC that can be noted are polyp in the middle meatus (Fig. 4.7), or mucoidal discharge in the middle meatus (Figs 4.5 and 4.8), purulent discharge in the middle meatus (Fig. 4.9). Frontal recess area is visualized to look for any discharge from the frontal recess. Swelling may be seen at the attachment of middle turbinate in case of frontoethmoidal mucocele.

Other Methods

Gustafson (1989) used a different technique. The scope is carefully passed along the floor of the nose while the septum, inferior meatus, inferior turbinate, middle turbinate and nasopharynx are inspected. The telescope is then gently raised to expose the face of sphenoid, the sphenoid ostium and spheno-ethmoid recess. The telescope is then rolled up

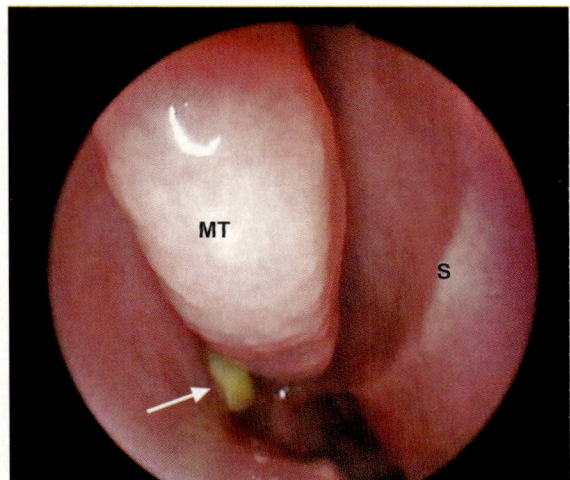

Fig. 4.9: Middle turbinate (MT), septum (S) and the white arrow pointing purulent discharge in the middle meatus

over the posterior tip of inferior turbinate into the posterior aspect of middle meatus. As the telescope is withdrawn anteriorly, visualize the structures in middle meatus.

The inspection of maxillary sinus mucosa through a postoperative middle or inferior meatal antrostomy is facilitated by angle telescope (70°) of 2.7 mm size.

The endoscope can be passed along the floor of the nasal cavity till the nasopharynx. The scope is withdrawn between the inferior and middle turbinates to evaluate middle meatus. The scope enters the middle meatus in a posterior inferior direction and moved anterosuperiorly to evaluate hiatus semilunaris, bulla ethmoidalis and nasofrontal recess. At this point, the scope is passed medial to the middle turbinate, posterosuperiorly to observe the superior meatus sphenoethmoidal recess and sphenoid ostium (Huerter 1992).

Kennedy advises gentle medial subluxation of middle turbinate or the use of a cannula placed under middle turbinate to help the introduction of 4 mm scope in middle meatus.

Nasal Endoscopy in Children

Performing nasal endoscopy in a child can be a very difficult problem and in many cases, we may have to resort to GA.

Chait, et al. (1991) have described their technique for successful paediatric examinations.

a. The environment of the examination room should be calm and the approach to the child must be gentle.
b. 2% cocaine solution (instead of 5%) is applied gently to the child's nostril 8–10 sprays are administered. Nasal cottonoids are not used.
c. Cocaine will produce a bitter taste and the child should be forewarned of this.
d. Introduce the scope gently into the nose shielding the light from child's eye.

Role of flexible endoscopy: Flexible endoscope of 3.5 mm and/or 2.5 mm flexible endoscopes can be quite effective in evaluating nasal cavity in children and in those younger than 8 years, even though the endoscopic view is of poor quality and inferior compare to rigid endoscopic evaluation after application of topical anaesthetic sprays (Berlucci, et al. 2011).

Diagnostic and therapeutic use: The use of nasal endoscopy in children can become very handy specially for evaluating sinus pathology, diagnosing adenoid hypertrophy, impacted foreign bodies deep inside the nasal cavity (Fig. 4.10). These foreign bodies can be removed safely by using a hook while avoiding injury to the nasal mucosa.

Limitations of Nasal Endoscopy

1. Gross septal deviation can make endoscopy difficult and unrewarding.
2. Localized disease within the infundibulum, frontal recess and maxillary sinus ostium is difficult to diagnose.
3. Due to the optical illusionary effect, a beginner may find it difficult to orient the anatomy especially when using different optical views.
4. Depth perception is not there because of absence of binocular vision.
5. Gives no information regarding position and status of vital relations of sphenoethmoids.

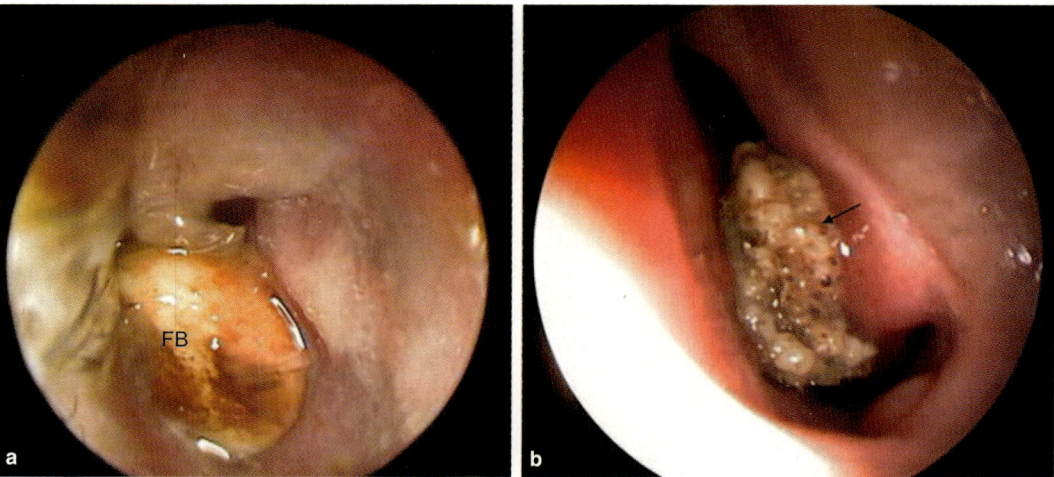

Fig. 4.10: Endoscopic picture showing foreign body (FB) in the nose: **a.** Stone, **b.** Rubber

6. Exact extent of disease within the spheno-ethmoid is difficult to be made.

These limitations can be overcome by CT imaging of OMC.

BIBLIOGRAPHY

1. Aracely Fernandes Duarte, Rita de Cássia Soler, Francis Zavarezzi Rev Bras. Nasal endoscopy associated with paranasal sinus computerized tomography scan in the diagnosis of chronic nasal obstruction. Otorhinolaryngol V.71, n.3, 361–3, May/June 2005.

2. Berlucchi M, Pedruzzi B, Sessa M, Nicolai P. Diagnostic and Therapeutic Sinonasal Endoscopy in Pediatric Patients in "Advances in endoscopic surgery" edited by Enacu C, Published by InTech.

3. Chait DH, Lotz WK. Successful pediatric examination using nasoendoscopy. Laryngoscope, 1991 101 (9): 1016–1018.

4. Duarte AF, et al. Nasal endoscopy associated with paranasal sinus computer tomography in the diagnosis of chronic sinusitis. Rev Bras Otorhinolaringology V71, N-3, p 361–363, May/June 2005.

5. Gustafson RO, Kern EB. Office endoscopy when, why, what, and how. Otolaryngol Clin North Am 1989 Aug; 22(4):683–89.

6. Haytham Kubba, Brian JG Bingham. Endoscopy in the assessment of children with nasal obstruction. Journal of Laryngology and Otology 2001;115:380–384 Cambridge University Press.

7. Huerter JV. Functional endoscopic sinus surgery and allergy. Otolaryngol Clin North Am 1992;25(1):231–238.

8. Kennedy DW. Arch Otolaryngol 1985;111:643–98.

9. Levine SB, Gill AJ, Levinson SR, Coffey TK. Diagnostic nasal endoscopy and functional endoscopic sinus surgery: An update and review of complications. Conn Med 1991 Oct; 55(10):574–76.

10. Stammberger H, Wolf G. Headaches and sinus disease: The endoscopic approach. Ann Otorhinolaryngol 1988 Sept–Oct 134:3.

11. Frank S, Brown SM, Capriotti JA. In vitro effect of povidone iodine nasal antiseptic for rapid inactivation of SARS-CoV-2. JAMA Otolaryngol-Head and Neck surgery. doi:10.1001/jamaoto.2020.3053

12. Tajudin DA, Kennedy DW. Thirty years of endoscopic sinus surgery. World J of Otolaryngology-Head and Neck Surgery 2017;3:115–21.

Indications for Endoscopic Surgery of the Nose and Paranasal Sinuses

DR Nayak, P Hazarika, KK Samantray, A Bhandarkar

Endoscopy has revolutionized the diagnosis and management of inflammatory sinus disease where mucosal preservation is the key for the successful treatment outcome (Palmer, et al. 2012). Functional endoscopic sinus surgery is a relatively minimally invasive technique and the goal of this procedure is to restore sinus ventilation and normal function (Stammberger 1991). It is more successful in patients who have recurrent acute or chronic infective sinusitis. Initially the indication for endoscopic sinus surgery was confined to the management of chronic sinusitis refractory to medical treatment, but over the years the indications for endonasal endoscopic surgery have extended to encompass a wide variety of diseases other than just chronic sinusitis. The effectiveness of standard surgical techniques for inflammatory diseases of nasal and paranasal sinuses has been well established for more than a century. With the recent popularization of endoscopic sinus surgery, however, many of these techniques are now considered radical (Friedman 1989).

Endoscopic sinus surgery is most commonly performed for inflammatory and infectious sinus disease although endoscopic approach is gaining acceptance for selected neoplastic disease and skull base lesions. Tabulated below are all the indications and extended indications for endoscopic nasal and sinus surgery.

Indications for Endoscopic Sinus Surgery

1. Chronic sinusitis refractory to medical management (Figs 5.1 and 5.2)

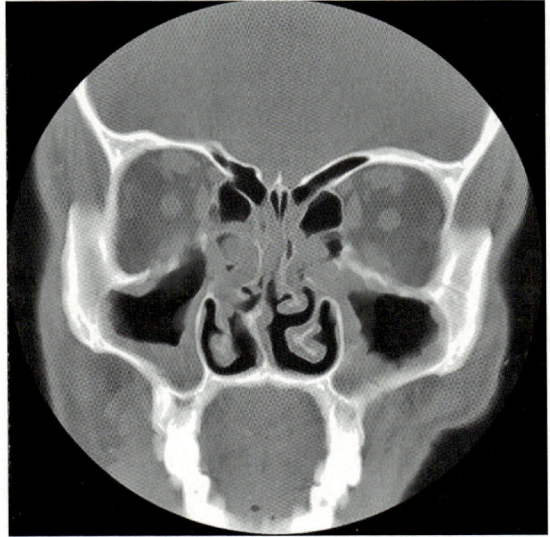

Fig. 5.1: Chronic pansinusitis associated with bilateral ostiomeatal complex disease

2. Recurrent sinusitis
3. Fungal sinusitis
4. Nasal polyposis
5. Excision of concha bullosa
6. Partial turbinectomy
7. Allergic fungal sinusitis
8. Epistaxis
9. Synechiae release
10. Endoscopic reduction of inferior turbinates
11. Sinus mucoceles/pyocele

Extended Indications for Endoscopic Sinus Surgery

1. Cerebrospinal fluid leak
2. Optic nerve decompression

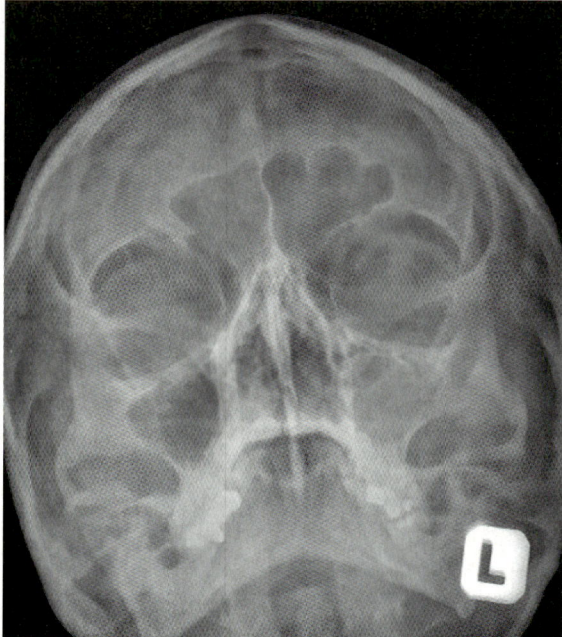

Fig. 5.2: X-ray PNS (Waters' view) showing complete opacity of the left maxillary sinus and mucosal thickening of the right maxillary sinus. Also there is haziness of the right frontal sinus suggestive of chronic sinusitis

3. Orbital cellulitis/abscess (for orbital decompression)
4. Foreign bodies from the paranasal sinuses
5. Osteoma nasal cavity/PNS

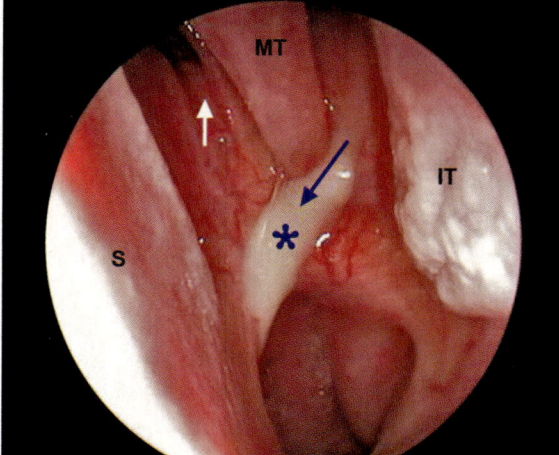

Fig. 5.3: Mucopurulent discharge from left middle meatus moving towards nasopharynx (blue arrow and asterix). Also seen are middle turbinate (MT), posterior end of inferior turbinate (IT) and nasal septum (S) and white arrow pointing sphenoethmoidal recess

6. Meningoceles/meningoencephalocele
7. Contact headache/neuralgia

Indications for Endonasal Endoscopic Surgery

1. Endoscopic septoturbinoplasty
2. Endoscopic medial maxillectomy, craniofacial resection, etc. and skull base surgery
3. Atrophic rhinitis
4. Dacryocystorhinostomy
5. Pituitary tumours (endoscopic hypophysectomy)
6. Adenoidectomy
7. Congenital choanal atresia
8. Rhinosporidiosis
9. Vidian neurectomy
10. Nasopharynx biopsy
11. Inverted papilloma
12. Sphenopalatine ganglion block
13. Meningoceles/meningoencephalocele
14. Impacted foreign bodies in the nose

Chronic sinusitis usually involves the anterior ethmoids and maxillary sinuses. Pansinusitis, involvement of all the sinuses, almost always including the posterior ethmoidal cells with or without the sphenoid and frontal sinuses.

Recurrent sinusitis is defined as periodic episodes of acute sinusitis with complete clearance of disease in between. As a result of frequent infection and confinement of the disease to the anterior ethmoids, it is mandatory to undergo endoscopic surgery especially when the disease interferes with our daily routine work.

Fungal sinusitis is usually associated with immunocompromised patients and can be treated successfully through endoscopic sinus surgery. Clearance of the disease is possible under direct endoscopic vision and repeated inspection of the FESS cavity. Allergic fungal sinusitis can be associated with polypoidal changes and polyp formation in the middle meatus whereas polypoidal oedematous middle turbinate alone is seen in allergic rhinosinusitis (Figs 5.4 to 5.7).

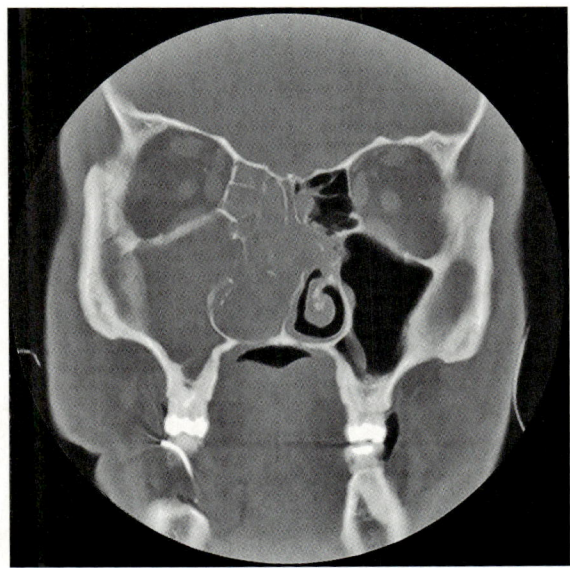

Fig. 5.4: Coronal CT scan of ostiomeatal complex showing gross involvement of right maxillary sinus and ethmoids in a case of allergic fungal sinusitis

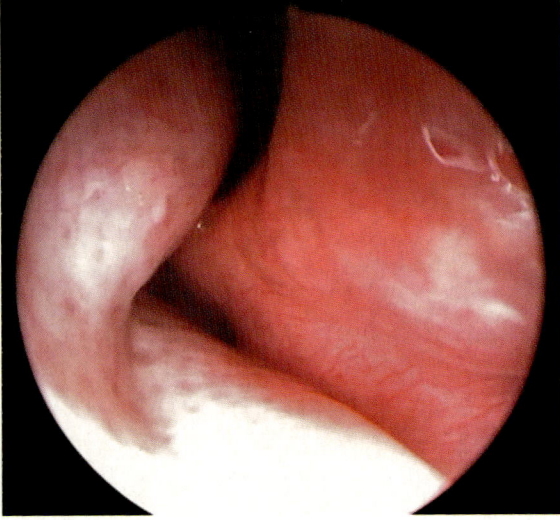

Fig. 5.6: Video endoscopic photograph showing septal spur in contact with right lateral nasal wall

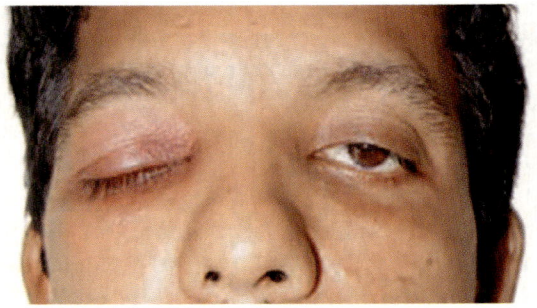

Fig. 5.5: Right orbital cellulitis due to invasive aspergillosis of PNS

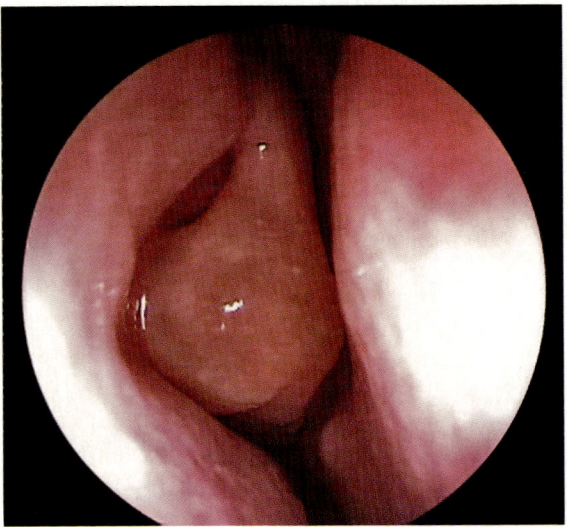

Fig. 5.7: Video endoscopic photograph showing polypoidal middle turbinate

Nasal polyposis (Fig. 5.8) can be surgically removed by endoscopic surgery. Polyps seen in the younger age group can avoid extensive procedures like external ethmoidectomy which leave a scar, thus causing psychological trauma. For antrochoanal polyp, Caldwell-Luc operation is a morbid procedure, if the facial skeletal growth and dentition is not complete.

Intranasal glioma can be safely excised through endoscopic approach (Fig. 5.9).

Persistent nasal obstruction due to concha bullosa or extensive hypertrophied inferior turbinates can be resected endoscopically to relieve the obstruction and also additional septal surgery can be done to prevent a roomy cavity. Synechiae formation after extensive intranasal polypectomy or multiple nasal surgeries can be relieved. A dental wax plate can be inserted to prevent synechiae in such cases.

Posterior nasal bleeds occur from the sphenopalatine vessels, which can be easily identified and cauterized. Hypertrophied, oedematous inferior turbinate, particularly the

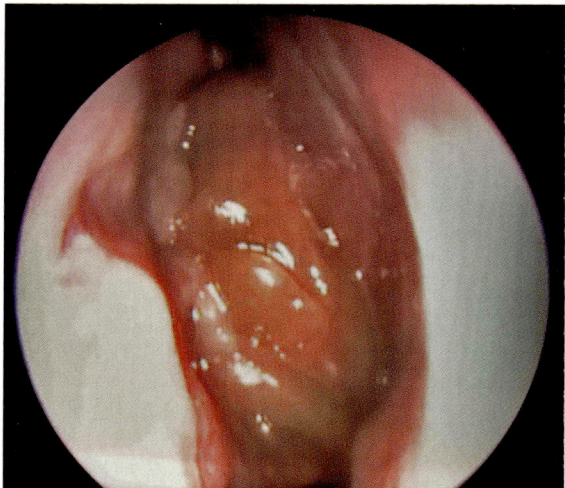

Fig. 5.8: Video endoscopic photograph showing ethmoidal polyposis

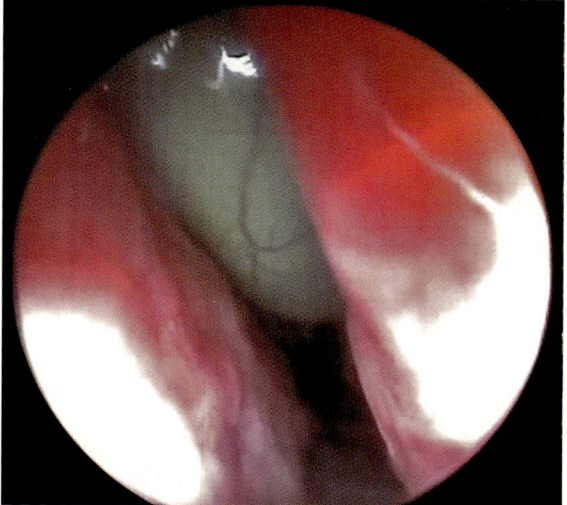

Fig. 5.9: Video endoscopic photograph showing intranasal glioma

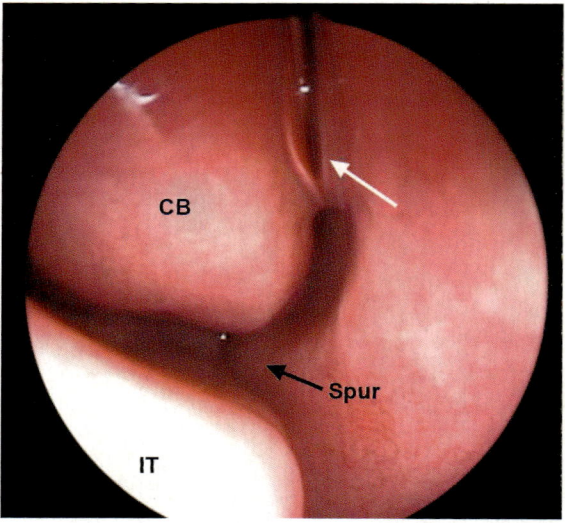

Fig. 5.10: Endoscopic picture showing septal spur (black arrow), concha bullosa (CB) and clear discharge between middle turbinate and the septum in a case of CSF rhinorrhoea (white arrow)

Cerebrospinal fluid leak is commonly caused by trauma and leak into the floor of the nasal cavity through the cribriform plate. Clear watery discharge between middle turbinate and septum should be suspected for such cases (Fig. 5.10). Endoscopic repair is possible by using a temporalis fascia muscle graft and placing it at the leaking site. The graft is further supported by abdominal fat and gel foam.

Orbital decompression has its indications. By endoscopically removing the lamina papyracea and floor of the orbit, the orbit can be decompressed providing excellent results. Orbital cellulitis and abscess can be drained by opening the lamina papyracea and incising the orbital periosteum. Even optic nerve decompression can be achieved by endoscopic sphenoid sinus surgery. The lateral wall of the sphenoid sinus is exposed and drilled, thus relieving the compression on the optic nerve.

Foreign bodies in the paranasal sinuses are rare, more so in the sphenoethmoidal complex. Penetrating wound caused by a ricocheted air gun pellet lodged the posterior ethmoid labyrinth has been successfully removed by endoscopic intranasal ethmoidectomy. Nasal foreign bodies can be shown endoscopically.

posterior part which may occlude the posterior choana, can be endoscopically cauterized by a bipolar cautery, or reduced by laser.

Frontal and ethmoidal mucoceles commonly associated with rhinosinusitis and are more common than maxillary and sphenoidal mucoceles. Mucoceles and pyoceles can be treated successfully by endoscopic sinus surgery thus preventing a radical external approach and maintaining the normal physiological features and drainage pathway of the sinus.

Endoscopic dacryocystorhinostomy is performed to connect the lacrimal sac directly to the nasal cavity when there is an obstruction either in the sac or in the nasolacrimal duct (Chapter 14). Osteomas are bony tumours commonly seen in the frontal sinus. Endoscopically one can reduce or resect these osteomas with a drill.

Sphenopalatine ganglion block as a primary mode of pain therapy is clinically used for a variety of disorders of the head and facial regions. Endoscopically, the sphenopalatine foramen is identified between the posterior ends of the middle and superior turbinates. The sphenopalatine ganglion is located lateral to the sphenopalatine foramen. A long-acting local anaesthetic (0.25% bupivacaine) is administered repeatedly. Vidian neurectomy has been endoscopically performed with promising results.

Congenital choanal atresia can be treated by endoscopic intranasal or endoscopic sublabial transnasal approach. A portex naso-tracheal tube stent is left *in situ* for a period of two to three weeks.

Postoperative cavities following medial maxillectomy or craniofacial resection are inspected regularly for any infection or recurrence by nasal endoscopes. Post-operative assessment of the nasal mucosa for atrophic rhinitis in modified Young's opera-tion is possible by endoscopes, thus helping to determine the optimum time for reversal of Young's procedure.

Using a 30° endoscope, the entire naso-pharynx may be examined. In addition to the eustachian tube orifice, presence of any abnormal mass or early nasopharyngeal malignancy can be taken for biopsies. Recurrent epistaxis due to rhinosporidiosis can be located in the hidden areas of the nose such as inferior meatus, middle meatus, roof of the nasal cavity and the roof of the nasopharynx. It can be visualized, cauterized from its base and removed in Toto endo-scopically.

Recently endoscopic approach has been adopted to perform endoscopic medial maxillectomy and anterior skull base surgery for removal of benign tumours like inverted papilloma (Fig. 5.13), haemangioma, glioma, angiofibroma, etc. of the nasal cavity, paranasal sinuses and nasopharynx. Malignant tumours of the nasal cavity and paranasal sinuses without gross intracranial involvement can be removed by exclusive endoscopic/endoscopic assisted minimally invasive surgery depending on the extent of the disease in selected cases. Dural defects can be repaired with fascia lata graft and septal flap (Hadad flap).

Pituitary tumours can be approached endoscopically through transsphenoidal route. Meningocele and meningoencephalocele can be excised endoscopically. CSF leaks commonly associated with these surgeries can be repaired at the same sitting using the temporalis fascia, septal cartilage along with abdominal fat.

Endoscopic adenoidectomy has become popular nowadays because of minimal risk of complications. Nayak et al. first described endoscopic adenoidectomy in case of Scheie's syndrome and later described superiority of endoscopic adenoidectomy over traditional adenoidectomy. Microdebrider has been used for endoscopic adenoidectomy. Coblator has been used effectively for tissue ablation especially in endoscopic adenoidectomy (Figs 5.11 and 5.12) and also can be used for surface coagulation in angiofibroma.

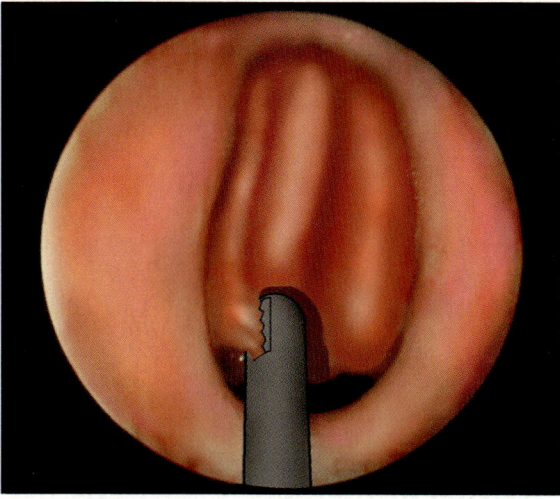

Fig. 5.11: Microdebrider-assisted endoscopic adenoidectomy in progress

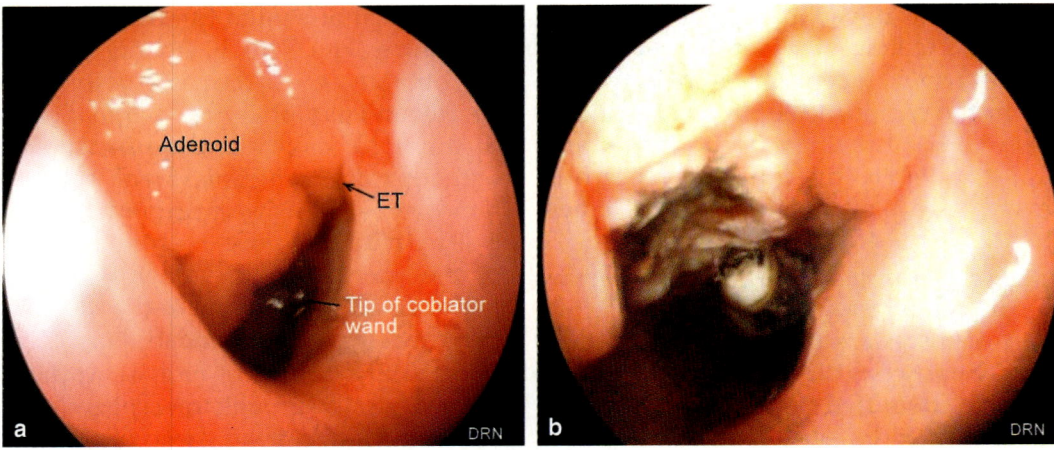

Fig. 5.12: Coblator-assisted endoscopic adenoidectomy in progress. Please note the tip of the coblator wand and the position of the eustachian tube (ET) orifice

Endoscopic septoplasty is performed to precisely correct only the deviated nasal septum and septal spur (Fig. 5.6), so that the endoscope can pass freely into the nasal cavity, thus enabling a functional endoscopic sinus surgery to be preformed. Nayak *et al.* (1998, 2001) described various endoscopic abnormalities of nasal septum and the associated lateral wall pathology and their management by ultraconservative septoturbinoplasty.

Other conditions: In selected nasal-ethmoidal tumours with brain invasion, endoscopic resection with transnasal craniectomy and subpial dissection can provide good local control, satisfactory survival, and limited morbidity (Matavelli, et al 2019). The advent of endoscopic extended transsphenoidal approach has expanded the indications for transnasal surgeries from pituitary surgery to craniopharyngioma, Rathkey's cleft cyst, arachnoid cyst, clival tumours, meningioma and extension of tumours from the paranasal sinuses, especially when there are not much adhesions (Garcia-Garigos, 2015 and Matsuo, 2014).

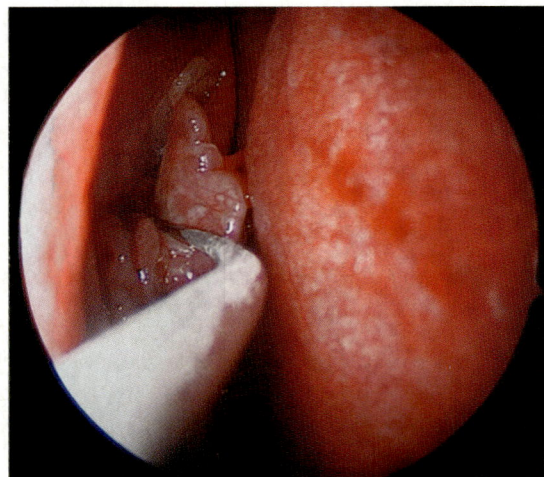

Fig. 5.13: Inverted papilloma right middle meatus

BIBLIOGRAPHY

1. Deepak Ranjan Nayak, Balkrishnan R, Murty KD. Turbinoplasty—letters to the Editor No. 2(reply) Ear, Nose and Throat Journal 2000.

2. Dipak Ranjan Nayak, Ramaswamy Balakrishnan, Deepak Murty K, Produl Hazarika. Endoscopic septoturbinoplasty: our update series. Indian Journal of Otolaryngology and Head and Neck Surgery, 2002:54(1):20–22.

3. Dipak Ranjan Nayak, Suresh Pillai, Balakrishnan R, et al. Traditional versus transnasal endoscopic adenoidectomy—a comparative study. Indian Journal of Otolaryngology and Head and Neck Surgery 2005: Special Issue 1: 383–87.

4. Nayak DR, Pillai S and Rao L. Rhinofacial Zygomycosis caused by conidiobolus coronatus. Indian Journal of Otolaryngology and Head and Neck Surgery 2004:56(3):225–27.

5. Friedman WH, Katsantonis GP. The role of standard technique in modern sinus surgery. Otolaryngol Clin North Am 1989; 22:759–77.

6. Kennedy DW, Zinreich SJ, Rosenbaum AE, Johns ME. Functional endoscopic sinus surgery: Theory and diagnostic evaluation. Arch Otolaryngol 1985; 111:576–82.

7. Kennedy DW. Functional endoscopic sinus surgery: Technique. Arch Otolaryngol 1985; 111:643–49.

8. Matavelli D, et al. Transnasal endoscopic surgery in selected nasal-ethmoidal cancer with suspected brain invasion: Indications, technique, and outcomes. Head and Neck 2019;41:1854–62.

9. Matsuo, et al. Indication and limitations of endoscopic extended transsphenoidal surgery for craniopharyngioma. Neurol Med Chir (Tokyo) 2014 Dec; 54(12): 974–82.

10. Murthy PS, Sahota JS, Nayak DR, Balakrishnan R, Hazarika P. Foreign body in the ethmoid sinus. International Journal of Oral and Maxillofacial Surgery 1994:23; 74–75.

11. Nayak DR, Balakrishnan R. Exclusive endoscopic/endoscopic-assisted minimaly invasive surgery for sinonasal neoplasm—our experience. J Neurol Surg; B 2012; 73-A015.

12. Nayak DR, Balakrishna R, Murthy KD. Endoscopic physiologic approach to allergy associated chronic rhinosinusitis—a preliminary study. ENT Journal 2001: 80(6):392–403.

13. Nayak DR, Balakrishnan R, Adolph. Endoscopic adenoidectomy in Scheie's syndrome (MPS IS). International Journal of Pediatric Otolaryngology 1998: 44; 177–81.

14. Nayak DR, Balakrishnan R, Murthy KD. An endoscopic approach to deviated nasal septum—a preliminary study. Journal of Laryngology and Otology 1998:112; 934–39.

15. Nayak DR, et al. Oncological outcome analysis of transnasal minimally invasive endoscopic resection of sinonasal malignancy not transgressing the dura: A single centre study. Orissa J Otolaryngology Head Neck Surgery 2017 June; 11(1):16–24. DOI: 10.21176/ojolhns. 2017.11.1.3

16. Nayak DR, Satish R, Shah Parul, Poojary K, Balakrishnan R. Endoscopic dacryocystorhinostomy and retrograde nasolacrimal duct dilatation with canulation—our experience. Indian Journal of Otolaryngology and Head and Neck Surgery 1999–2000: 52(1): 23–7, ISSN 0019–5421.

17. Nayak DR. "Paecilomyces infection of the paranasal sinuses in a child—a case report". International Journal of Pediatric Otolaryngology, 2000:52:183–87.

18. Rice DN. Endoscopic dacryocystorhinostomy: a cadaveric study. Ann of Rhinol, 1998;2:127–8.

19. Stammberger H. Functional endoscopic sinus surgery: The Messerklinger technique. Philadelphia: Decker, 1991:283.

20. Wigand ME. Endoscopic surgery of the paranasal sinuses and anterior skull base. New York: Thieme Medical Publishers, 1990:1–2.

21. Palmer O, Moche JA, Mathews S. Endoscopic surgery of the nose and paranasal sinus. Oral Maxillofac Surg Clin North Am. 2012 May; 24(2):275–83.

6
Preoperative Imaging Studies of the Nose and Paranasal Sinuses

DR Nayak, P Hazarika, N Periaswamy, KC Mallick

Inflammatory disease of the paranasal sinuses is a common but serious health problem that can be associated with life-threatening complications at times. Endoscopic sinus surgery has become a popular and effective surgical technique for treating patients with refractory inflammatory sinus disease.

The knowledge of the dominant role of the ethmoid sinus and the microarchitectural pathway between the sinuses and the nasal cavity in the pathogenesis, has paved the way for effective management of various nasal and paranasal sinus pathologies. The success of functional endoscopic sinus surgery is facilitated by a clear understanding and an accurate display of the anatomy of the nasal cavity and of the paranasal sinuses and their drainage pathways (especially the ostiomeatal unit) in a plane correlating to the surgical orientation (Melhem, 1996).

Functional endoscopic sinus surgery even though is effective and popular is not always safe. This is because of the proximity of the sphenoethmoid complex to the various vital structures, making them vulnerable to injury. Thus proper preoperative evaluation is mandatory. The CT scan imaging and diagnostic nasal endoscopy give complementary information and remain the mainstay of preoperative evaluation of such cases. Direct coronal computed tomography (CT) of sinonasal anatomy displayed by using intermediate window and level settings (window 511700 Hounsfield units [HU], level 52300 HU) has been established as the imaging technique of choice for examining patients before functional endoscopic sinus surgery as it gives simulation of the surgical orientation, adequate depiction of bony and soft-tissue landmarks, and ability to show disease processes (Kennedy, et al. 1985, Zenreich, et al. 1987).

Melhem, et al. (1996) proposed an optimal scanning protocol for the examination of the paranasal sinuses. Using a direct coronal plane with a scanning angle not exceeding 108 from the plane perpendicular to the hard palate, 3 mm thick contiguous sections, exposure factors of kV(p) 5–120, mA 5–80, detail reconstruction algorithm, and intermediate window settings (window 5–11700 HU, level 5–2300 HU). This protocol will provide excellent anatomic definition and orientation of the paranasal sinuses while significantly decreasing the radiation dose equivalent to patients. Improper selection of CT windows is one of the major cause for misdiagnosis of pathological changes in the paranasal sinuses. Therefore, it is reasonable to use CT windows dedicated for the sinuses or bones to avoid missing inflammatory findings (Cebula, et al. 2017).

Role of Plain Radiographs

Clinically, maxillary and frontal sinusitis is seen more frequently than the ethmoid sinus disease. Also the standard plain radiographs of the paranasal sinuses readily demonstrate the maxillary and frontal disease but not the ethmoidal disease, even though it is crucial in the pathogenesis.

Advantages of Plain Radiographs

a. Quick, non-invasive and relatively inexpensive.

b. It is possible to evaluate the maxillary, frontal, sphenoid sinuses and to some extent the posterior ethmoid and lower third of nasal cavity.

c. Along with the clinical data, it helps to distinguish three types of sinonasal inflammatory disease, viz. rhinitis, rhinosinusitis and polyposis.

d. Helps in optimal medical and conservative treatment including antral lavage and thus in attaining a more quiescent state of disease necessary for CT imaging.

Disadvantages of Plain Radiographs

1. Gives no information regarding the ethmoid sinus–ostiomeatal complex disease.

2. Gives no information regarding the position and status of the various vital structures related to the sphenoethmoids like the orbit, anterior cranial fossa, optic nerve and the internal carotid artery.

3. Extent of disease within the sphenoethmoids is not well delineated (Fig. 6.1).

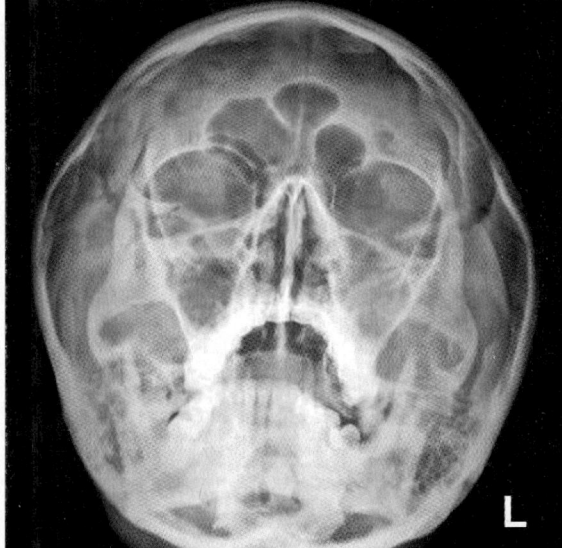

Fig. 6.1: Plain radiograph of paranasal sinuses (Waters view) showing haziness of left maxillary antrum

Role of CT Imaging

In contrast to the plain radiographs, the CT imaging gives information regarding all the above mentioned under the disadvantages of plain radiographs. CT is most useful for structures involving thin bony structures like PNS and orbit. CT imaging is superior to MRI in this region. MRI has the distinct advantage over other imaging techniques because of superior tissue contrast (Sievers, et al. 2000).

Advantages of CT Imaging

1. CT imaging provides a precise knowledge of various sinus involved and thus allows the surgeon to tailor his surgery to the affected sinuses. When posterior ethmoids and sphenoids are found to be normal, there is no need to exenterate these, thus reducing the possibility of potential complications (Figs 6.2a and b).

2. CT scan provides information regarding the various anatomical and pathological variations in the ostiomeatal complex. Apart from detecting the variations in the uncinate process, middle turbinate, paradoxical middle turbinate (Fig. 6.3) and bulla ethmoidalis, the CT scans also help in detecting the overpneumatized agger cells, frontal cells and Haller cells (Figs 6.2c and 6.4a,b). Haller and the Onodi cells are not detectable otherwise. The Haller cells are the infraorbital ethmoid cells which being in close relation to the maxillary sinus ostium could narrow the infundibulum (Figs 6.2a to c and 6.5).

3. Most crucial role of CT imaging is to provide the surgeon, information regarding the position and status of the vital structures in relation to the sphenoethmoids. The dehiscence in the papery thin lamina papyracea (Fig. 6.4) either developmental or due to previous surgery is easily picked up by the coronal CT scans. Low position of fovea ethmoidalis or cribriform plate is a potentially dangerous anatomical variation. A possible CSF leak can be averted by detection of this. Fovea ethmoidalis could also be dehiscent, and when so, is usually in its descending medial part. The position

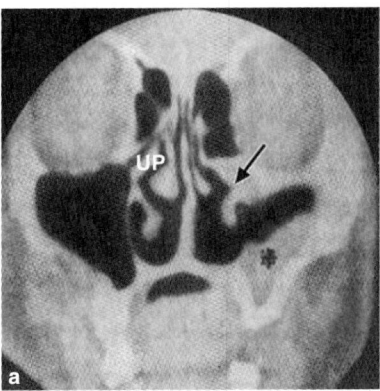
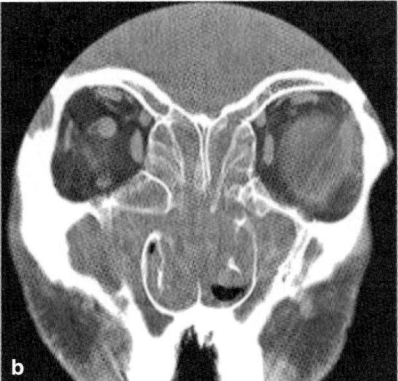
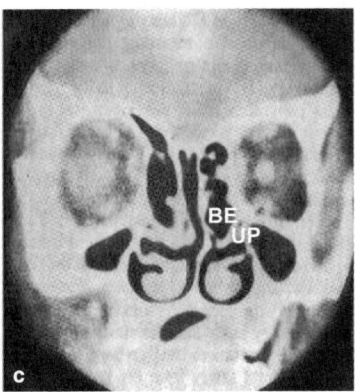

Fig. 6.2: a. CT imaging showing right maxillary disease (*) in spite of a patent intranasal antrostomy (INA), infundibular disease and obstruction due to overpneumatized bulla and medially turned uncinate process (UP) are also seen (black arrow), **b.** CT picture in ethmoidal polyposis, **c.** CT scan showing overpneumatized bulla ethmoidalis (BE) and medially bent uncinate process (UP)

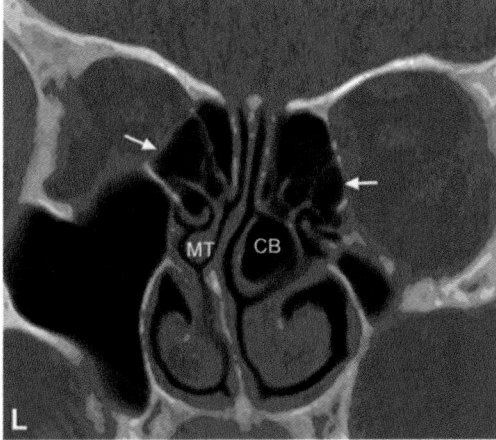

Fig. 6.3: CT scan showing paradoxically turned MT (middle turbinate) (left) and CB (concha bullosa) (right) and also note dehiscence fovea ethmoidalis and lamina papyracea (white arrows)

of anterior ethmoidal artery is an important landmark as it is considered high-risk area in endoscopic sinus surgery (Fig. 6.4).

Overpneumatization of the posterior ethmoids and/or the sphenoid increases the vulnerability of the optic nerve and the internal carotid artery, as they bulge into the sinuses in the lateral walls. In rare instances, the thin bone separating the internal carotid artery from the posterior ethmoid and sphenoid may be dehiscent. Overpneumatized sphenoid may give rise to various recesses like the anterior clinoid recess, pterygoid recess. Recess into the nasal septum or even into the greater wing of sphenoid. More the pneumatization, more is the chance for complications (Fig. 6.5b).

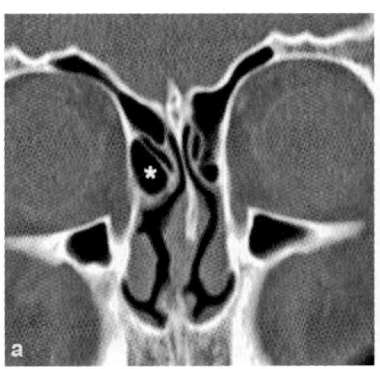
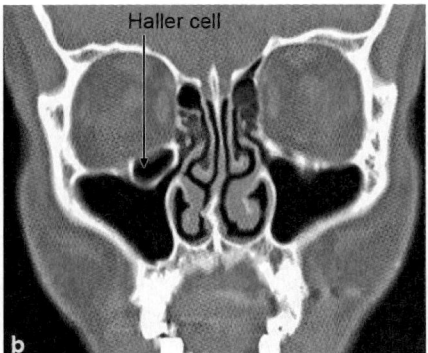
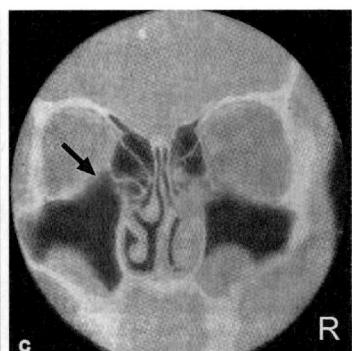

Fig. 6.4: a. CT scan showing overpneumatized agger cells (*), **b.** CT scan showing Haller cells, **c.** CT scan showing a dehiscent lamina papyracea (left side) associated with the right ostiomeatal complex disease and bilateral antral polyp

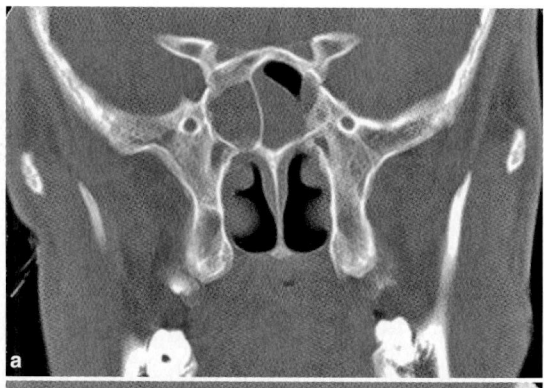

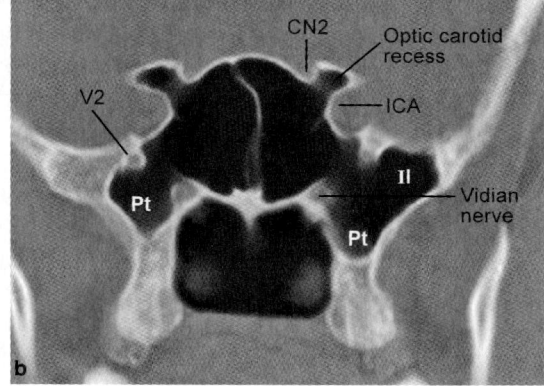

Fig. 6.5: a. CT scan showing sphenoidal sinusitis with fluid level on left side, **b.** CT scan showing bilateral pterygoid recesses (Pt), with an inferolateral recess on it (II) extending into the floor of the left middle cranial fossa in continuity with the pterygoid recess. Also note optic nerve (CN2), maxillary nerve (V2), internal carotid artery (ICA)

Identification of an asymmetric intersphenoid septum is important because the posterior extension of this partition usually marks the location of the internal carotid artery canal. Acute infection within the sphenoid can extend to the neighbouring vital structures (Figs 6.5a, b and 6.6). The classification of sphenoid sinus was first described by Hammer & Radberg in 1961 into conchal, presellar and sellar based on its pneumatization. The sellar type was further modified into incomplete and complete by Guldner, et al. (1912). The follwing is the modified classification (Fig. 6.6c).

Type 1: Conchal (completely missing or minimal sphenoid sinus),

Type 2: Presellar (posterior wall of sphenoid sinus is in front of the anterior wall of the sella).

Type 3a: Sellar incomplete (posterior wall is between the anterior and posterior walls of the sella), **Type 3b:** Sellar complete (posterior wall of sphenoid sinus is behind the posterior wall of the sella).

Marked lateral deviation or even fusion of uncinate process to the medial orbital wall may endanger the orbit while the uncinectomy is being performed.

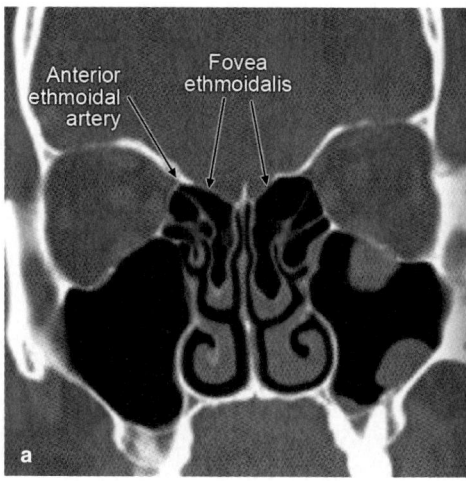

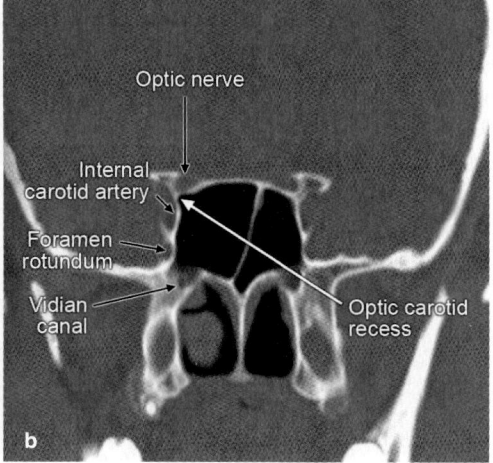

Fig. 6.6: a. CT scan showing dehiscence fovea ethmoidalis with polyps in left maxillary sinus. Also note the entry of anterior ethmoidal artery, **b.** CT scan showing the recess between the bulge of the optic nerve and carotid artery within the sphenoid sinus. Also note foramen rotundum and the vidian canal

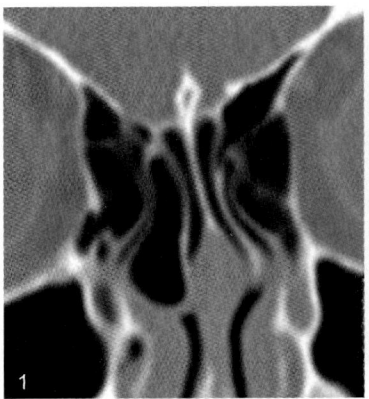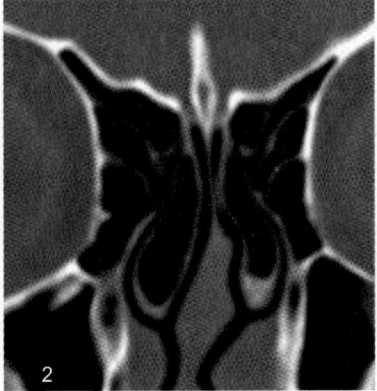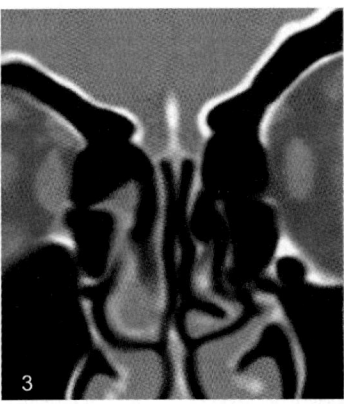

Fig. 6.6c: Coronal CT showing level of cribriform plate and olfactory fossa, Keros type 1–3 (*see* Fig. 9.12)

The Onodi cells are the most posterior ethmoid cells that extend posterolaterally, and surround the optic canal and optic nerve. These cells may extend more posteriorly and protrude into the sphenoid sinuses as well as migrate to reach the anterior wall of the sella (parasphenoidal posterior ethmoid) (Fig. 6.8).

4. CT scan imaging is a rapid, non-invasive and convenient investigation.
5. Helps in documentation and education.

Disadvantages of CT Imaging

1. Relatively expensive investigation.
2. Radiation dose to the sensitive lens and cornea is particularly high when axial cuts are taken nearly 185 times the dose to the sensitive cornea and lens than that recorded for plain radiographs. This can be reduced by careful positioning of the patient in the scanner and by favouring more coronal cuts.
3. Artefacts due to extensive dental fillings. Here again coronal sections are better than axial sections.

Coronal Versus Axial Cuts

Coronal CT scans are preferred as it displays structures in a plane closest to the endoscopist. Also the anatomical and pathological variations in the OMC are well delineated in the coronal cuts. The relation of cribriform plate, fovea ethmoidalis, the lamina papyracea, the optic bulge and ICA bulge are better appreciated in coronal cuts.

The coronal CT scan of the paranasal sinuses is performed with the patient in the prone position with the head hyperextended, 3 mm of thin coronal section are obtained from the frontal sinus to sphenoid sinus. The CT scan images should be photographed on bone (average 2000 H windows) setting as well as soft tissue (average 250 H windows) settings.

The coronal CT allows to study the level of the cribriform plate and the olfactory fossa as described by Keros (1962). This includes—(a) Keros Type-1: Olfactory fossa 1–3 mm deep, Type-2: Olfactory fossa 4–7 mm deep, Type-3: Olfactory fossa 8–16 mm deep (Fig. 6.6c).

The anterior and posterior walls of frontal sinus, the anatomical relationship between the posterior ethmoid and sphenoid sinuses and relationship of optic nerve to posterior ethmoid/sphenoid and pterygopalatine fossa are best evaluated in the axial planes. The axial cuts also help in delineating well the frontal sinus drainage pathway (frontal recess) and sphenoethmoidal recess.

Newer MDCT scanner allows taking 64 slices with each scanner rotation permitting high resolution multiplanner reformatted images. Use of this multiplanner reformation (sagittal and coronal) has been shown to improve preoperative understanding of the frontal recess. Review of sagittal images significantly helps in identifying and measure the frontal recess and assessing the obstructing anterior ethmoid (Kew, et al. 2002). Three-dimensional, reformatted images of frontonasal anatomy enable improved

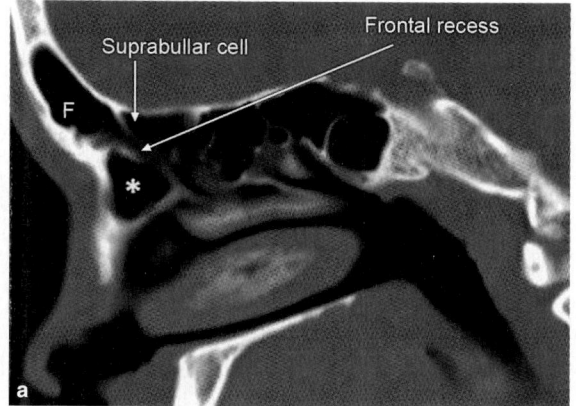

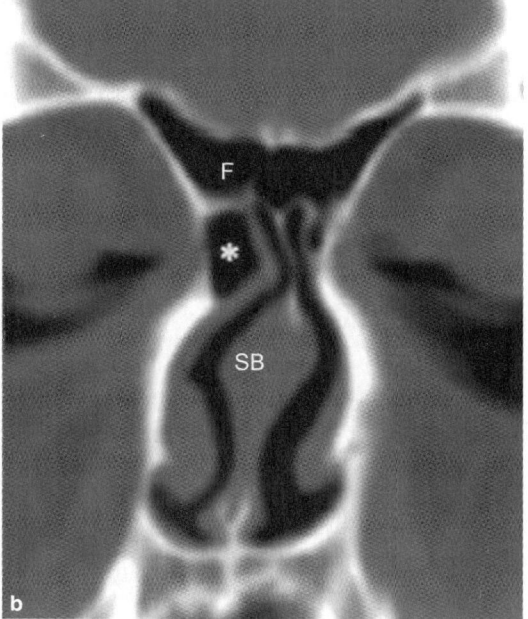

Fig. 6.7: a. Sagittal reconstruction, **b.** Coronal section ostiomeatal complex CT of paranasal sinus with prominent agger nasi cell (*). Also note frontal recess and suprabullar cell shown in fig(a) and frontal sinus (F)

under-standing of the frontal sinus drainage pathway, anatomy and of the spatial relationships between ethmoid air cells in this region (Fig. 6.7). Such images may provide a useful adjunct to surgical planning.

Axial cuts may be taken along with coronal and sagittal reconstruction. CT evidence of hyperattenuation within sphenoethmoid should raise suspicion of allergic fungal sinusitis. MRI helps in soft tissue delineation especially in orbital/intracranial complica-tions of sinusitis. It also readily differentiates mucus from the mucosal disease.

Cost-Effectiveness of CT Imaging

Keeping in mind the possibility of major complications that could result following an endoscopic sinus surgery, like blindness, orbital haematoma, CSF rhinorrhoea, major ICA/cavernous bleeding, etc. CT scan is definitely a cost-effective investigation.

The cost-effectiveness of CT scan imaging can be increased by:
a. Lowering the cost (by reducing the number of films).
b. Increasing the effectiveness.

Many efforts are made to achieve this by taking lesser but strategically placed cuts (The mini series technique of White, et al. 1990 and the limited scanning technique White, et al. 1991). Selective coronal and axial cuts are taken in the above technique. With improve-ment in software technology (DICOM viewing software, and CT technology like spiral CT scan, traditional CT films are replaced can be directly accessed in the PC in coronal, axial and sagittal planes.

Prerequisite before CT Imaging

As the objective of the CT imaging is to detect the subtle changes in the OMC causing the chronic sinusitis, and not the result of it the CT scan should be taken only after maximal medical therapy including intranasal cortico-steroids, oral antibiotics, mucolytic agents and saline irrigations (Lund 2006 and Huang, et al. 2020) to treat the disease in the major sinuses. The CT scan should be taken in a more quiescent state of the disease. A short course of steroid is helpful.

Technique (Zenreich, et al. 1987) (Table 6.1)
• Position: Prone with hyperextended head for coronal sections.
• CT specifications as per table.
• Window width around 2000 preferred and window centred to 200.
• When patient is unable to resume hyper-extended head position, axial cuts are taken and coronal indirect reconstructions can be made.

Table 6.1: Technique for CT of paranasal sinuses

Imaging parameter	Imaging plane	
	Coronal	**Axial**
Patient position	Prone	Supine
Gantry angulations	Perpendicular to IOML (infraorbital meatal line)	IOML
Extent of study	From anterior frontal sinus to posterior sphenoid sinus	From hard palate through frontal sinus
Section thickness (mm)	4	4
Table incrementation (mm)	3	3
kVp	125	125
mAs	450	450
Scan time (sec)	5	5

- Initially, a sagittal scout section is taken and the coronal cuts are strategically placed between the frontal and sphenoid sinuses. About 12 coronal cuts are usually sufficient. Infraorbital meatal line is drawn and cuts taken in the perpendicular or parallel to it for coronal and axial cuts, respectively.

Reporting of CT Films

A proforma followed by our institute for recording the findings is given below.

Proforma

1. *Extent of the disease (T: Mucosal thickening, O: Complete opacity, C: Cloudiness)*
   a. Max. sinus (polyp/fluid level)
   b. Frontal sinus
   c. Anterior ethmoids
   d. Middle ethmoid
   e. Posterior ethmoids
   f. Sphenoid
   g. Infundibulum
      (Patent = N; Partial occlusion = +;
      Total occlusion = + +)
   h. Middle meatus (N/Narrow)
   i. Polyps (+/−)
   j. Frontal recess (status of agger nasi and frontal cell/cells)
   k. Sphenoethmoidal recess
   l. Sinus lateralis
   m. Focal or diffuse area of attenuation.
   n. Other changes (bone/mucocele, etc.).
2. *Anatomical and pathological variations*
   a. Agger nasi cells
   b. Haller cells
   c. Overpneumatized bulla
   d. Uncinate process—medially turned, laterally turned, up bulla.
   e. Middle turbinate—concha bullosa, bulky MT, paradoxically turned MT
   f. Onodi cells
   g. Septal deviation
   h. Post-traumatic structural variations (including surgical, if any).
   i. Others
3. *Danger points*
   a. Cribriform plate
   b. Fovea ethmoidalis
   c. Lamina papyracea (can be involved due to extensive ethmoidal polyposis) (Fig. 6.2b)
   d. Relation of ICA/optic nerve to posterior ethmoids and sphenoids.
   e. Lacrimal bone/duct.

Friedman's CT Staging of Chronic Hyperplastic Rhinosinusitis

Stage I : Single focus disease.
Stage II: Multifocal disease responsive to conservative therapy.

Stage III: Diffuse disease partially responsive to medication.

Stage IV: Diffuse disease with bony changes and poorly responding to conservative therapy.

The staging is said to be useful in outlining operative strategies and a reliable prognostic indicator of the disease process. To summarize, CT imaging is a useful and essential tool to the rhinologist for performing endoscopic sinus surgery. It allows the surgeon to tailor his surgery to the affected sinuses, treat adequately and effectively the casual anatomical variation and pathological changes in the OMC and at the same time alarms the surgeon of the possibility of an avertable complication due to FESS, thus making the surgery both effective as well as safe and thus an efficient one.

MRI

An imaging modality that uses the response of the biological tissues to an applied and changing magnetic field to generate images. It is useful mainly in the evaluation of soft tissue masses of the nasopharynx and paranasal sinuses. It has excellent sensitivity and specificity. It supersedes CT in its ability to differentiate inflammatory changes from neoplastic changes and better demonstration of extranasal extension, thus helping in better assessment of the extent of the lesions (Lloyd 1989). The MRI of the paranasal sinuses must include T1-weighted images (spin-lattice relaxation) and T2-weighted images (spin-spin relaxation) of not only the nasal cavity and paranasal sinuses but include the orbit, anterior skull base and the adjacent intracranial compartment. The images are usually taken in axial and coronal plane with the sagittal images added where necessary. Contrast enhanced images (Fig. 6.8) are obtained by the administration of gadolinium-chelated contrast agents (iodine-based contrast agents are used in CT).

The presence of seven unpaired electrons in the outer ring of gadolinium produces a high magnetic moment, resulting in enhancement of areas of high vascularity on T1-weighted images (Lohrke, et al 2016).

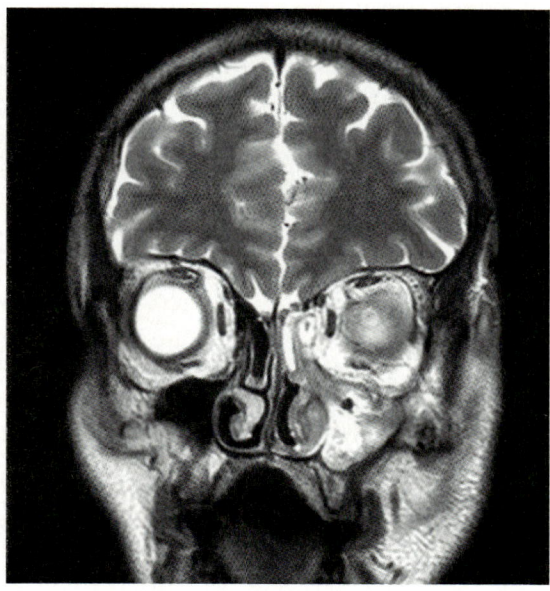

Fig. 6.8: Contrast enhanced MRI of the nose and PNS showing irregular mucosal thickening in the left maxillary sinus with few linear areas of diffusion restriction with orbital involvement in a case of acute invasive fungal sinusitis

However, fat also appears enhanced in these images. Hence, fat-saturated T1-weighted images make the lesions more enhanced and precision in the identification of perineural spread and intracranial spread.

In case of an inflamed mucosa, characterized by increased submucosal oedema and surface secretions which is predominantly water (95%), the appearance is dark on T1-weighted images and bright on T2-weighted images (Fig. 6.9a and b). In case of a tumour which is more cellular than normal with lesser water content, they appear dark in both T1- and T2-weighted images (Fatterpekar 2008).

Applications in Various Pathologies

In acute rhinosinusitis, MRI is mainly used when complications are suspected. MRI can identify subperiosteal abscesses and vascular complications like superior ophthalmic vein occlusion and cavernous sinus thrombosis, intracranial complications like meningitis.

In chronic rhinosinusitis, the oedematous mucosa appears uniformly bright on T2 and dark on T1 images.

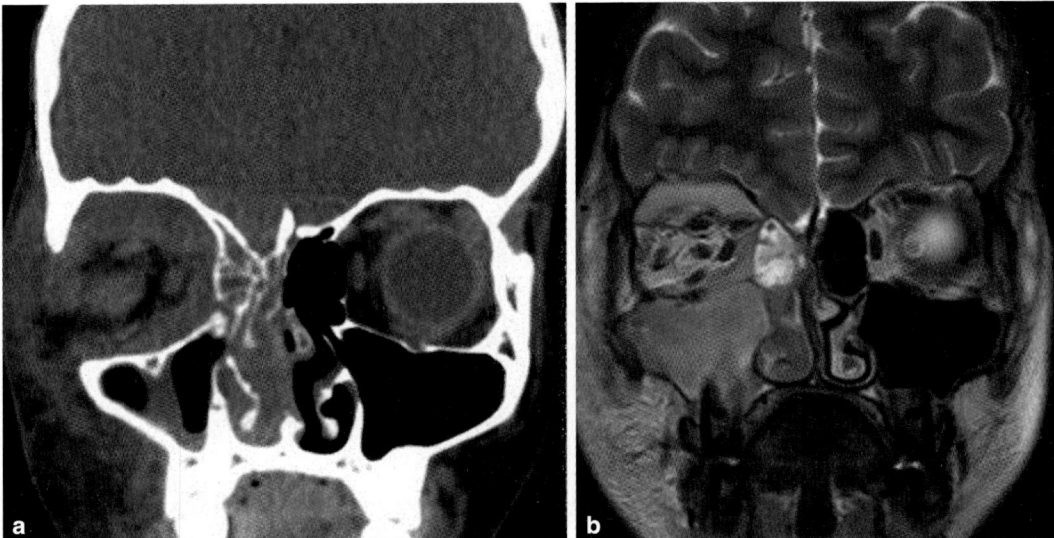

Fig. 6.9: a. Coronal CT showing mucosal thickening in the right maxillary sinus with gross involvement of right ethmoid and right orbital abscess; **b.** MRI (T1 + contrast) in the coronal plane showing fluid in the maxillary sinus, gross mucosal thickening of right ethmoid and right preseptal abscess with extension into intraconal space

In antrochoanal polyp, the intramaxillary part is cystic and appears dark on T1 and bright on T2, whereas the solid intranasal portion appears dark on both T1 and T2.

In fungal ball and eosinophilic fungal sinusitis due to the high mineral content in the fungal hyphae, they appear hypointense and show signal voids on T1 and T2 images of MRI. In acute invasive fungal rhinosinusitis including mucormycosis, due to the evolving tissue ischaemia, they produce variable tissue intensities on T2 images. However, their role in the early detection of extranasal involvement is essential (Lloyd, et al 1987). MRI plays an important role in the diagnosis of rhinocerebral and rhino-orbital mucormycosis.

In fibro-osseous benign lesions of the nose and paranasal sinuses, CT plays a more important role than the MRI (Som 1988). In the management of sinonasal tumours, the role of MRI is not in the differentiation of benign and malignant lesions, but it is the mapping of the extension of the lesion. The soft tissue lesions exhibit certain distinct patterns on MRI (Koeller 2016):

- Juvenile nasopharyngeal angiofibroma—finger-like projections with sharp lobulated margins. Postoperatively plays a role in excluding unresected persistent disease.
- Inverted papilloma—septate striated appearance/convoluted pattern/ceribriform pattern.
- In sinonasal malignancies:
  - Orbital extension—a thin and regular hypointensity is seen between neoplasm and orbital fat on T2 images indicates intact orbital periosteum.
  - Intracranial extension—an uninterrupted hypointense signal on T1 and fat suppressed T1 indicates intact bone and periosteum (extracranial tumour).
  - Interruption of the hypointense signal indicates erosion of the cribriform plate.
  - Uninterrupted hyperintense dura indicates, intracranial, extradural extension.
  - Replacement of the hyperintense dura by the signals of the tumour indicates intracranial intradural extension.
  - Oedema indicates involvement of the brain parenchyma (Lloyd, et al 1987).

BIBLIOGRAPHY

1. Bolger, et al. Paranasal sinus surgery—anatomic variations and mucosal abnormalities. CT

analysis for endoscopic sinus surgery. Laryngoscope 101 Jan. 1991; 56–64.

2. Cebula M, et al. Impact of window computed tomography (CT) parameters on measurement of inflammatory Changes in paranasal sinuses. Pol J Radiol 2017;82:567–70.

3. Dale H Rice. Basic surgical techniques and variations of endoscopic sinus surgery. OCNA Vol 2 No. 4 Aug. 1989;713–726.

4. Elias R. Melhem, Patrick J Oliverio, Mark L Benson. Optimal CT evaluation for functional endoscopic sinus surgery. Am J Neuroradiol January 1996;17:181–188.

5. Friedman CT staging of PNS in Chronic hyperplast rhinosinusitis. Laryngoscope 100 Nov. 1990; 1161–1165.

6. Girish M. Fatterpekar, Bradley N. Delman, and Peter M. Som, Imaging the Paranasal Sinuses: Where We Are and Where We Are Going, The Anatomical Record 2008;291:1564–1572.

7. Hammer G, Radberg C. The sphenoidal sinus: An anatomical and roentgenologic study with reference to transsphenoid hypophysectomy. Acta Radiol 1961 Dec;56:401–22.

8. Hiremath BS, et al. Assessment of variations in sphenoid sinus pneumatization in Indian population: A multidetector computed tomography study. Acta Radiol. 1961 Dec; 56:401–22.

9. Huang Z, Ma J, Sun Y, et al. Maximal medical therapy for chronic rhinosinusitis: A survey of Chinese Otolaryngologist. Ear Nose Throat J 2020 Mar;99(3):159–64.

10. Jessica Lohrke, Thomas Frenzel, Jan Endrikat, Filipe Caseiro Alves, et al. 25 years of contrast-enhanced MRI: Developments, current challenges and future perspectives. Adv Ther 2016; 33: 1–28.

11. Kennedy, et al. FESS-part I-theory and diagnostic evaluation. Arch Otolaryngol Vol 111 Sept. 1985, 576–82.

12. Keros P. On the practical value of differences in the level of the lamina cribrosa of the ethmoid. J Laryngol Rhinol Otol 1962;41:809–13.

13. Kew J, et al. Multiplanar reconstructed computed tomography images improves depiction and understanding of the anatomy of the frontal recess and frontal sinus. Am J Rhinology 2002, 16(2):119–23.

14. Koeller KK. Radiologic features of sinonasal tumours. Head and Neck Pathol 2016;10:1–12.

15. Lloyd GA. Magnetic resonance imaging of the nose and paranasal sinuses. JR Soc Med 1989 Feb; 82(2):84–87.

16. Lloyd GA, Valerie J Lund, Peter D Phelps, David J Howard. Magnetic resonance imaging in the evaluation of nose and paranasal sinus disease. The British Journal of Radiology 1987; 60:957–968.

17. Llyod, et al. CT of paranasal sinuses and FESS. A critical analysis of 100 symptomatic patients. JLO, March 1991;Vol 105;181–5.

18. Lund VJ. Maximal medical therapy for chronic rhinosinusitis. Otolaryngologic Clinics of North America 38(6):1301–10.

19. Mafee MF. Preoperative imaging anatomy of nasal ethmoid complex for FESS. RCNA Vol. 31, No. 1, Jan. 1993;1–20.

20. Melhem ER(1), et al. Optimal CT evaluation for endoscopic sinus surgery. Am J Neuroradiol 1996 Jan;17(1):181–88.

21. Paul S White. Limited CT scanning techniques of the PNS. JLO Jan. 1991 Vol. 105;20–3.

22. Sievers KW, Greess H, Baum U, et al. Paranasal sinuses and nasopharynx CT and MRI. European Journal of Radiology, Vol 33, Issue 3, 185–202.

23. Som PM, Shapiro MD, Biller HF, Sasaki C, Lawson W. Sinonasal tumors and inflammatory tissues: Differentiation with MR imaging. Radiology 1988;167(3):803–8.

24. Zenreich, et al. Paranasal sinuses—CT imaging requirements for endoscopic surgery. Radiology 1987;163:769–75.

Premedication, Preoperative and Intraoperative Management

DR Nayak, PSN Murthy, R Singh, N Mathew

Proper preoperative counselling and adequate preparation of the patient prior to endoscopic sinus surgery is mandatory for smooth and effective conduction of endoscopic sinus surgery. Serious complications usually result from impaired visibility due to excessive bleeding during surgery.

To avoid such complications, endoscopic sinus surgery can be performed either with local anaesthesia with vasoconstrictors (Friedman 1996), or under general anaesthesia supplemented with controlled hypotension (Heermann 1999). The preparation should be done in the following lines:

1. Adequate control of active infection by appropriate topical antibiotics, topical corticosteroids (fluticasone furoate, mometasone furoate) and oral antihistaminics. Persistent positive culture suggests bacterial biofilm formation. Topical antibiotic application like moxifloxacin is quite effective in this regard to control infection (Desrosiers 2007).

2. More quiescent the state of the disease, less is the possibility of haemorrhage intraoperatively, thus allowing the endoscopic sinus surgery to be more effective. Oral antibiotics like doxycycline have anti-inflammatory effect on chronic rhinosinusitis and can be given preoperatively (Kim and Douglass, 2012)

3. In case of polyposis, oral steroids, like prednisolone 5 mg tid for a week prior to surgery, will help in either reducing the size of polyp or at times even causing

disappearance of the polyp. With this, the intraoperative bleeding will be less and the surgeon can completely exenterate the ethmoids.

4. Preoperative evaluation should concentrate towards finding out the other causes which could lead to intraoperative bleeding like hypertension, bleeding diatheses, history of concommitant aspirin or warfarin therapy, etc. ESS should be performed after tackling the above factors. The routine work-up of the patient should hence include:

   a. A complete blood picture like Hb, PCV, total and differential count, etc.

   b. Estimation of bleeding, clotting and prothrombin times, and

   c. Urine analysis for albumin and sugar.

5. A xylocaine sensitivity test is advocated prior to surgery.

Patient is ideally hospitalized a day prior to surgery for the preparation and investigations. Oral diazepam 5–10 mg is given at night previous day to the surgery and also in the morning next day about 4 hrs before surgery. This helps in reducing anxiety and thus preventing a possible rise in blood pressure. The patient is advised to stay Nil per oral overnight prior to surgery.

Premedication for FESS under Local Anaesthesia

The following premedication is given 45 minutes prior to surgery:

1. Inj. Pethidine 1–1.5 mg/kg body weight (approximately 75–100 mg in an average adult patient). Instead of pethidine, pentazocine 30 mg (Fortwin), an opioid, can be administered.
2. Inj. Phenergan 25 mg (an antihistaminic acts as sedative and antiemetic).
3. Inj. Atropine 0.6 mg (an anticholinergic to reduce secretions).

These are given together deep intramuscular about 45 minutes before the surgery. Pethidine is a very potent narcotic analgesic, the action of which is synergised by phener-gan. Phenergan in addition combats the side effect of nausea and vomiting due to pethidine. Increased dose of pethidine is preferred rather than use of largactil, a tranquilliser, as it gives better analgesia and patient will have fewer hallucinations.

Atropine helps in reducing the nasal secretions, thus giving a dry operative field. Also being a vagolytic, it is cardioprotective. Oral opioids are commonly prescribed after sinus surgery but are associated with adverse effects, including gastrointestinal and neurologic symptoms which can be avoided unless absolutely necessary. Premedication with both phenergan and atropine have been reported to cause postoperative agitation due to crossing of blood–brain barrier and can be minimized by the use of atropine substitute glycopyrrolate (Elsersy & Ahmed 2017). Nonopioid analgesics have been suggested to offer similar pain control efficacy with fewer adverse effects.

Premedication for FESS under GA

Clonidine, a potent suppressor of sympathoadrenal activity, has been given orally before operation to augment the hypotensive action of isoflurane. The antihypertensive drug, clonidine, is a centrally acting alpha 2 agonist, useful as a premedication because of its sedative and analgesic properties and provides a clear field. It also reduces bleeding effectively during intraoperative period during endoscopic sinus surgery (Jabalameli, et al. 2005).

On Table Preparation

Cottonoid strips are made by cutting the soft roll rayon pads available commercially, into strips of 3 × 1.5 cm and a black cotton or silk thread about 1 foot long is stitched to one end of the strip as in Fig. 7.1. Such strips are made into a bundle and are sterilized by autoclaving. These cottonoid strips are dipped in a solution containing 10 ml of 4% xylocaine and 1 ml of 1:1000 adrenaline thus making the dilution of adrenaline into 1:10,000. The strips are squeezed and 4–5 such strips are used per nasal cavity for preoperative packing, after sparying the nasal cavity with 4% xylocaine spray. The packs are placed by direct visualization using nasal endoscope. Sites of placement are as follows:

1. Posteriorly in the middle meatus and as close to the sphenopalatine foramen as possible (Fig. 7.2a)
2. Between the lateral wall and middle turbinate anteriorly
3. Between the middle turbinate and septum
4. Between the inferior turbinate and the septum (1 or 2 strips) (Fig. 7.2b).

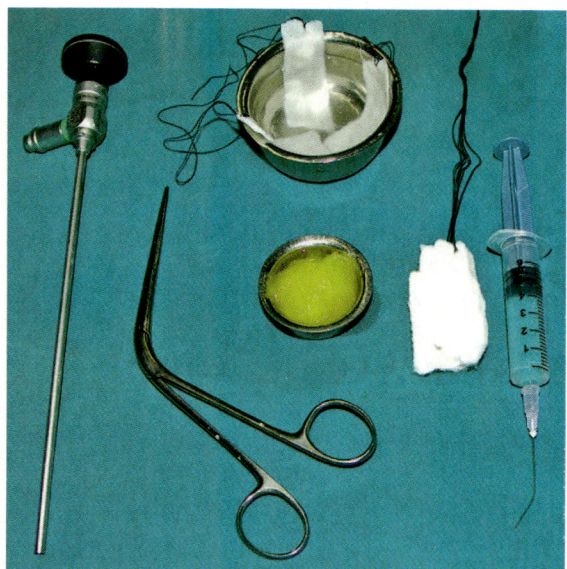

Fig. 7.1: 10 ml 4% xylocaine with 1:1000 adrenaline solution cottonoids strip nasal endoscope and nasal dressing forceps required for placement of strips in the middle meatus and nasal cavity, syringe for 2% xylocaine with 1:100000 adrenaline for infiltration

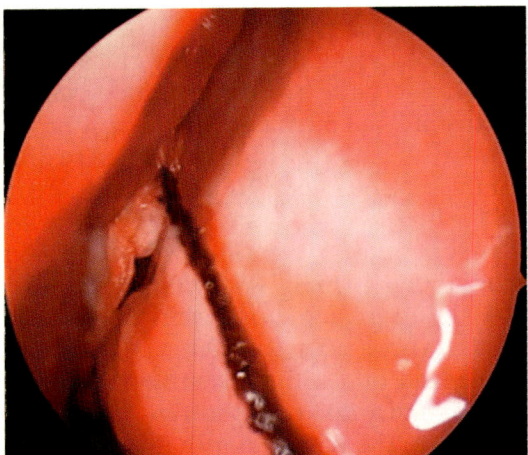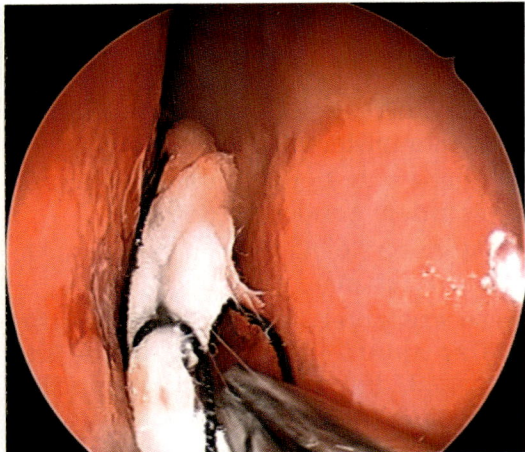

Fig. 7.2: Placement of 4% xylocaine with 1:1000 adrenaline solution-soaked cottonoid strips being placed in the middle meatus in a systematic manner

This gives good surface anaesthesia as well as decongests the turbinates, increasing the exposure of the operative field. Thus handling of the nasal endoscope and other instruments is made easy and less painful.

Antifog solution like savlon or sterile dilute soap water solution is used to prevent fogging of the tip of nasal endoscope.

Intraoperative treatment: Saline irrigations were found to significantly reduce the amount of *S. pneumoniae* found within the maxillary sinus mucosa. No difference was found for *H. influenzae* in bacterial load reduction which was noted between the pressurized saline flushes and manual saline rinse methods (Kristine, et al. 2011). During the COVID-19 pandemic, endoscopic sinus surgery has become a major challenge for the surgeons. Povidone-iodine nasal antiseptic solution at concentration of 1.25% and below can effectively be used as an adjunctive in mitigating viral transmission (Frank, et al. 2020).

Data analysis has shown significant improvement in early postoperative healing in sinonasal cavities receiving triamcinolone-impregnated absorbable nasal packing following ESS and is also associated with significantly improved healing up to 6 months postoperatively (Cote and Wright, et al. 2010). The author (DRN) in his personal experience also found significant improvement in healing while using hydrocortisone and dilute povidone-iodine/antibiotic impregnated absorbable nasal packing. In the recent past, drug-eluting stents have become popular. These steroid impregnated dressings and implants appear to be safe, but have increased posibility of systemic absorption compared to topical nasal steroids (Hauser JL, et al. 2017).

BIBLIOGRAPHY

1. Christopher A, *et al*. Rofecoxib versus hydrocodone/acetaminophen for postoperative analgesia in functional endoscopic sinus surgery. Laryngoscope. 116(4):602–606, April 2006.
2. Cote DWJ, Wright ED. Triamcinolone-impregnated nasal dressing following endoscopic sinus surgery: A randomized, double-blind, placebo-controlled study. Laryngoscope 2010; 120(6):1269–73.
3. David WJ Cote, Erin D Wright. Triamcinolone-impregnated nasal dressing following endoscopic sinus surgery: A randomised double blind placebo control study. Laryngoscope, 2010;(120)1269–73.
4. Desrosiers M, Bendouah Z, Barbeau J. Effectiveness of topical antibiotics on *Staphylococcus aureus* biofilm *in vitro*. American Journal of Rhinology 2007;21(2):149–53.
5. Elsersy HE, Ahmed AA. Factors affecting postoperative agitation in adults following functional endoscopic sinus surgery: A randomized, double-blinded controlled trial. Anaesth Crit Care Med J 2017;2(2):000123.

6. Friedman M, Venkatesan TK, Lang D, Caldarelli DD. Bupivacaine for postoperative analgesia following endoscopic sinus surgery. Laryngoscope 1996;106(11):1382–85.

7. Functional Endoscopic Sinus Surgery: A Randomized, Double-Blinded Controlled Trial. Anaesth Critic Care Med J 2017;2(2):000123.

8. Hauser JL, Turner JH, Chandra RK. Trends in the use of stents and drug-eluting stents in sinus surgery. Otolaryngol Clin North Am 2017;50,3:565–71.

9. Heermann J, Neues D. Intranasal microsurgery of all paranasal sinuses, the septum and the lacrimal sac with hypotensive anesthesia. Ann Oral Rhinol Laryngol 1999;95:631–38.

10. Jabalameli *et al*. Oral clonidine premedication decreases intraoperative bleeding in patients undergoing endoscopic sinus surgery. Journal of Research in Medical Sciences 2005;1:25–30.

11. Kim RJT, Douglass RG. Perioperative care for functional endoscopic sinus surgery. The Otorhinolaryngologist 2012;5(1):27–30.

12. Kristine, *et al*. Effect of intraoperative saline irrigation on bacterial load within the maxillary sinus. International Forum of Allergy and Rhinology, 2011;V-1(5):351–355.

13. Frank S, Brown SM, Capriotti JA, et al. In vitro efficacy of a povidone-iodine nasal antiseptic for rapid inactivation of SARS-CoV-2. JAMA Otolaryngol-Head Neck Surg. 2020;146(11):1054–1058. doi:10.1001/jamaoto.2020.3053

DR Nayak, PSN Murthy, CS Ray

Instrumentation for Diagnostic Nasal Endoscopy and Endoscopic Sinus Surgery

(Figs 8.1 to 8.3)

1. 7210 A. Hopkins II Forward-Oblique Telescope 30°, 70°, 90°, diameter 4 mm, length 18 cm. Used for diagnostic nasal endoscopy and during surgery in the frontal recess and maxillary sinus ostium (Fig. 8.1).

2. 7210 AA. Hopkins II Straightforward Telescope 0°. Diameter 4 mm, length 18 cm. Used for endoscopic sinus surgery (Fig. 8.1).

3. 723770 Stammberger telescope handle for use with telescope for giving stability and preventing bending of the endoscope, that can damage the optics (Fig. 8.2).

4. 27018 A. Hopkins Straightforward Telescope 0°, diameter 2.7 mm, length 18 cm. Used for endoscopic sinus surgery in paediatric age group patients.

5. 27018 B. Hopkins Forward-Oblique Telescope 30°, diameter 2.7 mm, length 18 cm. Used for diagnostic nasal endoscopy in paediatric age group patients also available 70° and 90° angled endoscope used in frontal sinus surgery (Fig. 8.1).

6. 722830. Suction tube, inch finger cut-off, working length 14 cm, size 3 mm.

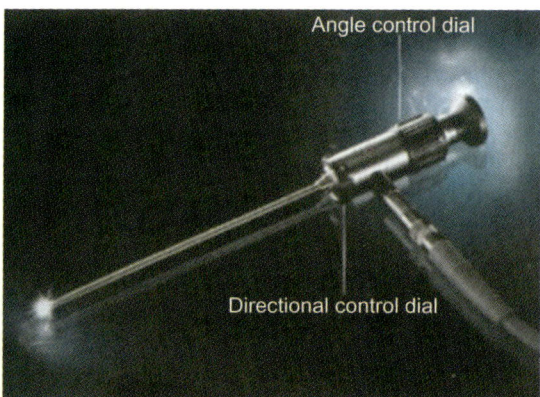

Fig. 8.1b: Multiangle endoscope

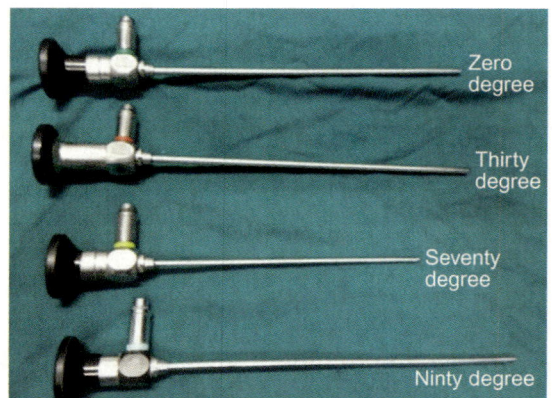

Fig. 8.1a: Hopkins 0° straightforward and 30°, 70°, 90° oblique telescopes

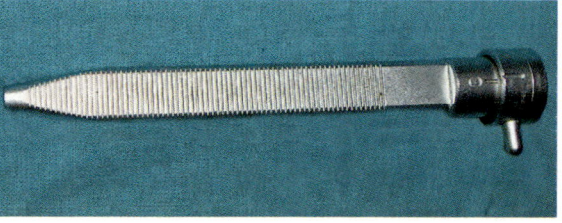

Fig. 8.2: Stammberger telescope handle

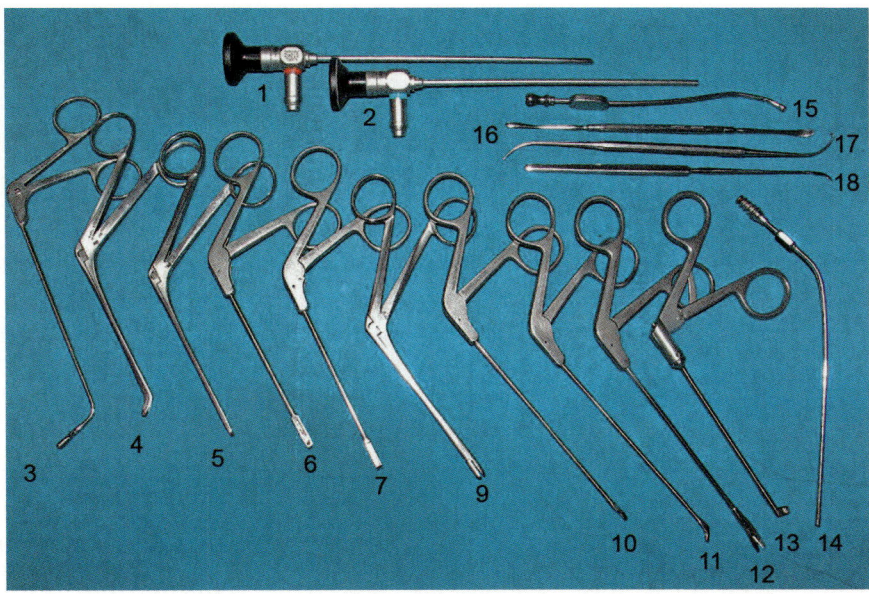

Fig. 8.3: 0° and 30° endoscopes (1 and 2), 90° upturned Stammberger (Giraffe) forceps (3), Blakesley 45° and 0° forceps (4 and 5), Stammberger antrum puncture back biting right and left (6 and 7), Takahashi nasal forceps (9), Heuwieser through cutting tissue sparing forceps (10 and11), Rhinoforce nasal scissors (12), Stammberger antrum punch down and forward cutting (13), Frazier suction tube (14), Curved suction cannula for frontal sinus (15), Mucoperichondrial elevator (16), Kuhn-Bolger frontal ostium seeker (17), Sickle knife (18)

7. 586230. Suction tube, short curved, 15 cm, size 3 mm.
8. 456001 B. Rhinoforce Blakesly nasal forceps, straight, 19 cm, working length 10 cm, size 1.
9. 457001 B. Rhinoforce Strumpel-Voss nasal forceps, 45° upturned, working length 10 cm, size 1.
10. 455000 B. Rhinoforce Takahashi nasal forceps, straight, working length 10 cm.
11. 449201 Rhinoforce nasal scissor, working length 13 cm, straight.
12. 459011 Rhinoforce Stammberger antrum puncture, working length 10 cm, right side backward cutting.
13. 459012 Rhinoforce Stammberger antrum puncture, working length 10 cm, left side backward cutting.
14. 628001 Sickle knife, pointed, 19 cm.
15. 474000 Freer elevator, double ended, length 20 cm.
16. 723772 Stammberger telescope handle, round.

17. 20112001 Cold light Fountain Halogen 150.
18. 20112025. Spare reflector lamp 150 W, 15 V.
19. 495 NB. Fibreoptic light cable. Size 4.8 mm, length 180 cm.
20. 486030 V. EICKEN antrum cannula, 15 cm long curved, OD 3 mm, Luer-lock. (Fig. 8.3).
21. 723005 A. Trocar and cannula for sinuscopy, OD 5 mm. Length of cannula 8.5 cm, fenestrated beck (Fig. 8.4).
22. Stortz endoscopic video camera and cable system (Fig. 8.5).
23. Xomed microdebrider system (Fig. 8.6a and b).
24. Colour monitor

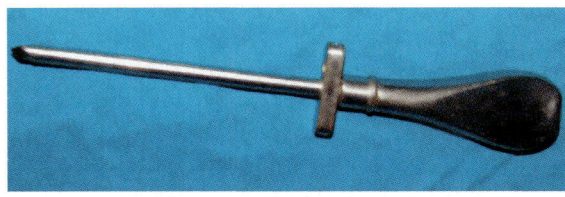

Fig. 8.4: Trocar and cannula for sinuscopy

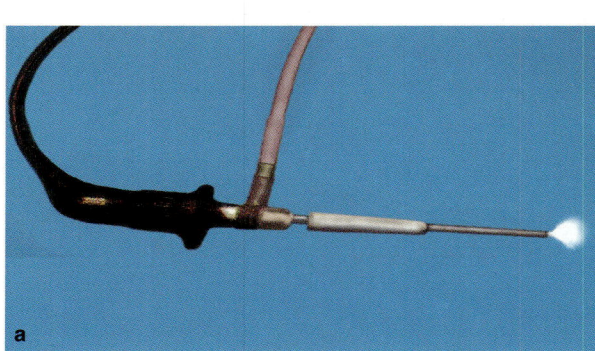
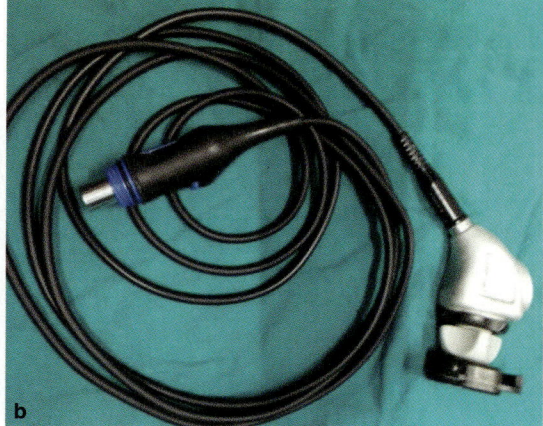

Fig. 8.5: a. Endoscope with camera attachment for video endoscopy (single chip), **b.** Preferably HD camera

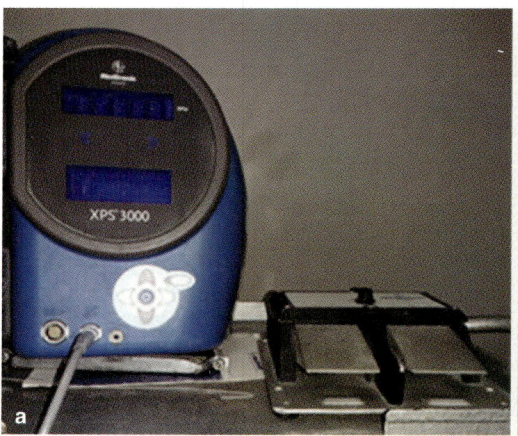
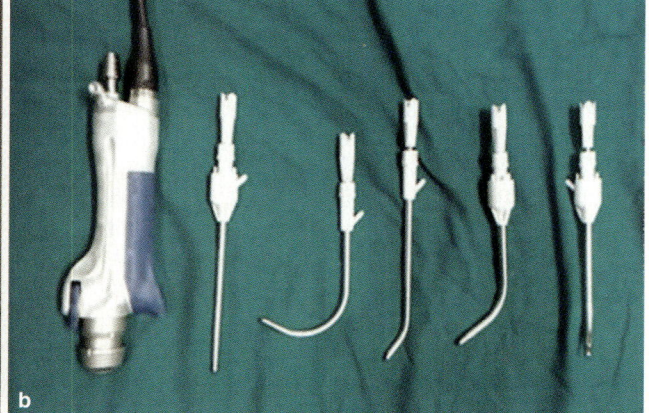

Fig. 8.6: a. Xomed microdebrider system for endoscopic sinus surgery, **b.** Handpiece cable and blades

Set-Up

1. Patient's table
2. Double level instrument table: Upper level—cottonoids, lower level—light source.
3. Mayo stand for the instruments and kidney tray filled with saline.
4. Adjustable stool for the surgeon.
5. Floor should be carpetted or padded; in case an endoscope or instrument falls, it will not get spoilt.

Handling the Instruments

Endoscope

It is held in the left hand like a pen. Extra grip can be attained by using the telescope handles (optional). The last 3 fingers of the left hand should rest on the patients face for proper stability. The tip of the endoscope is dipped in defogging solution, excess solution is wiped off, and then the endoscope is inserted into the nasal cavity. The surgeon should instruct the patient not to move his or her head and to inform him, if the patient has pain or feels like sneezing. This is important as the patient's movements can damage the delicate endoscopes and instruments besides injuring himself. Nowadays endoscopic cameras are being used frequently while doing surgery. This makes the endoscope little heavier. One has to be careful while mounting the camera onto the endoscope and should ensure that it is properly fitted before using to prevent damage to the camera lens. For long duration surgery, especially when dealing with skull base lesions and transsphenoidal surgery including pituitary, a two surgeons and four hand technique is advisable for better control.

Powered Instrument System

The shaver (powered instrument) system offer different handpieces, knives, irrigation and modes (rotating or oscillating). Shaver (microdebrider) is a combination of suction and cutting round knife working together. It was first patented in 1969 for acoustic neuroma surgery. Setliff and Parsons introduced microdebrider (shaver) to endoscopic sinus surgery. Knives of different shapes are put into handpiece. Shaver surgery is precise in soft tissue resection, so the most advantages to power the system is in rhino-surgery, polypectomy with extension to pansinus surgery (Dalke, et al. 2006). Microdebrider is a very useful tool to do polypectomy with precision and achieves a relatively bloodless field during endoscopic surgery although the precision depends on the surgeon's anatomical knowledge and operative skills (Singh, et al. 2011). At present, navigation controlled shaver is available and the first clinical application was done by Strauss, et al. in 2008 and was found to be superior to conventional pointer based navigation (image gidance system).

Image Guidance Systems for Sinus Surgery

Image-guided endoscopic sinus surgery is one of the most significant advancement developed since mid-1980s. Although it was first adopted in neurosurgery but gained leading acceptance by the endoscopic surgeon throughout the world (Citardi & Batra 2005). The electromagnetic-based Insta Trak® system and the optical-based Stealth-Station are commonly used for endoscopic sinus surgery. Each system was noted to have limitations. The presence of metallic objects in the operative field interfered with functioning of the electromagnetic system, whereas the optical system required a clear line of sight to be maintained between the infrared camera and surgical handpiece. Both systems required specialized headsets to be worn by patients during surgery to monitor head position. The electromagnetic system also required these headsets to be worn during the preoperative computed tomography scan. Although both these two image guidance systems proved valuable for anatomic localization during sinus surgery, individual preferences can be based on distinct differences in their design and operation.

The LandmarX ENT Image Guidance System (Xomed Surgical Products, Jaksonville, FL, USA) consists of a monitor (Fig. 8.8), a computer, an optical camera (Fig. 8.7a), a reference head frame (Fig. 8.7c), and specialised optical probes (Fig. 8.7b). It uses real-time surgical navigation with the help of pre-operative computed tomographic images. The computer software restructured the computed tomography images and displayed them (Fig. 8.8) on the screen in different perspectives (axial, coronal and sagittal and three-dimensional model). The reference frame and the optical probes contain infrared emitting diodes that transmit infrared light which are identified by the optical (infrared) camera and are finally relayed to the computer which detects exact position of the tip of the probe (Fig. 8.7a). After the process of "co-registration", green and yellow circles illustrated the regions within which the localisation error deviated 1 mm or less (green) and 2 mm or less (yellow). After reference frame attached to the patients head, landmark points are selected from the computer images and then corresponding points selected from patient's external anatomy with the help of optical probe. Computer software can build a map by analyzing these information. Intra-operative navigation can be done by identifying various critical points like sphenoid sinus, optic nerve, carotid artery, etc. with the help of optical probe and the corresponding area in the CT images in three different planes can be matched. This system is a valuable tool for experienced endoscopic surgeon for performing complex endoscopic

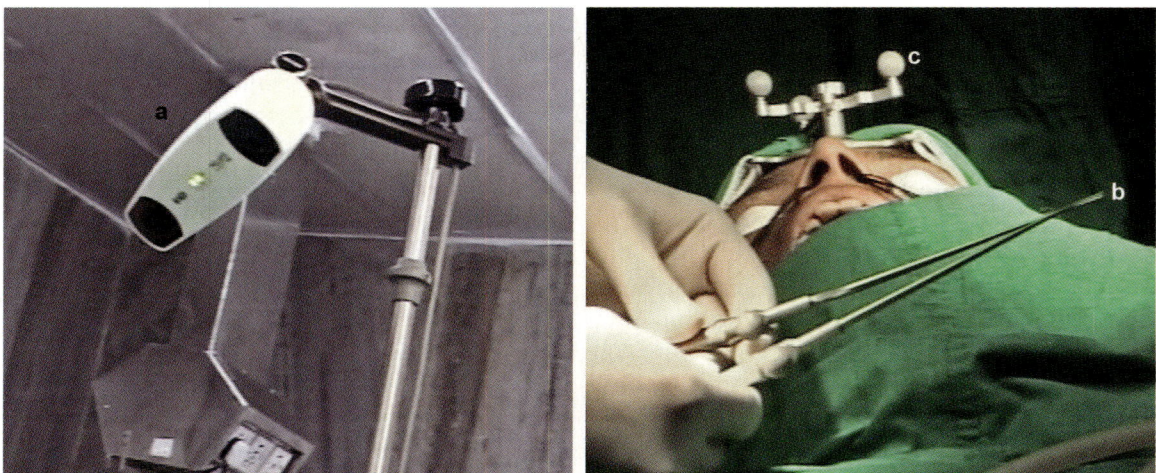

Fig. 8.7: (a) Infrared camera, (b) Instrument tracker reflective spheres (optical probe) and (c) Patient tracker reflective spheres (head band)

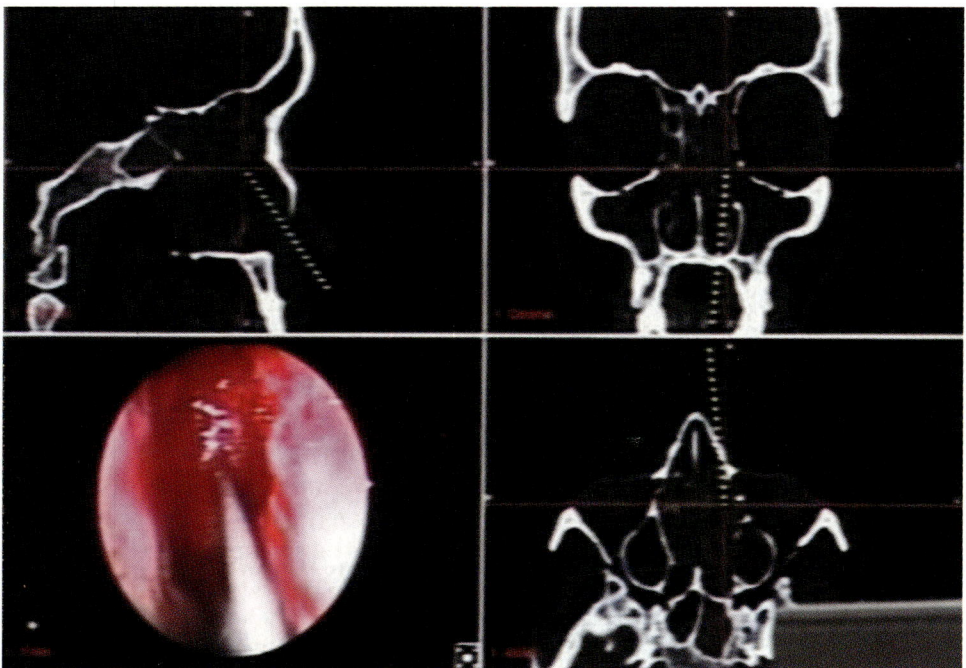

Fig. 8.8: Optical probe identifying the surgical landmark in the monitor through endoscopic camera and the corresponding position is shown in sagittal, coronal and axial CT imaging

surgery and minimal invasive procedure in the nose and paranasal sinuses (Eliashar, et al. 2003). Recent introduction of navigation controlled shaver system has replaced the optical probe so that surgeon need not have to check repeatedly the targeted area and the information can be directly accessed while performing surgery (Strauss, et al. 2008).

Multiangle endoscope: This endoscope, developed by Acclarent Cyclops, has a shaft which rotates, giving an angle of view from 10° to 90°. It is useful in minimally invasive sinus surgery and endoscopic skull base surgery avoiding repeated changing of scopes for angle vision (Fig. 8.1b) besides, giving a custom desired angle of view.

Risk of Infection and Its Prevention

Continuous diagnostic and therapeutic endoscopy in the out patient or operation setting for patients with multiple users can be associated with nosocomial infections due to contamination (Kramer, et al. 2015). Often endoscopy is associated with mucosal trauma that can facilitate entry of pathogen form the surface or endoscope itself and even can spread from the environment. Nasal vestibule is one of the common site for organisms like *Stapheilla*, *Candida albicans,* etc. that can cause nosocomial infection in susceptible patients. Thus basic principles of infection prevention needs to be followed (Hossemann and Draf 2013). Disinfection of hands and surfaces used near the patient, which are important sites of contamination during routine nasal endoscopy, is important to maintain proper hygienic environment. For endoscopic therapeutic procedure including FESS, operation theatre must be sanitized well after shifting the previous patient which may have undergone surgery in an infected setting. Cleaning of instruments also caries the risk of infection transmission and the sister or technician doing the job must have proper protection. The instruments and endoscope must be cleaned properly to remove organic matter before sending them for sterilization in the disinfectant solution (glutaraldehyde). Non-fibreoptic metalic instruments like forceps, curette, probe, etc. should be autoclaved. Microdebrider handpieces are sent for gas sterilization.

Disinfection of the Instruments

High-level disinfection provides a reasonably effective method of reducing bacterial and fungal contamination of fiberoptic nasal endoscope. Appropriate surveillance technique should be used in each clinical setting with flexible and rigid fiberoptic scopes to ensure adequate disinfection effectiveness.

This is done by using a 2% W/V solution of glutaraldehyde (Cidex®). Addition of the activator to this solution turns it bright green (activated solution). This can be used for a maximum period of 2 weeks, clean, rinse and rough dry the endoscopes and instruments before immersing in the activated solution. Cleanse and rinse the lumens of the suction tubes before filling with activated solution. Immerse completely for a minimum of 10 minutes (Fig. 8.9). This destroys the vegetative organisms, pathogenic fungi and viruses. Remove the equipment from the activated solution and rinse thoroughly with sterile water prior to use.

Before using the endoscopic system in each case, one has to inspect the entire system for any damage, loosening kinking of cable, etc. It is always better to know in detail of instruments from product specific manual provided with the system and their handling instructions. One should first make overall inspection followed by inspection of telescopes for their proper functioning, light guide cable, HF cable and electrodes for secure fixation, any cut or damage, proper insulation, etc.

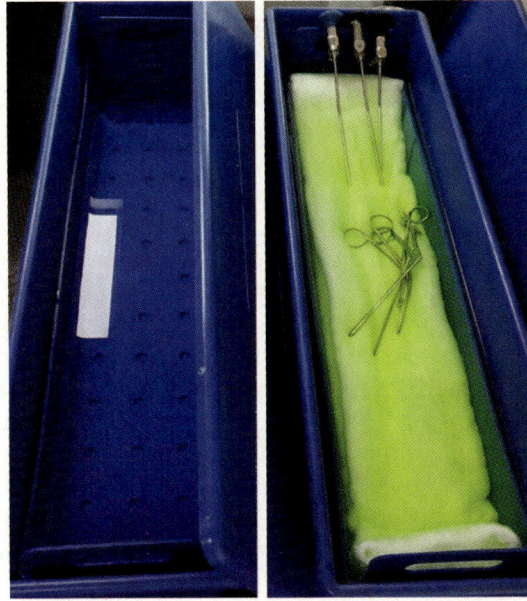

Sterile water to rinse   Cidex (2% Glutaraldehyde)
instrument

Fig. 8.9: Sterilization trays for endoscope and endoscopic instruments

Electrical hand instruments like cautery and bipolar should also be inspected in a similar way as per the product manual. Video equipment should be inspected with respect to wiring and functioning as per the product information and handling manual. It is always better to have a trained personnel like endoscope technician to handle these equipment after installation by the supplier and after proper demonstration of handling of these equipments. After completion of surgery, after performing the surgery, one should separate and dispose the single use products as per legal requirements from reusable products. The reusables should be transported carefully to the processing area for cleaning immediately after use and each instrument should be handled and disassembled, cleaned and sterilized as per the product instruction provided. Endoscopic instruments after prier cleaning should be disinfected with proper certified solution recommended by the company like Cidex (2% glutaraldehyde) for Stortz instruments to achieve high level disinfection with respect to mycobacteria, bacterial spores and viruses (Fig. 8.9). Then the instruments should be rinsed with sterile water and dried with sterile cloth. Some instruments may require proper lubrication for their functioning besides protect them from corrosion and eroding. Optical instruments should be cleaned with 70% alcohol.

Taking care of nasal endoscope is extremely important while performing the surgery. The tip of the nasal endoscope gets frequently soiled with blood. Unless cleaned regularly, the dried blood clot can decrease the longevity of the endoscope. The author prefers to clean the tip with normal saline, which is kept in a bowl with cotton being kept at the bottom. Recently endo-scrub 2 lens cleaning sheath has been introduced. This helps in continuing the surgery without withdrawing the endoscope for repeated cleaning. This system also prevents fogging, while performing endoscopy and endoscopic surgery.

BIBLIOGRAPHY

1. Dalke, et al. Rotation suction-knife (shaver) in otorhinolaryngological surgery. Otolaryngol Pol 2006; 60(1):37–40.
2. Hosemann W, Draf C. Danger points, complications and medico-legal aspects in endoscopic sinus surgery. GMS Curr Top Otorhinolaryngol Head Neck Surg. 2013;12:Doc06. doi: 10.3205/cto000098.
3. Citardi M, Batra PS. Image-guided sinus surgery: Current concepts and Technology. Otol Clin North Am 2005;38,3:439–52.
4. Kramer, et al. Principles of infection prevention and reprocessing in ENT endoscopy. GMS Curr Top Otorhinolaryngol Head Neck Surg 2015; 14: Doc10.
5. Metson, Ralph MD. Laryngoscope. 108 (8, Part 1): 1164–1170, A Comparison of Image Guidance Systems for Sinus Surgery August 1998.
6. Neil Bhattacharyya MD, Lynne J Kepnes RNP. The effectiveness of immersion disinfection for flexible fiberoptic laryngoscopes Otolaryngology—Head and Neck Surgery, June 2004; Vol 130, Issue 6; 681–85.
7. R Eliashar, Sichel JY, Gross M, et al. Image guided navigation system—a new technology for complex endoscopic endonasal surgery. Postgrad Med J 2003;79:686–90.
8. Setliff RC, Parsons DS. The "hummer": New instrumentation for functional endoscopic sinus surgery. Am J Rhinol 1994;8:275–78. doi: 10.2500/105065894781874232.
9. Singh R, Hazarika P, Nayak DR, et al. A Comparison of microdebrider assisted endoscopic sinus surgery and conventional endoscopic sinus surgery for nasal polyp. Indian J Otolaryngol Head Neck Surg 2013 Jul; 65(3): 193–96.
10. Stortz the world of endoscopy, endoscopes and instruments for ENT, 6th Edition.
11. Strauss G, Hofer M, Fischer M, et al. First clinical application of a navigation-controlled shaver in paranasal sinus surgery. Surg Technol Int 2008;17:19–25.

Technique of Functional Endoscopic and Minimal Invasive Sinus Surgery

DR Nayak, R Balakrishnan

Introduction

Functional endoscopic sinus surgery (FESS) has become the standard of care since its introduction by Messerklinger in 1978. He studied the mucus movement of the major sinuses in fresh cadaver obtained within first 24 hours through endoscopic time lapsed photography and found that direction of mucus movement occurs towards natural ostium of the sinuses, the process which now is recognized as mucociliary clearance. This study also showed that compromised narrow transition space due to mucosal contact involving the ethmoidal infundibulum can lead to retention of secretions that can ultimately lead to chronic persistent infection. This facilitated the development of FESS (functional endoscopic sinus surgery). Simple clearance of disease from the transition space depending on the extend of disease can reverse the mucosal changes in the major sinuses (Stammberger, 1986).

MESSERKLINGER'S TECHNIQUE

Anaesthesia

This can be done either under local anaesthesia or general anaesthesia, but local anaesthesia is preferred. There is difference of opinion among otolaryngologists about the safest way to administer anaesthesia during endoscopic sinus surgery. Most of the surgeons maintain that the risk of complications under general anaesthesia is greater because of greater blood loss and poor visualization than with local anaesthesia (Stankiewicz 1989), where vasoconstriction is better achieved. Moreover, the medial orbital wall, orbital periosteum and the thinnest part of the skull base are sensitive to pain, facilitate careful monitoring in an awake patient. Thus major complications can be avoided and vision can be monitored. Local injection of a solution containing a vasoconstrictor is required in all cases regardless of the anaesthesia chosen to minimize the bleeding. The surgical risk to the patient diminishes as the surgeon's ability to visualize the field increases.

General anaesthesia is given in children and in apprehensive patients. Topical anaesthetic agent like 4% xylocaine with 1:100,000 adrenaline soaked in cottonoids are used for initial vasoconstriction. The cottonoids should be kept in the middle meatus, between the septum and the turbinates. This facilitates in increasing the area of access to the operative field and allows smooth passage of instruments through the nose without causing much discomfort to the patient. After 5 minutes, the medial infundibular wall, anterior end of middle turbinate and ethmoidal bulla are injected with 2% xylocaine with (1:100,000) adrenaline under endoscope visualization (black dots shown in Fig. 9.2). In recent days with improved surgical technique and expanding indications, various endoscopic approaches have been developed requiring anaesthesia management. Hence, general anaesthesia is being preferred, limiting the use of local anaesthesia for minor endoscopic procedure. Recently total intravenous anaesthesia has been introduced in endoscopic sinus surgery. It has a distinct advantage over inhalant anaesthesia by creating a selective vasodilatation of arterial area because of calcium antagonist properties. The general anaesthesia is induced by remifentanyl (1 mg/kg) followed by propofol (1–2 mg/kg) (Tirelli, et al 2004).

Operative Technique

Position of the Patient

The patient should be placed in the supine position with the head slightly elevated and turned towards the surgeon. At present, a "15° reverse Trendelenburg position" is preferred to facilitate better endoscopic view as well as intraoperative blood loss. The patient should be asked to breath through mouth, if the operation is performed using local anaesthesia. A 0° nasal endoscope is used for most part of the surgery and this is the only endoscope to be used by the beginner as it gives a direct view. After getting well acquainted with the normal landmarks, one can start using angled endoscope (Fig. 9.1).

Steps of Surgery

Ethmoidal infundibulum: It is a three-dimensional space bounded anteriorly and inferiorly by the uncinate process and its attachment to the frontal process of maxilla, posteriorly it is bounded by bulla ethmoidalis and laterally is the hiatus semilunaris. Thus uncinate process plays a very key role in endoscopic sinus surgery and its removal (infundibulotomy), gives direct access to the ethmoidal infundibulum. The superior attachment of uncinate process determines the drainge of frontal recess, i.e. to the infundibulum or middle meatus.

Infundibulotomy (Uncinectomy)

After proper infiltration as in Fig. 9.2, the Kuhn Bolger frontal and maxillary sinus ball probe is used to check the swing door movement of uncinate process to look for its attachment and accordingly, the incision is given circumferentially over the mucosa following its attachment using a sickle knife. The tip of the knife should be directed inferiorly and parallel to the lateral nasal wall to prevent injury to the lamina papyracea (Fig. 9.3).

After the incision, the uncinate process is subluxed medially with the help of a straight perichondrial elevator from its superior and inferior attachment (Figs 9.4 and 9.5a to d).

The superior insertion of the uncinate process is then carefully grasped with

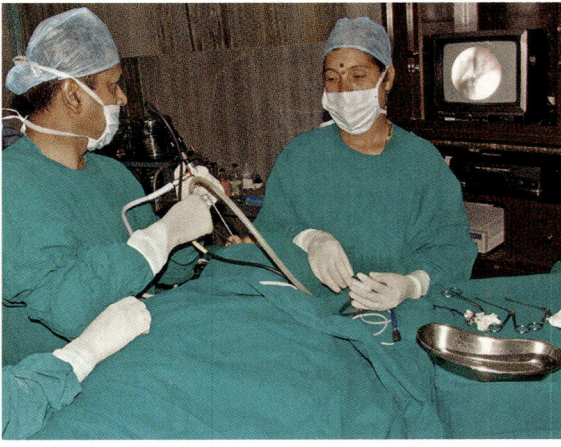

Fig. 9.1: Endoscopic assessment before starting FESS

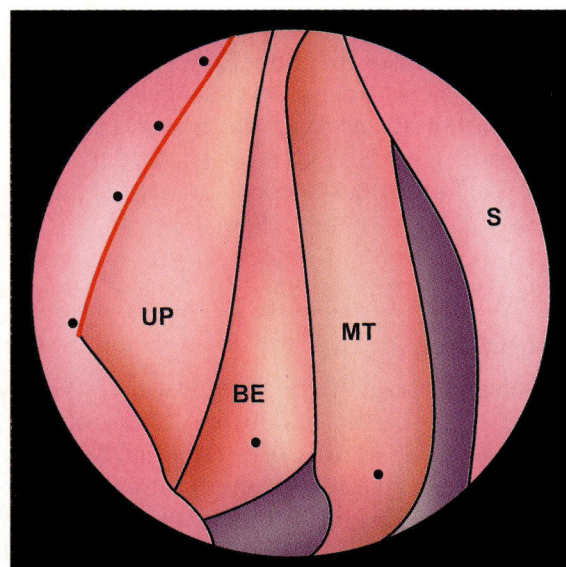

Fig. 9.2: Sites of local anaesthetic infiltration on the uncinate process (UP), bulla ethmoidalis (BE) and the middle turbinate (MT), septum (S) (after Stammberger)

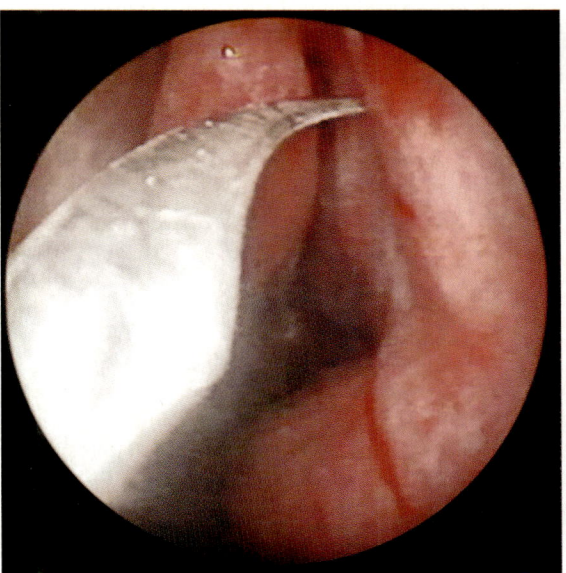

Fig. 9.3: Incision being given at the attachment of the uncinate process on the left side

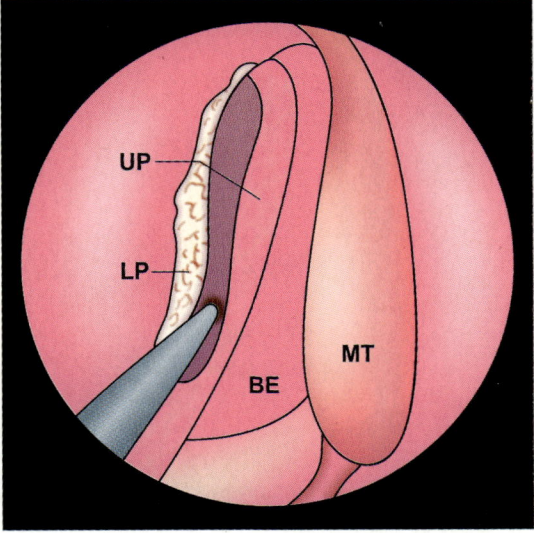

Fig. 9.4: The uncinate process (UP) being subluxed using an elevator on the right side exposing the lamina papyracea (LP). Also seen is middle turbinate (MT)

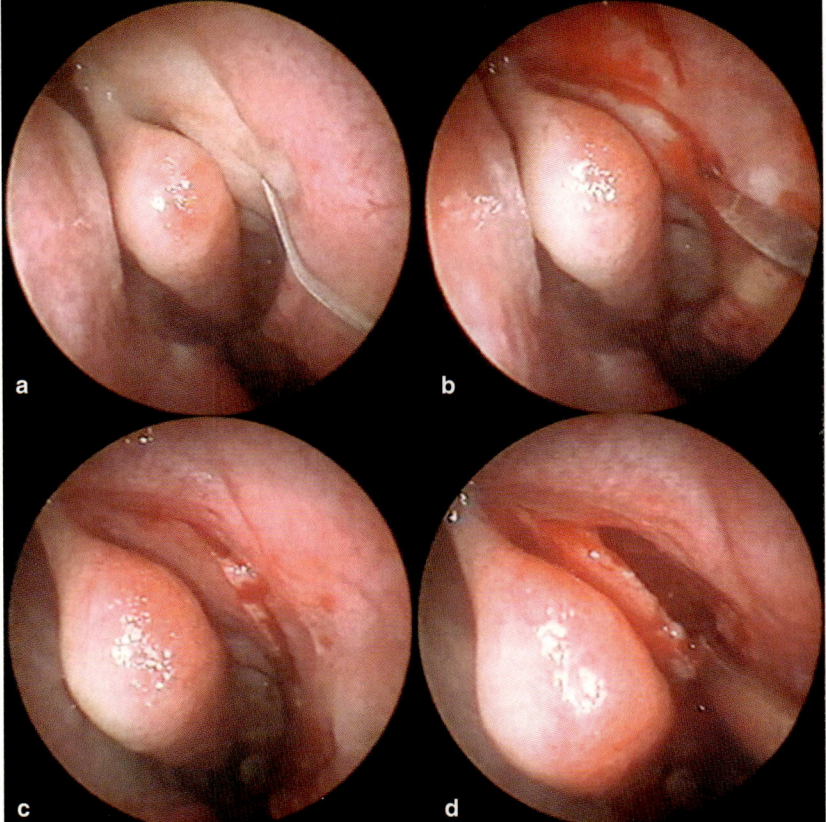

Fig. 9.5: Video endoscopic photograph showing the steps of infundibulotomy: **a.** Infiltration along the uncinate process, **b.** Incision is being given at the attachment site, **c.** The incised uncinate process before subluxation, and **d.** Subluxation of uncinate process is carried out by using a curved septal elevator (left)

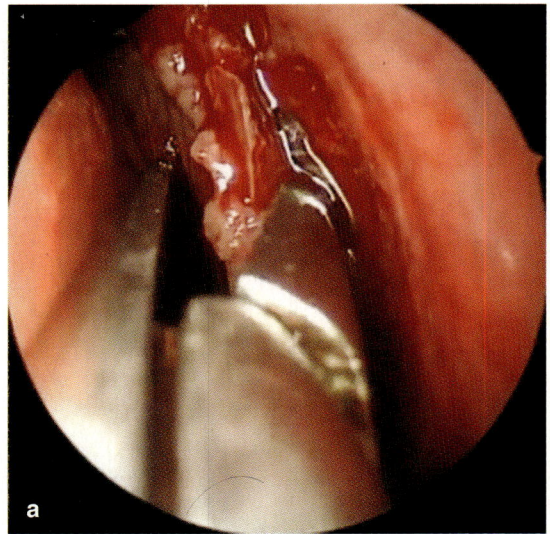

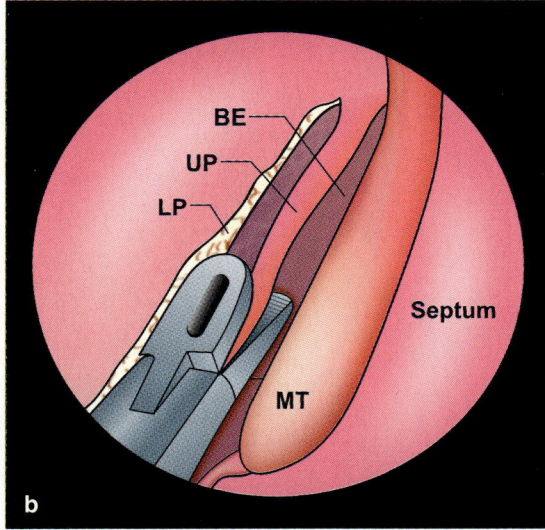

Fig. 9.6: a. Uncinate process being removed with Blakesley forceps after separation from lateral wall, **b.** The uncinate process (UP) is grasped using Blakesley forceps before removal. Other structures can be seen are bulla ethmoidalis (BE), lamina papyracea (LP), middle turbinate (MT), and septum

Blakesley-Weil forceps and is resected using endoscopic scissors and then separated from the lateral wall by a twisted motion of the forceps (Figs 9.6a and b).

Then the inferior portion is grasped and removed in a similar way. Alternately a cut can be made with paediatric back biting forceps at the level of lower border of bulla and then microdebrider can be used to resect rest of the upper part of uncinate. After infundibulum is opened, the surgeon can then

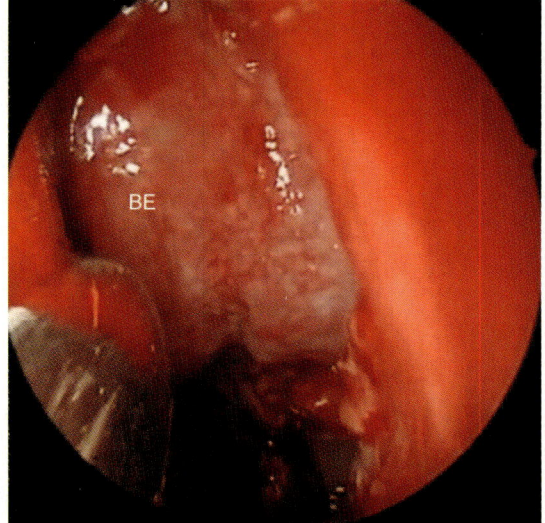

Fig. 9.6c: Exposed bulla after uncinectomy on left side

determine, if further procedure in the area of frontal recess or the ostium of the maxillary sinus is required.

Anterior Ethmoidectomy and Middle Meatal Antrostomy

Antrostomy

After infundibulotomy, the ostium of the maxillary sinus is frequently visible. Sometimes the posterior inferior remnant of the uncinate process prevents the visualization of the ostium and has to be removed. If the frontal sinus is involved, one has to open the frontal recess. But in case the disease involves the ethmoidal bulla or posterior ethmoid and sphenoid, the disease has to be cleared from these areas before approaching the frontal recess to prevent troublesome bleeding that can complicate the surgical process unnecessarily.

Opening of the bulla: The bulla ethmoidalis is opened inferiorly and medially with the help of a straight suction tip, Blakesley forceps. Some surgeons use the tip of the microdebrider/shaver blade to open, if they are using this powered instrument for the surgery. The anterior wall of the bulla can be removed safely and systematically by using a straight mushroom forceps, after bulla is opened (Figs 9.7 and 9.8). A beginner must

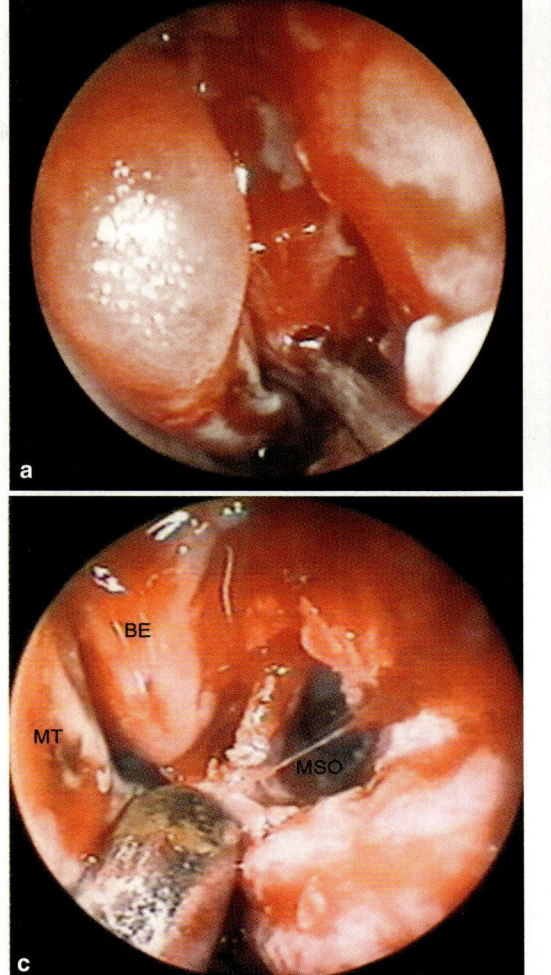

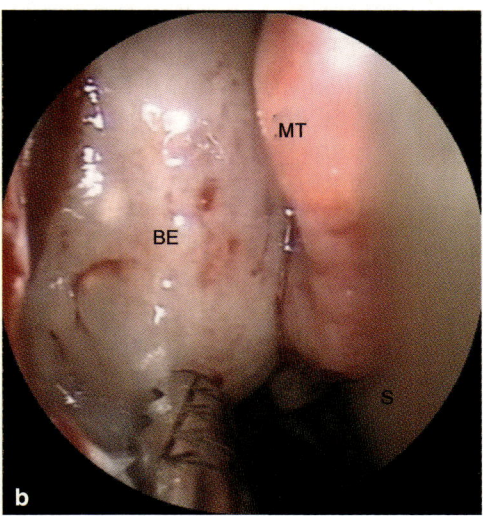

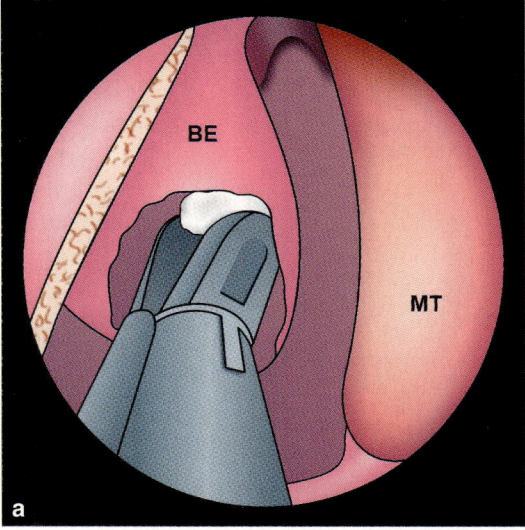

Fig. 9.7: a. Opened bulla ethmoidalis in its inferior medial portion (left) after uncinectomy is done with a straight curette, **b.** Opening of bulla (BE) with microdebrider in its inferior medial aspect on the right side. Also note middle turbinate (MT), septum (S). **c.** Maxillary sinus ostium visible after infundibulotomy

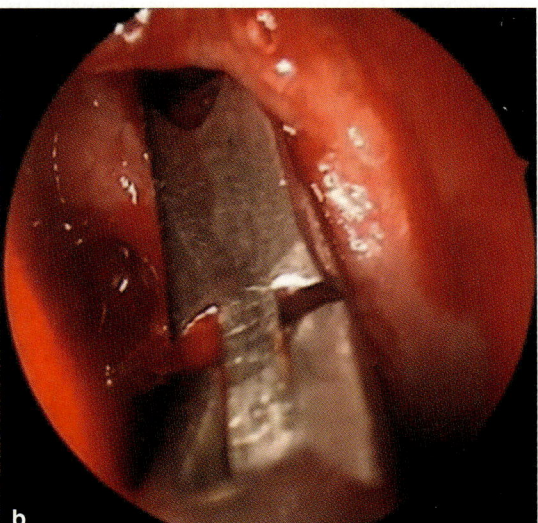

Fig. 9.8: Anterior ethmoidectomy is being performed after opening of the bulla (BE)

use a 0° scope for surgery of this region and should keep the upper attachment of the middle turbinate as the superior landmark, and should never go above that level to prevent injury to the dura. After identifying the lumen, the entire bulla can be resected step by step (Figs 9.9 and 9.10). Alternately bulla can be opened with a straight currete in a retrograde fashion by inserting the currete into the retrobullar space and then opening the bulla anteriorly. If there is no disease in the frontal sinus, the frontal recess is not explored. In such cases, the superior attachment of bulla should be preserved as a landmark and also to prevent stenosis in the frontal sinus drainage pathway.

Above and anterior to bulla, there are 2–3 small ethmoidal cells (agger nasi and frontal cells) and the sinus lateralis. These cells can be removed in a similar fashion, by using a currete. While clearing the disease from the roof of the ethmoid, the position of the anterior ethmoidal artery should be kept in mind (Fig. 9.11). It is always important to study the position of anterior ethmoidal artery in a coronal CT before dealing in this area. The artery is always posterior to the anterior wall of the bulla. Therefore, one should routinely preserve the upper attachment of bulla, if frontal recess and frontal sinus are not

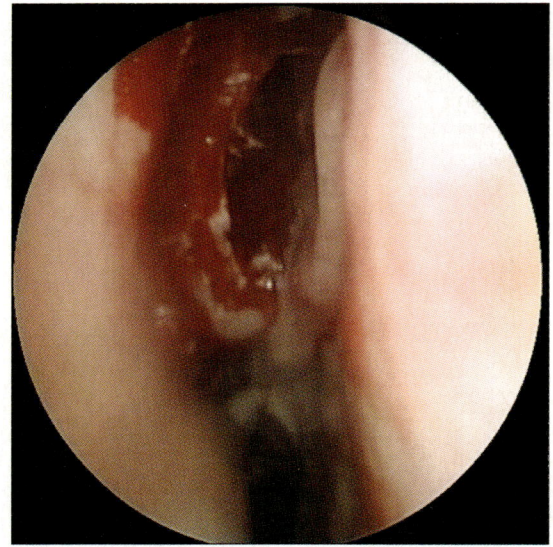

Fig. 9.9: Removal of right bulla in progress. Note the removal of anterior medial wall of bulla while preserving the superior attachment

addressed. If frontal recess and forntal sinus are diseased, it should be cleared first as described under frontal recess clearance and frontal sinusotomy before proceeding for anterior and posterior ethmoidectomy.

The vessel passes across the ethmoid immediately below the anterior skull base in a partial or complete bony ridge attached to the ethmoidal roof as an useful landmark. If

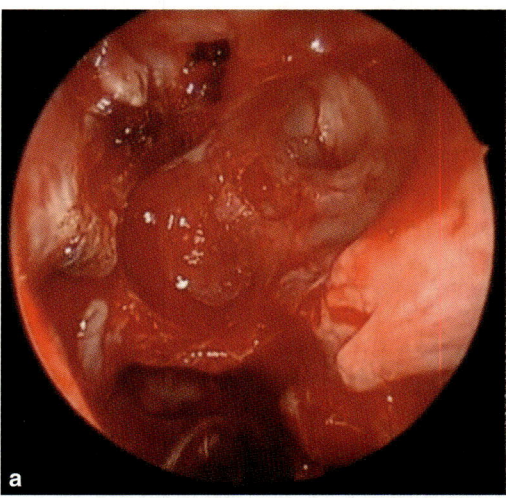
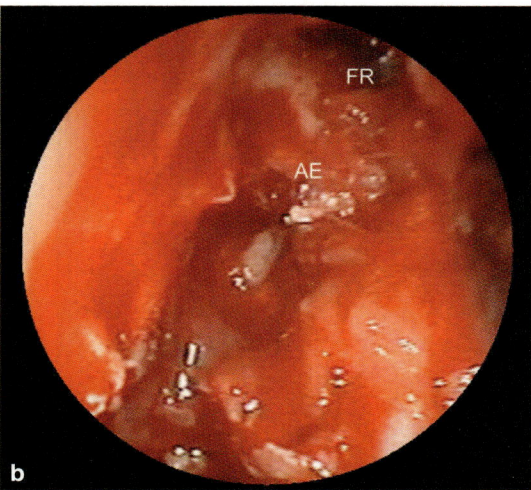

Fig. 9.10: a. Complete removal of bulla and anterior ethmoidectomy and exposure of ground lamella in its superior aspect, **b.** Anterior ethmoids have been opened completely exposing anterior ethmoidal artery (AE), fovea ethmoidalis and frontal recess (FR)

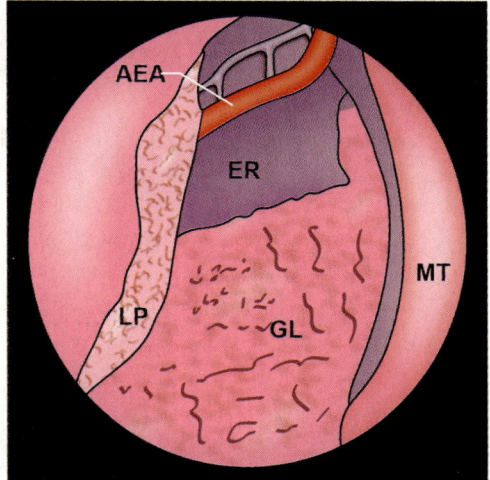

Fig. 9.11a: Exposure of ground lamella (GL) after anterior ethmoidectomy (right), showing anterior ethmoidal artery (AEA), ethmoidal roof (ER), lamina papyracea (LP), middle turbinate (MT)

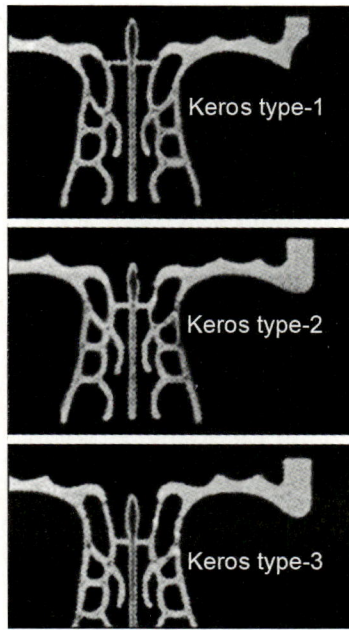

Fig. 9.12: Level of ethmoidal roof in relation to cribriform plate and middle turbinate (described in details under Chapter-1)

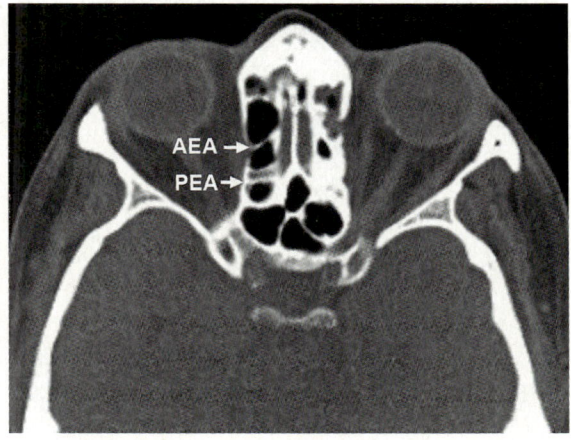

Fig. 9.11b: Axial CT showing relationship of anterior ethmoidal artery (AEA) and posterior ethmoidal artery (PEA) to orbit

the anterior skull base is not identifiable, surgery in this area is deferred until ethmoidal roof is identified within the posterior ethmoid or sphenoid. CT imaging showing level of ethmoidal roof and cribriform plate is very important while dealing with the ethmoidal roof (Fig. 9.12). Use of navigation is very helpful in this regard.

The maxillary sinus ostium is not enlarged routinely, if the ostium is well patent. In case of stenosis, the ostium is enlarged towards the anterior fontanelle by using back biting forceps (Figs 9.13a and b), after identification of the ostium by palpation with a bent spoon. Care is taken not to open the ostium anterior to the level of the middle turbinate to prevent injury to the nasolacrimal duct.

Exploration of the Frontal Recess and Frontal Sinusotomy

In case of limited or absence of disease in the ethmoid, the agger nasi cell is opened without opening the bulla. A curve ball probe/curve curette is passed behind the opened agger nasi cell gently to palpate frontal recess and frontal ostium. Then the agger nasi cell and frontal recess cells, if any, are excentereted and frontal ostium exposed while preserving the frontal sinus outflow tract (Fig. 9.15a and b). The frontal recess can be explored after the removal of anterior ethmoidal cells and bulla and identification of ethmoidal roof. An angled Blakesley forceps/microdebrider and 30/45/70 nasal endoscopes are used for this purpose. Microdebrider is an excellent instrument to clear polyps from the frontal recess while preserving the mucosa of the frontal recess (Figs 9.15 to 9.17). As there are a

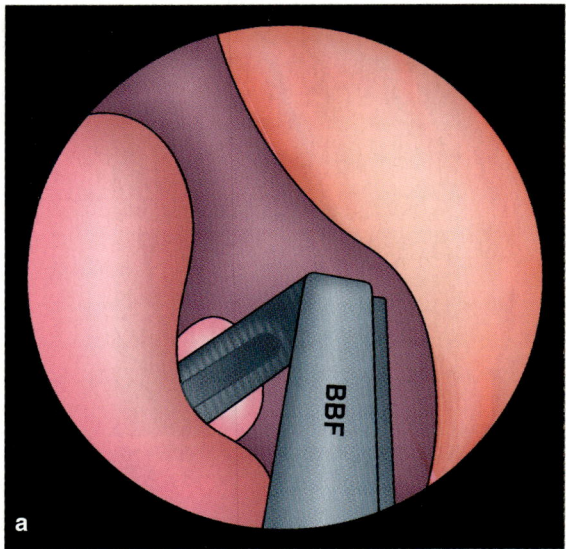

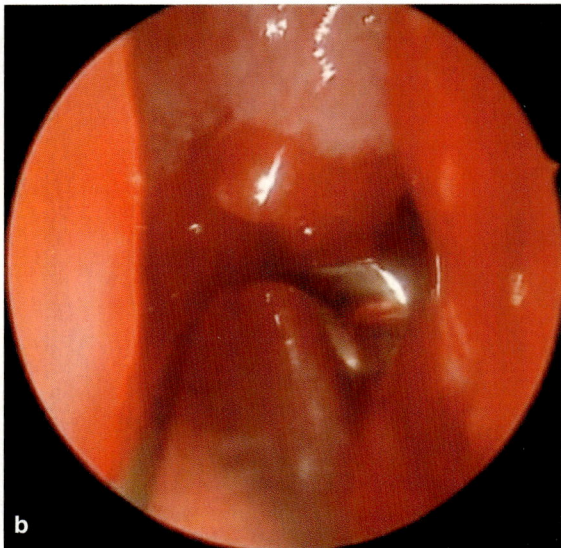

Fig. 9.13: Right **(a)**, left **(b)** middle meatal antrostomy being performed using a back biting forceps (BBF)

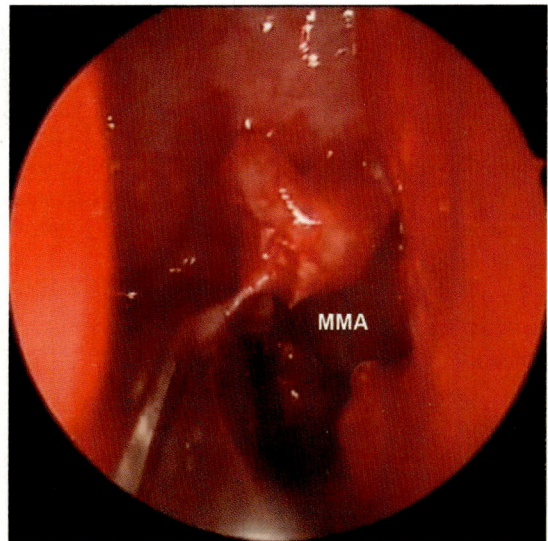

Fig. 9.13c: Completed middle meatal antrostomy (MMA) by joining accessory ostium with natural ostium

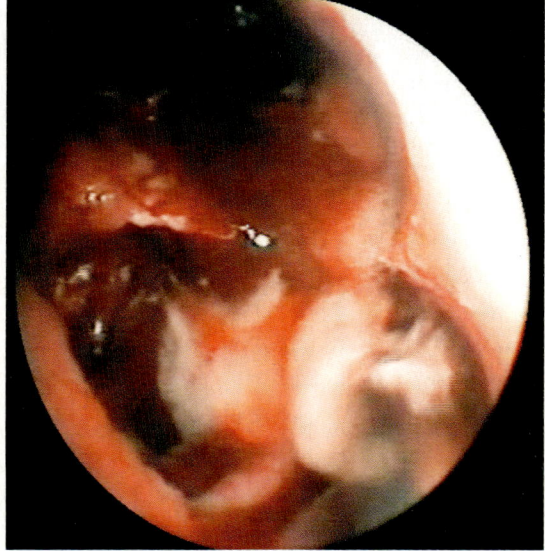

Fig. 9.13d: Fungal mass being removed from the maxillary sinus with suction after completed middle meatal antrostomy

lot of anatomical variations in this area, the exact technique varies. It is usually possible to view sinus after tracing the cranial extent of the uncinate process remnant on its posterior aspect where the agger nasi cell is encountered. The frontal recess lies between the posterior wall of agger nasi and anterior wall of bulla. One also should remember that the superior aspect uncinate may be pneumatized by agger cell. The superior

attachment of the bulla should be preserved before exploring frontal sinus as frontal recess lies always anterior and superior to that. Incomplete removal of cells or striping of mucosa are the common causes for stenosis of the frontal ostium. Preoperative spiral multi-slice CT including sagittal cuts is essential to analyze the anatomy of the frontal recess with

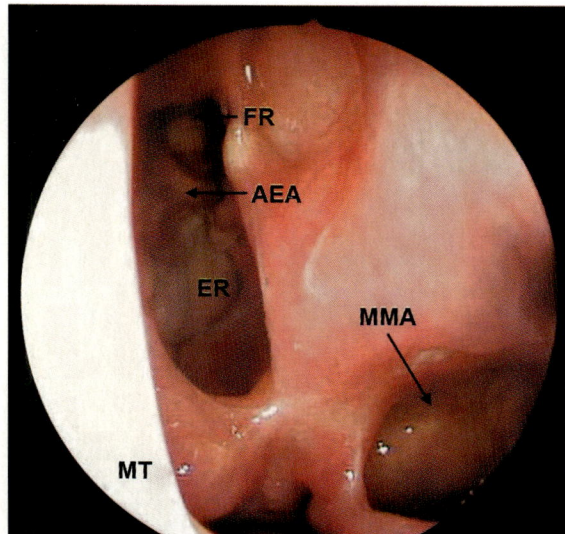

Fig. 9.14: Video endoscope picture showing the post-operative picture of maxillary ostium after middle meatal antrostomy (MMA) (left), frontal recess (FR), anterior ethmoidal artery (AEA), ethmoidal roof (ER), middle turbinate (MT)

the user friendly Kuhn's classification of frontal ethmoidal cells. A ball probe or a curved curette is an useful instrument to uncap and exenterate the frontal and agger nasi cells and should be done from the

posterior to anterior fashion under vision while preserving the mucosa of the frontal drainage pathway. At no stage, a curette or the probe should pass through the roof of a cell. If the bulla is removed completely especially in the previous surgery (Fig. 9.14), the anterior ethmoidal artery is identified using the 30°/70° scope to locate a small recess which usually opens into a supraorbital recess directly in front of the artery, and frontal ostium is further anterior (Fig. 9.18). Often there are difficulties in identifying the frontal ostium due to previous surgery or extensive disease in the frontal recess. In such cases, it is useful to raise an axillary flap described by Wormald (2002) similar to that for DCR of 7–8 square mm from lateral wall towards the middle turbinate to expose the anterior wall of the agger nasi. The anterior wall is then removed to identify the agger nasi cell by using a drill or Hajek-Kofler punch foreps (Fig. 9.19a). The agger nasi cell is carefully removed and other cells are identified. The frontal sinus drainage pathway is carefully identified with a curved ball probe.

The removal of frontal cells individually from posterior medial to anterior direction

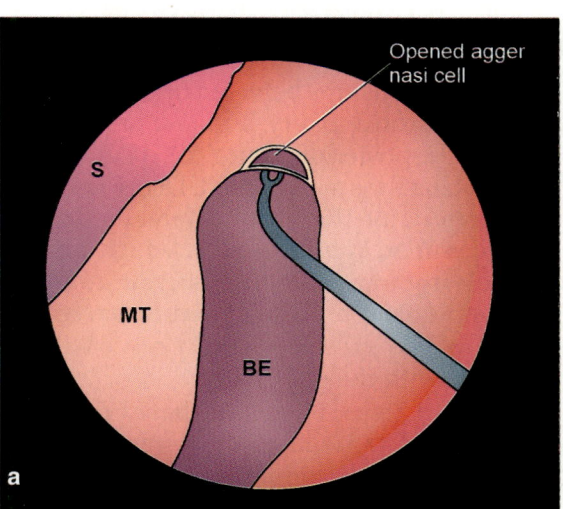

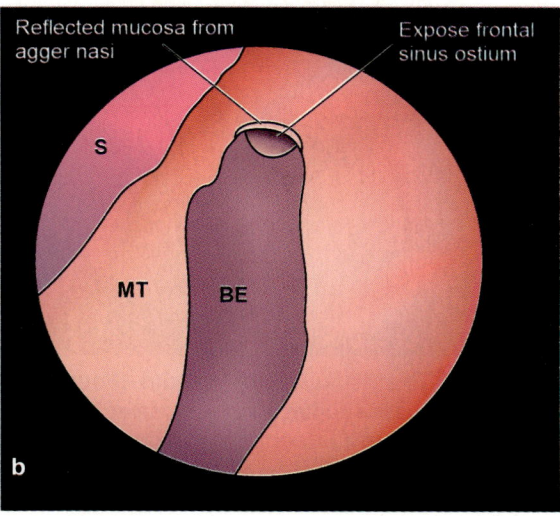

Fig. 9.15: a. Intact bulla technique. A curved curette being passed behind the opened agger nasi cell before exenteration to palpate the frontal recess and ostium, **b.** Frontal recess is cleared after exenteration of agger nasi cell completely while preserving the mucosa of the posterior surface to expose the frontal ostium and reflecting anteriorly overexposed bone while preserving frontal sinus drainage pathway. The landmarks including septum (s), middle turbinate (MT), intact bulla etmoidalis (BE) can be seen in both the pictures

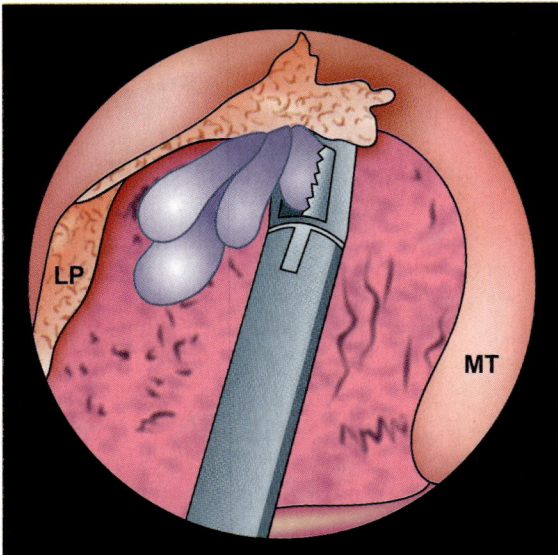

Fig. 9.16a: Endoscope photograph showing polyp being removed from left frontal recess with micro-debrider. Note the position of lamina papyracea (LP) and middle turbinate (MT)

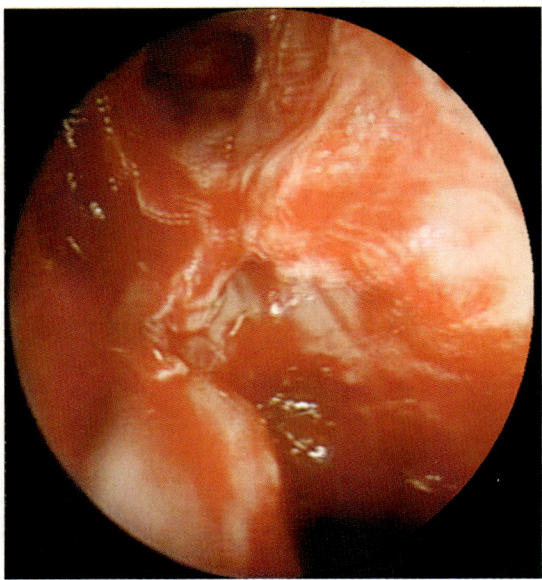

Fig. 9.16b: Exposure of frontal sinus ostium after clearance of frontal recess

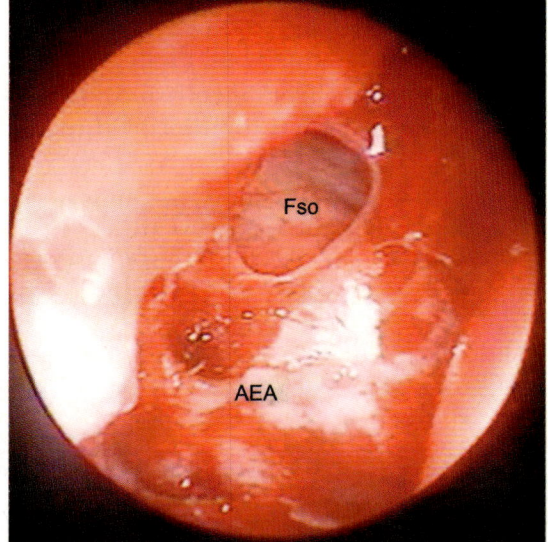

Fig. 9.17: The frontal sinus ostium (Fso) after clearance of the left frontal recess exposing the fovea ethmoidalis seen posterior to anterior ethmoidal artery (AEA)

without injuring the attachment of the middle turbinate finally allows the visualization of the frontal ostium (Fig. 9.19b). Enlargement of the ostium is done anteriorly while taking care to preserve the mucosa. The axillary flap

is placed into the cavity to cover the raw bony surface to maximize the healing (Fig. 9.19c). This completes Draf I procedure.

Posterior Ethmoidectomy and Sphenoidotomy

In any operation on the posterior ethmoidal or sphenoid sinus, it is a must to study the tomograms preoperatively to analyze the spatial relationships between optic nerve, the internal carotid artery and the sphenoidal sinus. If the posterior ethmoid is diseased, the ground lamella is approached. Dehiscence and perforations of the ground lamella are the most common route through which disease spreads from anterior to posterior ethmoid. After ethmoidal bulla has been removed, the course of the ground lamella can easily be followed with the endoscope.

Opening of ground lamella (basal lamella): The ground lamella is the lateral part of middle turbinate, which is inserted to the lamina papyracea behind the bulla ethmoidalis and divides anterior ethmoidal cells from the posterior ethmoidal cells.

To open the posterior ethmoid, the ground lamella should be opened as far medially and inferiorly as possible. The best place is 3 to

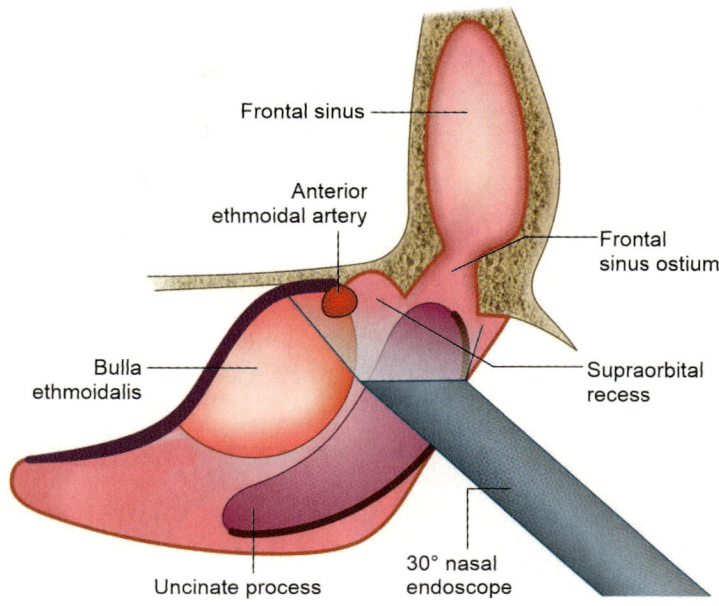

Fig. 9.18: Position of supraorbital recess, and frontal ostium

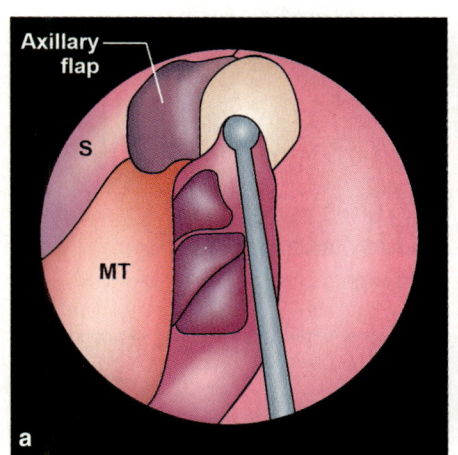

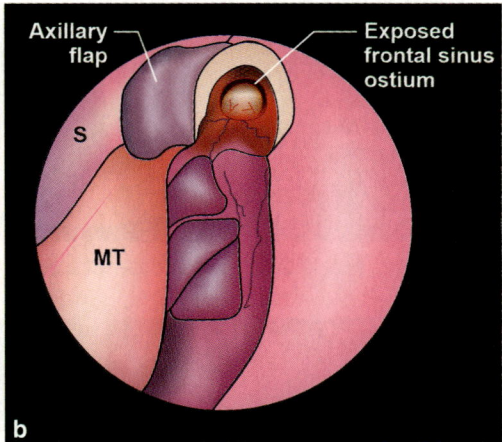

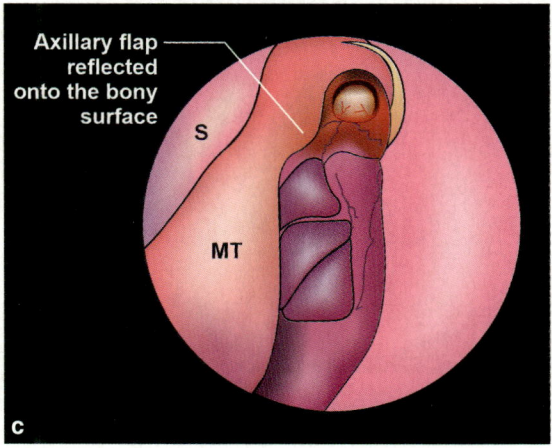

Fig. 9.19: a. Elevation and drilling of anterior wall of agger nasi cell of axillary flaps, **b.** Exenteration of agger nasi air cell and removal of frontal cell to expose frontal sinus ostium, **c.** Placement of axillary flap over raw bony surface. Other structures seen are middle turbinate (MT), nasal septum (S)

4 mm cranially from the point where the ground lamella turns superiorly from its horizontal course as the roof of the posterior one-third of the middle meatus, just behind the ethmoidal bulla (Figs 9.20 to 9.22). The entire ground lamella should never be removed totally as it can destabilize the middle turbinate instead the horizontal or inferior aspect of it, is preseved as it supports the middle turbinate. The larger cells and milder disease usually allow the skull base identification more easily. If skull base cannot

be identified as in extensive disease, it may be necessary to open the sphenoidal sinus initially before skull base is identified. In a markedly pneumatized posterior ethmoids, the optic nerve can be seen posteromedially as a convexity in the wall of the posterior ethmoid sinus.

If the sphenoidal sinus needs to be opened, the surgeon must remember that the path through the ethmoid does lead to the anterior wall of the sphenoid. The bulge of the sphenoidal sinus is evident in the inferomedial

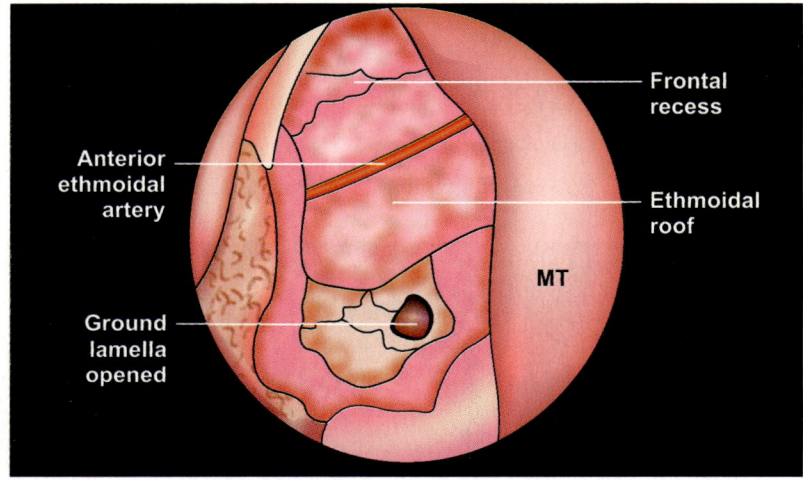

Fig. 9.20a: Ground lamella being opened (right)

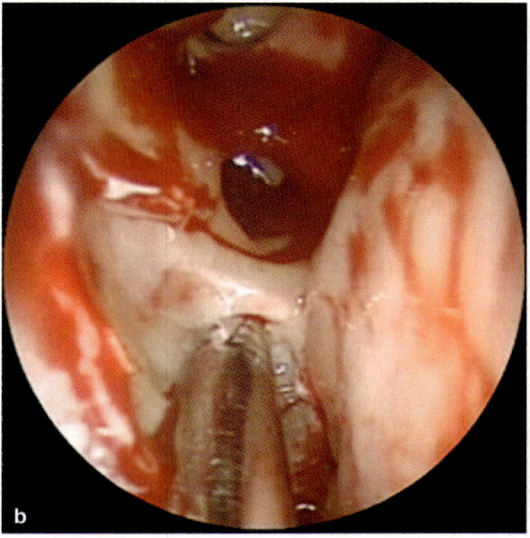

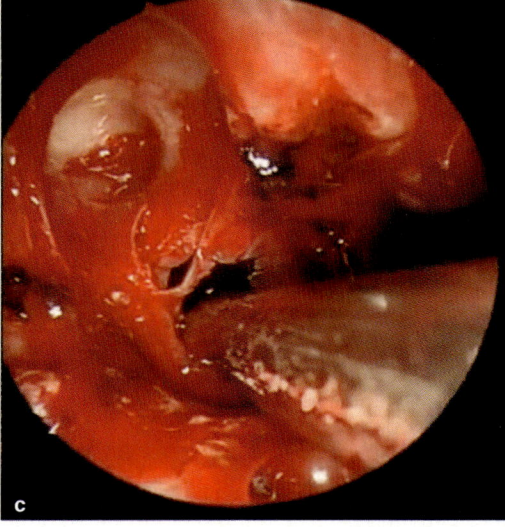

Fig. 9.20: b. Site of opening of ground lamella in the inferior medial aspect on the right side with microdebrider after anterior ethmoidectomy on right side. **c.** Ground lamella is opened on left side

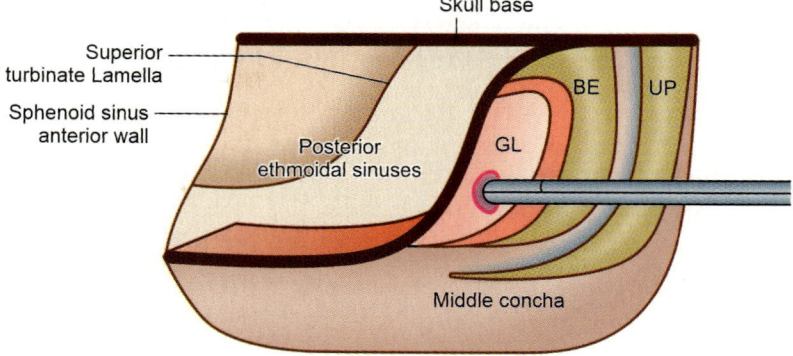

Fig. 9.21: Middle turbinate as seen from within the middle meatus are uncinate process (UP), the basal lamella/ground lamella (GL) being opened in its inferomedial aspect (after Stammberger) after bulla ethmoidalis (BE) has been removed

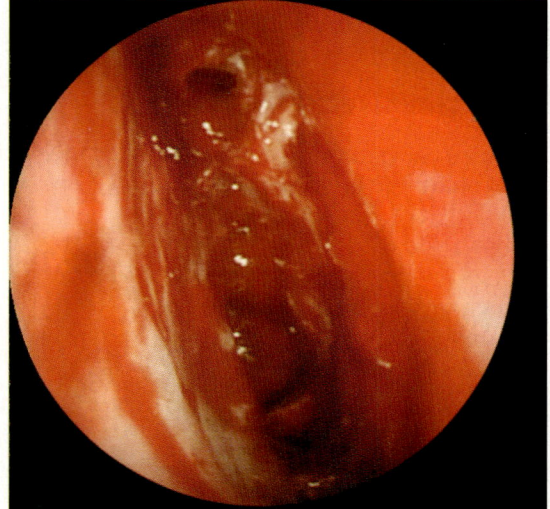

Fig. 9.22a: Complete clearance of posterior ethmoid

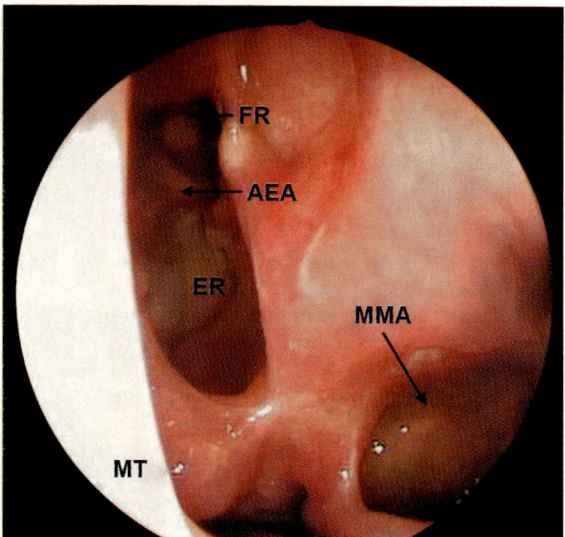

Fig. 9.22b: The frontal recess (FR), anterior ethmoidal artery (AEA) and ethmoidal roof (ER) can be appreciated after opening of anterior and posterior ethmoids. Maxillary ostium is seen laterally after middle meatal antrostomy (MMA) on the left side. The cavity is well epithelialized postoperatively

aspect of the most posterior ethmoid and should be opened under direct vision (Figs 9.23 and 9.24). The depth of penetration should also be measured using measuring probe or suction tip. Bulging of the optic nerve and internal carotid artery may be seen in the inferolateral aspect (Figs 9.25a and b) on a close-up view after opening the sphenoidal sinus.

As the dissection is performed from anterior to posterior direction, the surgeon will encounter four distinct bony laminas (Fig. 9.26). Identification and recognition of these landmarks during the dissection prevent the possibility of any intracranial and intraocular injury. In case of unfamiliar anatomy, previously operated case and for the beginner, a measuring probe should always be used to confirm the landmark. Bleeding is usually minimal under local anaesthesia with proper vasoconstriction, and trauma to the turbinate and vascular lateral nasal wall is avoided.

Wigand's Technique

This surgical approach is performed under hypotensive general anaesthesia.

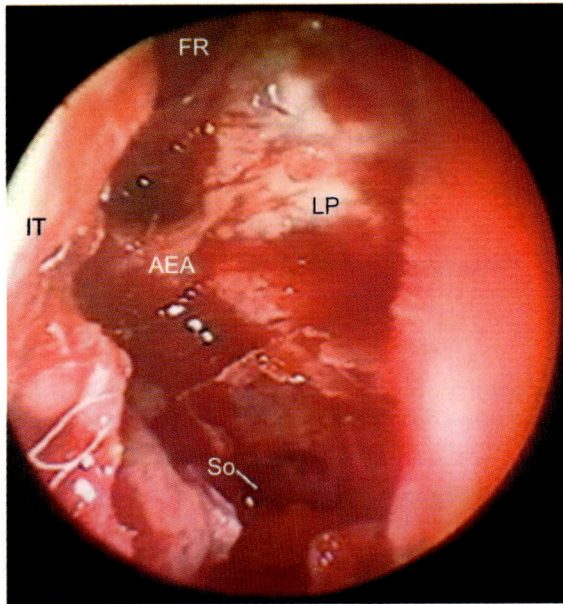

Fig. 9.23: Endoscopic photograph showing sphenoid ostium (So) being exposed through posterior ethmoid window after posterior ethmoidectomy. Also seen are frontal recess (FR), middle turbinate (MT), anterior ethmoidal artery (AEA), lamina papyracea (LP)

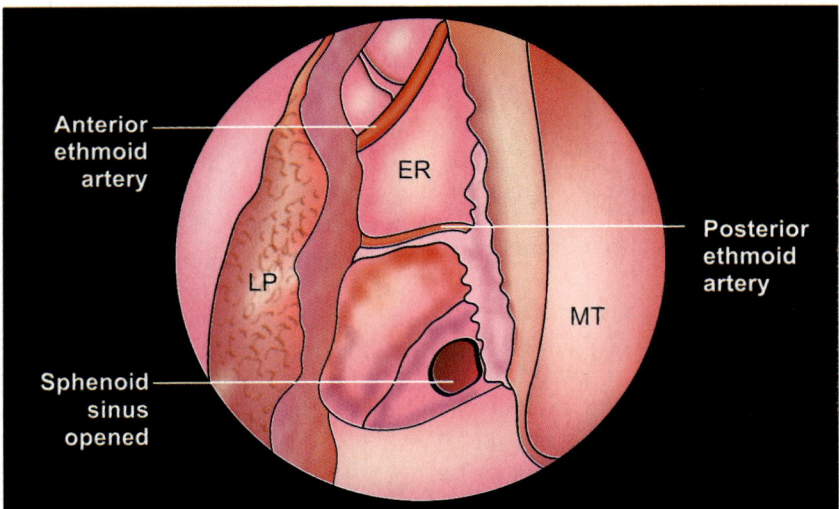

Fig. 9.24: Opening of the sphenoid inferomedially after complete ethmoidectomy on the right side. Also note lamina papyracea (LP), ethmoidal roof (ER), middle turbinate (MT)

The Steps of Surgery

1. Septal mobilization and partial middle turbinate resection.
2. Bipolar cauterization of sphenopalatine artery is required to control the bleeding.
3. The medial position of posterior ethmoidal sinus is taken down under direct visualization through a headlight.
4. Sphenoid ostium is located.

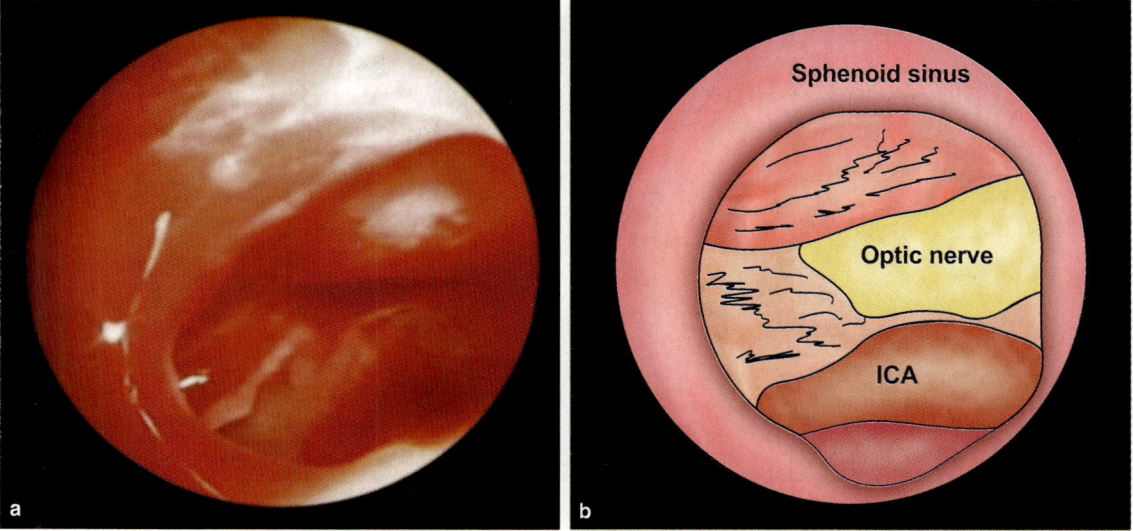

Fig. 9.25: a. Video endoscopic photograph showing optic nerve and internal carotid artery after sphenoid is opened (sphenoidotomy) **b.** Diagrammatic representation of the same

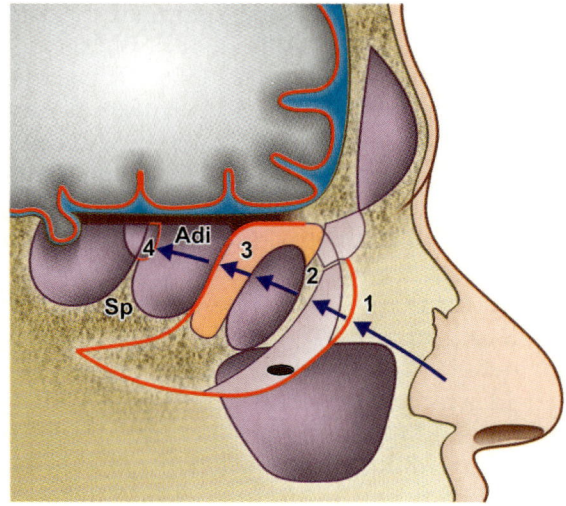

Fig. 9.26: Diagrammatic representation of the five lamellae that are encountered during an anterior to posterior dissection (1—uncinate, 2—Bulla, 3—Ground lamella, Adi—aditional lamella, 4—superior turbinate lamella, Sp—lamella of sphenoid)

5. Anterior wall of the sphenoid is removed.

6. The skull base is identified and the lateral wall of sphenoid is kept as landmark.

7. Dissection starts from that region towards a posterior anterior direction.

8. Agger nasi is removed for adequate visualization of frontal recess.

9. The 70° telescope is used to dissect the frontal recess and maxillary sinus.

10. A complete sphenoethmoidectomy is done.

Endoscopic Management of Ethmoidal Polyposis and Antrochoanal Polyp

Functional endoscopic sinus surgery (FESS) can be used effectively as a minimally invasive

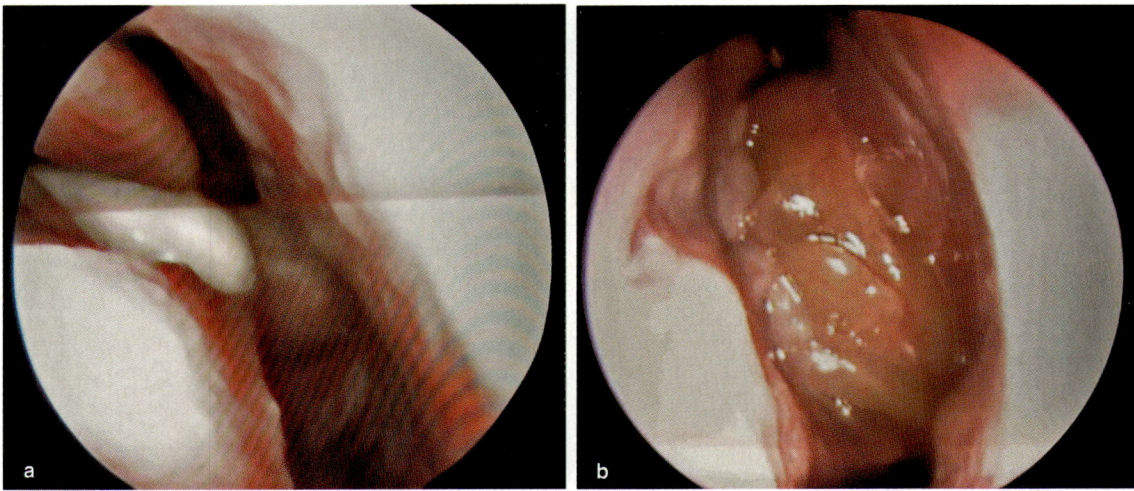

Fig. 9.27: a. Video endoscopic photograph showing right antrochoanal polyp, **b.** Left ethmoidal polyposis

technique. The endoscope is used to improve ventilation and drainage in addition to polyp removal as described already under Messerklinger's technique of endoscopic sinus surgery. The extent of surgery varies according to the extent of disease and surgeon's individual practice. Initially the steps include gross removal of polyposis with the help of a Luc's forceps or a microdebrider for proper visualization of middle meatus. Then the surgery is performed as done under conventional endoscopic sinus surgery with the help of a microdebrider (shaver) (Figs 9.28 and 9.29a). The endoscopic surgical technique has been used for more than a decade in treating sinonasal conditions. Advantages include a better view of the surgical field, a more precise and thorough clearance of the inflammatory changes. The use of microdebrider gives

added advantage of cutting and at the same time suctioning to facilitate clear field of vision which is required for safe and effective in getting functional outcome. The shaver was first applied in orthopaedic surgery. In the field of ENT, it was first used by Setliff (1994 and 1995). The shaver (powered instrument) system offers different handpieces, knives, irrigation and modes (rotating or oscillating). Shaver is a combination of suction and cutting round knife working together. Knives of different shapes are put into handpiece. They have outer sheath with a window, which protects the inner rotating blade. The blade is connected to suction and cutting tissue is removed from the operation field. In otolaryngology surgery, we mostly use the oscillation cutting mode which is the most sufficient. Shaver surgery is precise in soft

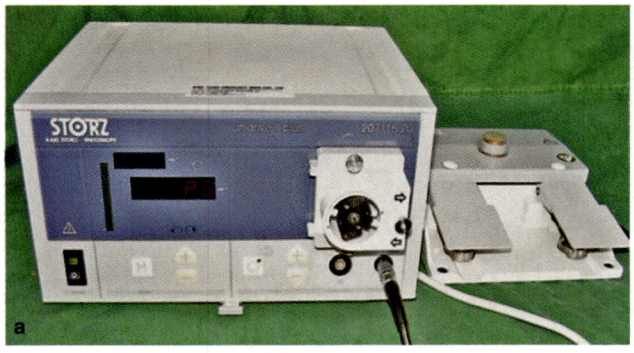

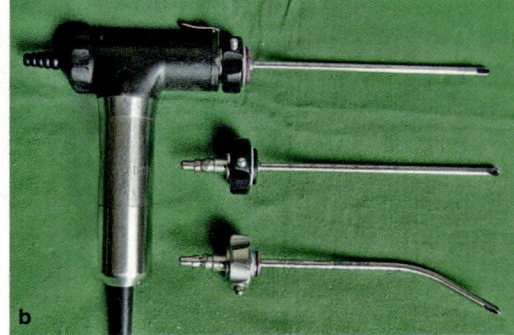

Fig. 9.28: a. STORZ microdebrider system, **b.** Handpiece and blades

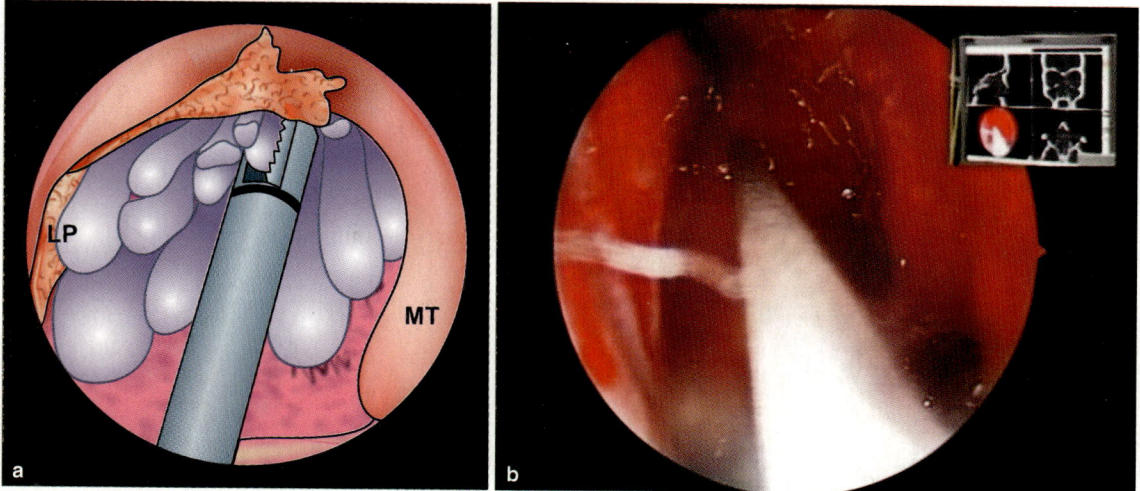

Fig. 9.29: a. Microdebrider-assisted endoscopic sinus surgery for ethmoidal polyposis, **b.** Image-guided endoscopic sinus surgery in progress. Reproduced with kind permission of editor OJOLHNS[12]

tissue resection, so the most advantages to power the system is in rhino-surgery, polypectomy with extension to pansinus surgery (Dalke, et al. 2006) (Figs 9.27 to 9.29).

The complications are few and recurrence rates are lower in comparison to conventional surgery in an experienced hand. Moreover, the shaver preserves the mucosa and submucosa overlying the bone and facilitate better healing after endoscopic sinus surgery following ethmoidal polyposis. The antrochoanal polyp is treated by using a forceps or a microdebrider to remove the polyp completely under endoscopic visualization from the antrum. Various types of angled handpieces are available for this purpose. Very rarely, an inferior meatal window/canine fossa window may be required for complete reoval from its attachment.

Image-guided Endoscopic Surgery

Image-guided surgery has recently been described in the literature as a useful technology for improved functional endoscopic sinus surgery localization. Image-guided surgery yields accurate knowledge of the surgical field boundaries, allowing safer and more thorough sinus surgery. The InstaTrak system is used for this technique with excellent results. Computer-aided endoscopic sinus surgery appears to be the wave of the future. Nevertheless, the modern endoscopic sinus surgeon must have thorough training in the basic anatomy of the paranasal sinuses as well as the various surgical techniques. This technique is useful in revision cases extensive disease with distorted anatomy and endoscopic skull base surgery. A prior CT scan is taken, which are then processed and downloaded onto the computer, where all the 2 sinus views (coronal, axial and sagittal) are displayed at the same time on the computer monitor. During surgery, the system is taken to the operating room and the same thing is viewed while the surgeon inserts a special probe in the nose that can be seen with standard surgical instruments.

Uncinate Process Preservation and Minimal Invasive Endoscopic Sinus Surgery

Nayak et al. (2001) were the first to introduce uncinate process preservation sinus surgery for patients having allergy associated rhinosinusitis. They found that limited endoscopic sinus surgery is more effective in managing postoperative problems than traditional FESS. This approach can also be used for patients having allergy associated ethmoidal polyposis and allergic fungal rhinosinusitis with gross bilateral frontal sinus

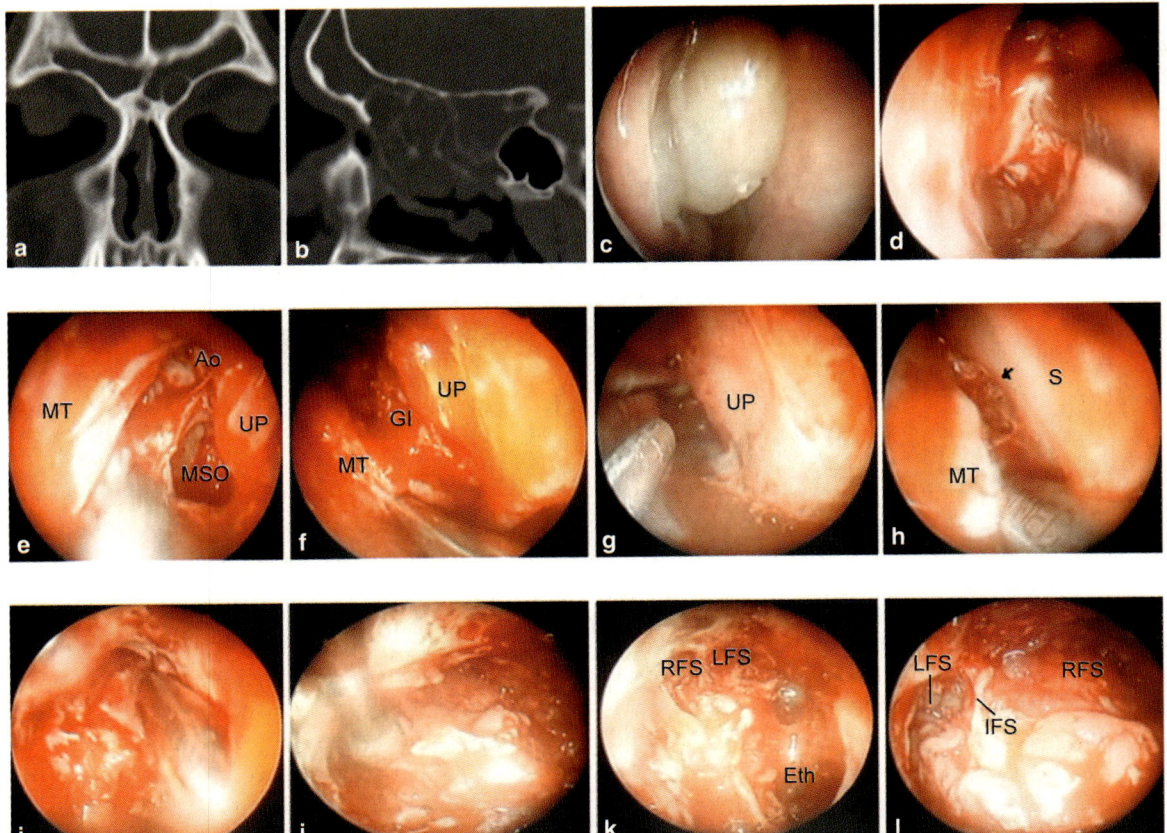

Fig. 9.30: Steps of uncinate preservation endoscopic sinus surgery with "inside out approach": Draf III for recurrent ethmoidal polyposis with gross frontal sinus and ethmoidal involvement and inferior turbinectomy on coronal and sagittal CT **(a & b). c.** Polyps in the right middle meatus with intact uncinate and missing middle turbinate, **d.** Left polypectomy in progress to skeletonize middle turbinate and to expose ethmoids and maxillary sinus ostium (MSO), also seen remnant of inferior turbinate, **e.** Polypoidal tissue from middle turbinate (MT) is removed, maxillary sinus ostium (MSO) is widened, uncinate process (UP) preserved, agger nasi cell (Ao) opened, **f.** Polypoidal middle turbinate (MT) is being trimmed. Also showing ground lamella (Gl), and uncinate process (UP), **g.** The axilla is being drilled, **h.** Septal window seen from right side (black arrow) showing cottonoid packed on the opposite side, also note septum (S), right middle turbinate (MT), **i.** Drilling of the left frontal beak and left frontal sinus, visible through septal window from right side, **j.** Drilling of frontal beak on the right side, interfrontal septum and left frontal sinus cavity, **k.** Left and right frontal sinus (LFS & RFS), ethmoid cavity, **l.** Right (RFS) and left frontal sinus (LFS) cavity and complete reduction of interfrontal septum (IFS) after completion of Draf III (modified Lothrop). Link Video DRN ENT Chapter–9 (Draf III)

disease by performing a Draf III procedure (Figs 9.30a–l). Uncinate process is preserved while performing the maxillary sinusotomy and can be done without opening the bulla when ethmoid is not diseased or transitional space is not compromised. A small opening is created in the posterior fontanelle in the absence of an accessory ostium which is then communicated with the natural ostium (Fig. 9.32). If transitional space is compromised

due to anatomical abnormalities or pathological changes like polyposis, the ethmoid is opened through a transbullar approach as done in FESS. Preservation of uncinate does not hamper clearance of frontal recess, rather it improves the transition space posterior to uncinate and facilitates drainage and ventilation. Posterior ethmoidectomy does in similar fashion. Middle turbinate trimming allows visualization of sphenoid ostium, that

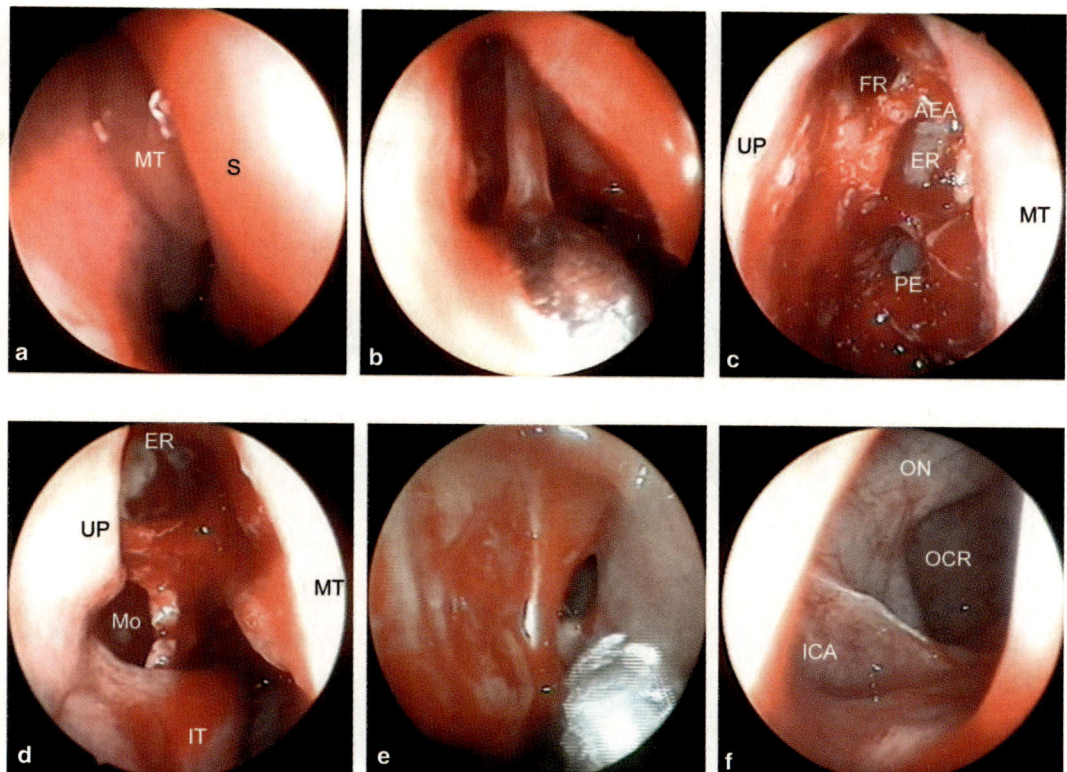

Fig. 9.31: Steps of uncinate process preservation endoscopic sinus surgery on right side: **a.** Polypoidal middle turbinate (MT), deviated septum (S), **b.** Mucopurulent discharge from frotal sinus after frontal recess (FR) is opened, **c.** After anterior ethmoidectomy, posterior ethmoid (PE) is opened; frontal recess (FR), anterior ethmoidal artery (AEA), ethmoidal roof (ER), middle turbinate (MT), uncinate process (UP) preserved, **d.** Enlarged maxillary ostium (Mo), inferior turbinate (IT), intact uncinate process (UP), **e.** Exposure of right sphenoidal ostium in the sphenoethmoidal recess, **f.** Interior of sphenoid sinus, optic nerve (ON), internal carotid artery (ICA), optic carotid recess (OCR)

can be enlarged further using straight mushroom punch forceps (Fig. 9.31a–f). Because of the address of nasal septum, lateral nasal wall including the sinus pathology in the same time as a comprehensive procedure, the author (DRN) terms the surgery functional endoscopic nasosinus surgery (FENS).[13]

Surgery for the frontal sinus can be done in similar way with preservation of uncinate process and bulla if not diseased. Similar draf technique is adopted as described under frontal recess exploration. The steps of sinus surgery includes:

Maxillary sinusotomy/sinuplasty (Fig. 9.32): The maxillary ostium is identified with a ball probe by passing it gently at the level of genu of the uncinate process/bulla without applying pressure. If it cannot be passed

without resistance, a partial uncinotomy is performed at the same level with a back biting forceps. This will allow smooth passage of the probe. At this point, the accessory ostium is joined with the natural ostium, if it is present. In case there is absence of accessory ostium, and maxillary ostium is necessary to be widened, an opening is made in the posterior Fontanelle and is then joined with the natural ostium. This approach prevents any damage to the natural drainage pathway of maxillary sinus (Nayak, 2015).

Frontal sinusotomy/sinuplasty: An axillotomy is performed by using the Hazek's/DCR punch forceps on a superior and lateral direction. The denuded fragments of bones are removed with the help of microdebrider. This opens the agger nasi from below. A frontal

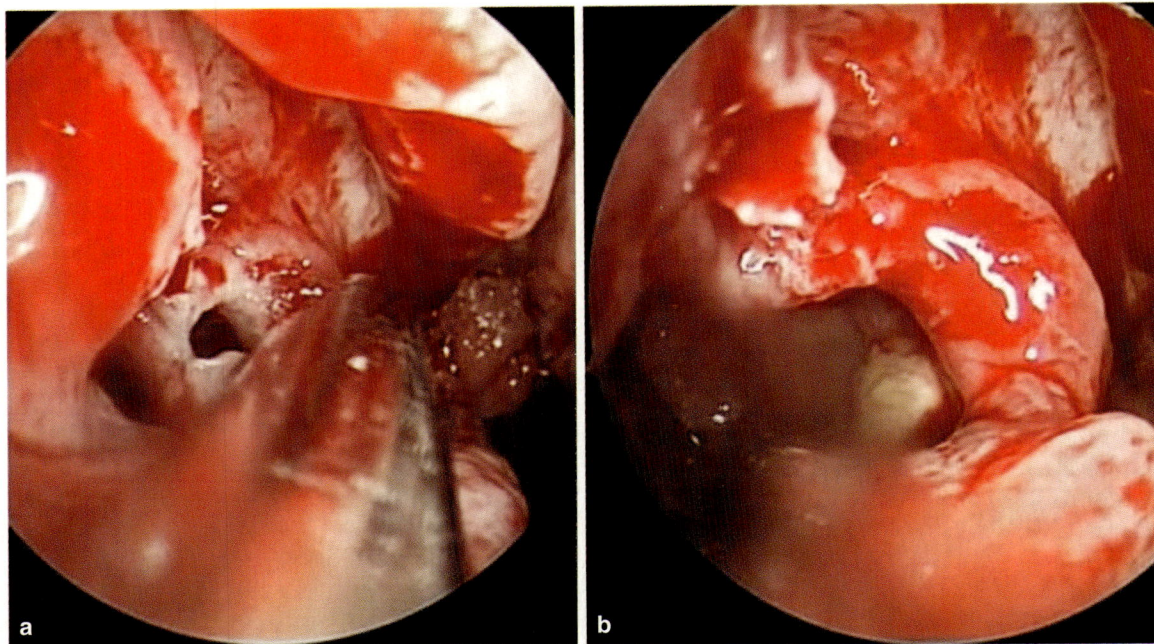

Fig. 9.32: a. Natural ostium and accessory ostium visible after partial resection of uncinate process with back biting forceps, **b.** Natural and accessory ostium being joined. Reproduced with kind permission of editor, OJOLHNS[12]

sinus probe is passed gently between posterior to the posterior wall of the agger nasi and anterior to the bulla, to confirm the drainage pathway of frontal sinus. After confirming the drainage pathway, the mucosa of the anterior and posterior wall of agger nasi and bone from the posterior wall is removed while preserving the mucosa posterior to the bone. A Foley's catheter fixed to the frontal ball probe is passed gently between the posterior wall mucosa and ethmoidal bulla and catheter balloon is inflated to dilate the frontal recess. This completes the procedure for frontal sinuplasty/Draf I. The ethmoidal bulla and uncinate process are preserved. The anterior and posterior ethmoidectomy is not done unless diseased and transitional space within the ethmoidal infundibulum related to maxillary ostium and frontal recess are not compromised. If diseased, they are dealt with through transbullar approach (Fig. 9.31) as described above under FENS (Nayak, et al 2001 and Nayak, 2015). Setliff (1996) described the involvement of transition space between the sinus ostia and nasal cavity responsible for

chronic rhinosinusitis. Relieving the contact areas through minimal surgical intervention in this space that can improve sinus drainage and ventilation rather than dealing with the ostium. Catalano (2004) advocated minimal invasive sinus technique (MIST) as an inital surgical intervation to manage chronic rhinosinusitis. In this technique, paediatric backbiting forceps was used to cut the uncinate process from hiatus semilunaris towards nasolacrimal duct anteriorly and then removing completely with powered instrument with less chance of damaging the lamina papyracea while sparing the mucosa. Maxillary ostium was kept untouched. Superiorly the retroagger space was widened by removing the posterior wall of agger. Then the medial wall of the bulla is removed to expose the anterior ethmoid ostium and increasing the transition space anteriorly. After completion of surgery, MeroGel® bioresorbable nasal packing was kept *in situ*. He considered MIST as an effective alternative to conventional endoscopic sinus surgery.

Three-dimensional endoscopic sinus surgery: Despite the progressive technological innovations in modern endoscopic surgery, the visualization that is currently used remains two-dimensional (2D). The development of a miniature stereoscopic camera and its adaptation to rigid endoscopes allows for performance of 3D endoscopic sinus surgery. It is hypothesized that incorporation of 3D visualization may enhance the spatial resolution required in advanced endoscopic approaches with a theoretical potential to improve outcomes. Future applications of this technology include the ability to fuse an MR scan with the endoscopic picture to enable surgeons to have a view beyond that which is normally visible. These merged images will likely in the future be able to work with the next generation of image-guidance systems to allow surgeons to continue to expand minimally invasive surgery intracranially (Brown, et al., 2008).

BIBLIOGRAPHY

1. Anon, Jack B. Computer-aided endoscopic sinus surgery. Laryngoscope 1998;108(7):949–961.

2. Brown, et al. Three-dimensional endoscopic sinus surgery: Feasibility and technical aspects. Otolaryngology–Head and Neck Surgery, 2008;138(3):40–42.

3. Byron and Bailey (Ed). Head and Neck Surgery—Otolaryngology, 1993.

4. Catalano P. Minimal invasive sinus technique—theory and practice. Otolaryngol Clin N Am 2004; 37:401–409.

5. Dalke, et al. Rotation suction-knife (shaver) in otorhinolaryngological surgery. Otolaryngol Pol 2006; 60(1):37–40 (ISSN: 0030–6657).

6. Draf W. Endonasal microendoscopic frontal sinus surgery: The Fulda Concept. Oper Tech Otolaryngol Head Neck Surg 1991;2:234.

7. Fried, Marvin P, et al. Image-guided endoscopic surgery: Results of accuracy and performance in a multicenter clinical study using an electromagnetic tracking system. Laryngoscope. 1997;107(5):594–601.

8. Friedman M, Landsberg R, Schults RA, et al. Frontal sinus surgery: Endoscopic technique and preliminary results. Am J Rhinol 2000 Nov-Dec;14(6):393–403.

9. Kenedy DW. Functional endoscopic sinus surgery technique Arch Otolaryngology 1985; 111:634.

10. Messerklinger W. Endoscopy of the nose. Baltimore: Urban and Schwarzenberg; 1978.

11. Kirtane MV. Functional Endoscopic Sinus Surgery 1993.

12. Nayak DR. A tailor made approach to endoscopic sinus surgery for chronic rhinosinusitis. OJOLHNS 2015;9:2:6–8.

13. Nayak, et al. Endoscopic physiological approach to allergy associated rhinosinusitis. ENT Journal 2001 June;80(5):392–403.

14. Decker BC, Stammberger Functional Endoscopic Sinus Surgery, Philadelphia 1991.

15. Stankiewicz JA. Complications in endoscopic ethmoidectomy: An update. Laryngoscope 1989; 99:686.

16. Ramadan HH. History of Frontal Sinus Surgery, Chapter-1 in "The Fraontal Sinus" Edited by Kountakis SE, Brent A, Draf W. © Springer-Verlag Berlin Heidelberg 2005.

17. Setliff RC. New concepts and the use of powered instrumentation (the hummer) for functional endoscopic sinus surgery. In: JA Stankiewicz (Ed.). Advanced Endoscopic Sinus Surgery, Mosby, St. Louis, 1995; pp. 161–70.

18. Setliff RC, Parsons DS. The "Hummer": New instrumentation for functional endoscopic sinus surgery. Am J Rhinnol 1994;8:275–78.

19. Setliff RC. Minimally invasive sinus surgery: rationale and technique. Otolaryngol Clin N Amer 1996;29:115–29.

20. Stammberger H. Endoscopic endonasal surgery—concepts in treatment of recurring rhinosinusitis. Part II. Surgical technique. Otolaryngol Head Neck Surg 1986;94(2):147–56.

21. Tirelli G, Brigarini S, Russolo M, et al. Total intravenous anesthesia in endonasal surgery. Acta Otorhinolaryngol Ital 2004; 24:137–44.

22. Messerklinger W. Background and evolution of endoscopic sinus surgery. ENT Journal 1994;73: 7449–55.

23. Wormald PJ. The axillary flap approach to the frontal recess. Laryngoscope 2002 March; 112(3):494–99.

10

Postoperative Care Following Endoscopic Surgery of Nose and Paranasal Sinuses

DR Nayak

Postoperative care is one of the most essential aspects of endoscopic sinus surgery and is just as critical as preoperative assessment and the intraoperative technique, in preventing complications. Proper postoperative care helps in promoting healing and early regeneration of sinus mucosa. It also helps to reduce localized infection and post-operative inflammatory changes. It reduces the postoperative crusting moisturizing the sinus cavity by regular use of alkaline nasal douching there by promote early return of ciliary function and prevent complications in the early postoperative phase that can avoid revision surgery (Rudmick and Smith 2012). The surgeon and the patient should both be fully committed to the postoperative cleaning and care including equipment inconvenience, discomfort and other factors required in achieving optimal results.

The most frequent and frustrating complication of functional endoscopic sinus surgery has been the tendency for scarring between the middle turbinate and the lateral nasal wall which leads to obstruction of the outflow at the ostiomeatal complex as a result of synaechia formation. Other examples of unsatisfactory healing that would compromise results include recurrence of polyps, stenosis of sphenoid or maxillary ostium and frontal recess or perioperative infection. After functional endoscopic sinus surgery mucociliary function at the ostiomeatal complex is impaired for approximately six weeks, until healing is complete. During this period, fibrosis, mucous secretion and blood clots tend to collect within the nasal cavity and ostiomeatal complex area causing patient discomfort and predisposing to perioperative infection and/or scarring.

The plan for postoperative care begins during the preoperative consultation. In general, the timing of care is individualized. However, in our institute, we have found that the following timetable for postoperative care is adequate for most patients. Usually the first postoperative cleaning is done on the 2nd postoperative day following surgery. The subsequent postoperative visits are after 1 week following surgery and then biweekly until the healing is complete which is usually by six weeks. Alternatively, particularly patient from far away place, we advice saline irrigation after the first day of surgery and then endoscopic cleaning on postoperative day-2 and one week after. Thereafter, the patient is advised to follow aggressive saline irrigation with the help of a 10 cc disposable syringe. Postoperative nasal douching is common and evidence supports their efficacy in improving outcome following FESS, which may avoid the need for frequent office debridement (Tysome 2007). Postoperative use of nasal douching with hypertonic saline alone has shown comparable outcomes in terms of symptom scores and synechiae (Fernandes, 1999).

Patients whose occupations are not physically demanding may return to work within 2 days of surgery but physical exertion should be avoided for 7 to 10 days after surgery. Patients are advised to avoid nasal irritants (fumes, excessive dust, etc.) until healing is complete. Patients may swim by 3 weeks after surgery but are advised against diving for 6 weeks postoperatively.

At the 1st postoperative visit after a week, the patient's nose is decongested and anaesthetized by placing pledgets of 4% xylocaine and 1% phenylephrine in the nose. After 10 minutes, the pledgets are removed and any early adhesions between the middle turbinate and the lateral wall in the frontal recess are released. Crusts of fibrin, mucus or blood are removed by gentle suctioning. This relieves the headache and nasal obstruction experienced by a few patients in the early postoperative period. If adhesions are extensive, they are released and a wax plate or steroid soaked nasopore is kept between the middle turbinate and lateral wall. At subsequent office visits, similar local anaesthesia and cleaning is again performed to remove loose crusts and clots. Aggressive debridement is avoided because it encourages bleeding and synechiae formation and delays healing. By 3 weeks, the mucosa in the ostiomeatal complex has usually healed. By the end of 6th week, the nasal mucosa begins to normalize and mucociliary flow has been re-established. At this point, a meaningful evaluation of symptomatic results can be obtained in most patients.

Much discussion has been made of the decision of whether or not to place intranasal packing immediately after endoscopic sinus surgery. Obviously, packing is required in cases of significant bleeding; however, in our experience, overnight nasal packing is very rarely needed and is done especially in cases where septal surgery is done simultaneously. We at times use a temporary pack of cottonoids soaked in 4% xylocaine with 1 in 10,000, adrenaline which is placed within the ostiomeatal complex and removed approximately 1 to 2 hours following surgery. We prefer a temporary pack, if adequate homeostasis is to be achieved as the discomfort of packing and stagnation of secretions is avoided.

To prevent the frequent complication of synechiae or lateralization of middle turbinate, various types of barriers are used within the ostiomeatal complex. Various stents and packs including silicone sheets, gelatin film wrapped around gelatin foam, telfa sheets, septal splints with wax plates, antibiotic soaked NasoPore and others are commonly used. We routinely use antibiotic with steroid soaked nasopore and at times wax plate which is placed between the middle turbinate and lateral nasal wall and separate splint for septum, if septoplasty has been performed in the same sitting (Nayak, et al. 1995). This is a temporary barrier and is removed at the 1st postoperative visit.

Stenosis of the maxillary ostium is occasionally seen in postoperative period. This is usually treated by enlarging the ostium under local anaesthesia. Narrowing of the nasofrontal duct and inflammation in this area is treated by removing sites of inflammation. The same is true for the sphenoid ostium and residual ethmoidal cells.

Routine postoperative medications include antibiotics, topical nasal (sprays) and systemic steroids. Topical steroids are used in the form of sprays or along with saline over a period of about 6 months and sometimes more, if there is associated nasal allergy. This is to prevent recurrence of polyps or oedema of sinus mucosa.

Postoperative care is extremely important for a successful surgery and more so in the paediatric patient. Obviously children cannot tolerate the discomfort of postoperative care and hence every postoperative cleaning has to be done under general anaesthesia. Therefore, children and parents are advised that endoscopic sinus surgery in children is a multistage procedure. Multistage procedure can be avoided, if a splint like dental wax plate is used between the lateral wall and the middle turbinate (Nayak, et al. 1998). Introduction of absorbable/biodegradable packing materials like MeroGel, NasoPore (synthetic polyurethane), etc. soaked with antibiotic and steroid may overcome this problem in paediatric patient.

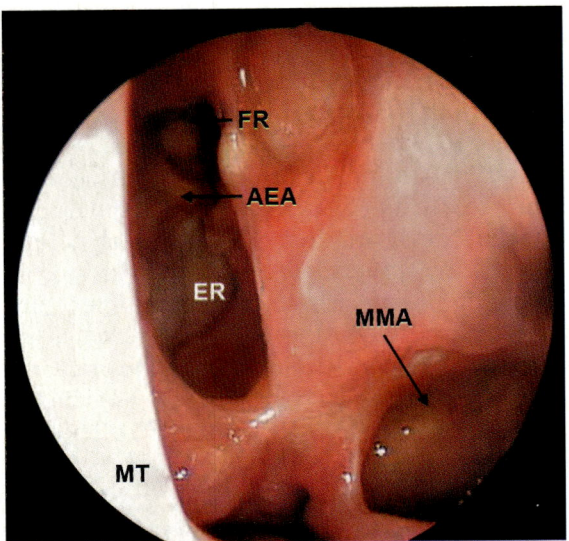

Fig. 10.1: Well-epithelialized operated cavity after FESS, FR (frontal recess), AEA (anterior ethmoidal artery), ER (ethmoidal roof), MMA (middle meatal antrostomy)

Aggressive postoperative care performed under local anaesthesia in the office setting can greatly increase the success rate of this procedure and diminish the need to return to the operating room for revision endoscopic sinus surgery (Fig. 10.1).

The patient should strictly be advised to the following guidelines:

- Patient requires frequent return visits to the clinic for sinus cleaning over a period of 4 to 6 weeks until appropriate healing of the sinuses is achieved.
- Normal to have some bleeding for several days after surgery. If bleeding occurs, tilt the head back slightly and ask the patient to breathe gently through the nose.
- Should not blow the nose for one week following surgery and following the removal of splint or pack. After one week, you may begin to blow your nose gently. Patient should sneeze with mouth open.
- For one to two weeks after surgery, use a saline nasal spray (non-decongestant) every 1–2 hours during the day to keep nose and sinuses moisturized.
- We prefer irrigation of homemade saline/alkaline solution to flush the accumulated blood clots and crusts from the nasal cavity. Nasal cavity should be rinsed twice a day following a day after surgery. Humidification of the postoperative cavities contributes to reduced crusting and has positive effects on the mucosa re-epithelialization (Watelet 2002).

- Antibiotics like ciprofloxacin can be continued for several weeks after surgery. Purulent nasal secretion can adversely affect the healing of sinus mucosa and a prescription of two weeks of antibiotics can facilitate better healing, while reducing the crusting and secretions. A broad spectrum antibiotic is useful in case of acute exacerbation (Eloy, et al. 2017). Biofilm can still pose problem in postoperative period with repeated crust formation and is always difficult to treat. Manuka honey, Johnson baby sampoo irrigation and several other measures have been tried with limited success (Lee, et al. 2017).
- A dose of analgesic at least 45 minutes to one hour before the first postoperative cleaning is helpful.
- Patient should strictly be advised not to take aspirin or aspirin-related products.
- All strenuous activity should be avoided for at least 2 weeks.
- Some dark brown nasal discharge may be noticed several weeks after the surgery that occurs as a result of old blood and mucus being cleared from the sinuses and is quite normal.
- Patient should consult the treating doctor as soon as possible, if he experiences any of the following:
  – Watery nasal discharge (CSF leak)
  – Swelling of the eyes or diminished vision
  – High grade fever
  – Persistent headache
  – Neck stiffness
  – GI upset
  – Epistaxis

During the postoperative healing period, oedema, crusting, secretions, and scarring are the major problems and need to be carefully managed to get a successful outcome after edoscopic sinus surgery. Postoperative nasal packings are often used to prevent postoperative haemorrhage and sometimes stent is used to prevent postoperative synechia formation and to facilitate better healing during this period. However, all these materials can cause severe discomfort to the patient and can be very painful on removal.

Jonnalagadda et al. (2011) found targeted topical pharmaceuticals have fewer side effect than systemic therapy and present an interesting option to treat chronic sinus disease. Techinque using bioabsorbable nasal sponges, such as NasoPore®, may introduce a feasible, safe, and effective methods of drug delivery, providing high concentrations of medication locally with lower sustainable concentrations systemically. Further study is necessary to elucidate the optimal concentration, dosing and effects.

Cote and Wright (2010) found a significant improvement in early postoperative healing in nasal cavities receiving triamcinolone-impregnated absorbable nasal packing following ESS and is also associated with improved healing up to 6 months postoperatively.

However, recent research shows promise with microporous polysaccharide haemospheres and chitosan gel having promising effects on haemostasis, and chitosan gel showing a significant adhesion prevention effect. The area of wound healing and adhesion prevention remains an area of active research and more prospective controlled trials are needed to define any benefits biomaterials may have (Rowan and Peter-John 2010).

The author of this book (DRN) uses biodegradable nasal packing like NasoPore® (polyganic) soaked with anti-infective agent along with prednisolone to pack the ethmoidal cavity and also in the region sinus ostium and found encouraging results in achieving healing and prevention of synechia (Fig. 10.2). Role of doxycline releasing stents by Medtronic has been studied and found to have reduced bacterial colonization and better postoperative healing compared to placebo (Huvenne, et al. 2008).

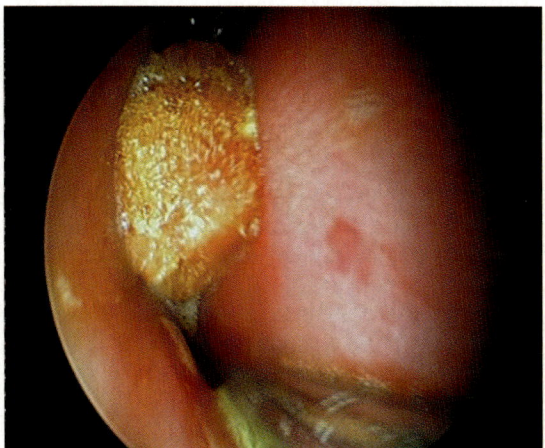

Fig. 10.2: Endoscopic picture showing dilute betadine (1%) and triamcinolone soaked NasoPore® placed in the middle meatus and is left *in situ* while the patient is asked to irrigate the nose with normal saline at home

BIBLIOGRAPHY

1. Cote DW, Wright ED. Triamcinolone-impregnated nasal dressing following endoscopic sinus surgery: A randomized, double-bline, placebo-controlled study. Laryngoscope 2010 June; 120(6):1269–73.

2. Dipak Ranjan Nayak, Ramaswamy Balakrishnan, Deepak Murty K, Produl Hazarika. "Endoscopic septoturbinoplasty: Our update series". Indian Journal of Otolaryngology and Head and Neck Surgery 2002:54 (1):20–22.

3. Eloy P, Andrews P, Poirrier AL. Postoperative care in endoscopic sinus surgery: A critical review. Curr Opin Otolaryngol Head Neck Surg. 2017 Feb;25(1):35–42.

4. Fernandes SV. Postoperative care in functional endoscopic sinus surgery. Laryngoscope 1999; 109:945–48.

5. Huvenne W, Zhang N, Tizsma E, et al. Pilot study using doxycycline-releasing stents to ameliorate postoperative healing quality after sinus surgery. Wound Rep Reg 2008;16:757–67.

6. Lee VS, Humphreys IM, Prucell PL, et al. Manuka honey sinus irrigation for the treatment of chronic rhinosinusitis: A randomized controlled trial. International Forum of Allergy and Rhinology 2017 Vol. 7, No. 4, 365–72.

7. Mair EA. Pediatric functional endoscopic sinus surgery: Postoperative care. Otolaryngol Clin North Am 1996;29:207–19.

8. Nayak DR, Balakrishnan R, Hazarika P. "An endoscopic approach to deviated nasal septum—a preliminary study". Journal of Laryngology and Otology 1998:112; 934–39.

9. Nayak DR, Balakrishnan R, Murty KD. "Prevention and management of synechia in pediatric endoscopic sinus surgery using dental wax plates". International Journal of Pediatric Otolaryngology 1998: 46; 171–78.

10. Nasal dressings after endoscopic sinussurgery: what and why? Valentine rowan, Wormland; Current Opinion in Otolaryngology and Head and Neck Surgery: February 2010 Volume 18-Issue 1-p 44–48.

11. Nayak DR, Balakrishna R, Murthy KD. Endoscopic physiologic approach to allergy associated chronic rhinosinusitis—a preliminary study. ENT Journal 2001;80(6):392–403.

12. Nayak, DR Balakrishnan R, Murty KD. Septal splint with wax plates". Journal of Postgraduate Medicine. "An endoscopic approach to deviated nasal septum—a preliminary study" 1995:41 (3); 70–71.

13. Rowan Valentine; Peter-John Wormald. Are routine dissolvable nasal dressing necessary following endoscopic sinus surgery? Laryngoscope 2010;120(12):2528–31.

14. Rudmik L, Smith TL. Evidence-base practice: Postoperative care in endoscopic sinus surgery. Otolaryngol Clin North Am 2012;45: 1019–1032.

15. Sashikanth Jonnalagadda, Vivian M Yu, Peter J. A feasibility study to evaluate a novel drug delivery technique through nasal/sinus mucosa using a biodegradable polymer in a guinea pig model. Catalano, Otolaryngology–Head and Neck Surgery 2011;144(6):978–81.

16. Tysome JR, Sharp HR. Current trends on pre- and postoperative management of functional endoscopic sinus surgery. The Internet Journal of Otolaryngology 2007.

17. Watelet JB, Bachert C, Gevaert P, Van Cauwenberge P. Wound healing of the respiratory mucosa: A review. Am J Rhinol 2002; 16:77–84.

Complications of Endoscopic Surgery of Nose and Paranasal Sinuses

DR Nayak, K Pujary, A Bhandarkar

Since its introduction endoscopic sinus surgery has revolutionized the treatment of sinus disease. But with advent of its popularity the number of documented complications has also risen due to the intimate relation of sinuses to the orbit and anterior cranial fossa (Neuman 1994). Knowledge of the surgical anatomy by the endoscopic surgeon is absolutely essential to prevent complications. Even the most experienced surgeon may encounter problems. Stankiewicz (1989) in his first series of FESS patients, he reported a complication rate of 29% and in his second series he reported a complication rate of 2.2%. The incidence of major perioperative complications was 0.85%, with cerebrospinal fluid (CSF) leak being the most common, the complication rate drops as on gain experience and training, handling endoscopes and instruments, thorough understanding of sinus anatomy including variations and pathological changes (Knanna & Sama 2019). With expansion in the scope in endoscopic surgery, including approach to anterior skull base and transsphenoidal approaches, catastrophic complications like injury to internal carotid artery can happen although rare.

The most common minor complications of ESS were those related to orbital penetration and middle turbinate adhesions; minor complications occurred in 6.9% (Levine, et al. 1994). Despite advances in endoscopic sinus surgery technique and instrumentation, serious ophthalmic complications may still occur. Inadvertent entry into the medial orbital wall can result in ocular motility

complications (Bhatti, et al. 2001). The risk of complications is most common in patients with revision surgery, extensive sinus disease like allergic fungal sinusitis, invasive fungal sinusitis, etc. associated with gross pathological changes dehiscences, anatomical variations in the skull base and lateral wall and use of powered instruments (Stankiewicz, et al 2011). Availability of navigation during surgery can minimize these complications. The compli-cations are characterized as:

Major

- Haemorrhage
- Blindness
- Injury to internal carotid artery
- Cavernous sinus—ICA fistula
- Intracranial haemorrhage
- Pneumocephalus
- Brain abscess
- Death

Minor

- Orbital haematoma
- Orbital surgical emphysema
- Nasolacrimal duct injury
- Antrostomy closure
- Synechiae

HOW TO AVOID COMPLICATIONS

Preoperatively

- Careful history of bleeding disorders

- Adequate medical treatment for chronic inflammatory conditions of paranasal sinuses before planning for surgery. This includes both antibiotics and steroids (local/systemic).
- Ophthalmological examination including visual status of the patient.
- Proper outpatient endoscopic assessment prior to surgery.
- Preoperative CT scan is extremely important to assess the anatomical and pathological abnormalities which should ideally contain both axial and coronal cuts. The coronal cuts give better information about anterior ethmoid, cribriform plate and frontal sinus in relation to the anterior cranial fossa, whereas axial cuts give more information about the posterior ethmoid, sphenoid and the orbit.

Perioperatively

- Use of adequate decongestant before starting surgery is extremely important.
- As a beginner, local anaesthesia should be preferred over general anaesthesia.
- 0° endoscope is the best to start with for a beginner.
- Angle endoscope should be avoided, if the surgeon is not able to appreciate the landmarks properly. Absence of surgical landmarks like dehiscent lamina papyracea, radically resected middle turbinate, not able to identify maxillary ostium due to extensive disease or previous surgery are the potential risk factors for complications. In such situation, a beginner should better avoid attempting such cases. Such cases should be handled by surgeon having enough expertise. Preoperative CT scan is very useful in such cases. Recently CT guided surgery has been introduced to tackle such cases.
- The concept of surgery suggests beginner should strictly follow the learning curve and start with endoscopic middle meatal antrostomy initially. Once the surgeon gain confidence and are well acquainted with endoscopic anatomy, he can venture into

posterior ethmoid and sphenoid sinuses. Finally the frontal recess should be tackled to prevent major complications.

COMMON PERIOPERATIVE AND POSTOPERATIVE COMPLICATIONS

Haemorrhage

Major complications following endoscopic sinus surgery account between 0.36 and 3.1% of patients, and including severe haemorrhage, injury to orbit and lacrimal system, CSF leak, and intracranial injury (Halderman 2015).

It is very important to assess the patient preoperatively for hypertension, bleeding disorder, current medications including aspirin and other nonsteroidal anti-inflammatory drugs, etc. If patient is on any such medications, it should be stopped at least for a week before doing surgery. Intraoperative bleeding can compromise visibility and may seriously hamper to identify landmarks. A reverse Trendelenburg position can significantly reduce perioperative bleeding. Controlled hypotension of 70 mm Hg can also reduce bleeding. Total intravenous anaesthesia is being used recently to control perioperative bleeding (Halderman, et al 2015).

Injury to internal carotid artery (ICA) varies from 0.1–0.3%. This catastrophic injury can be prevented by studying the axial and coronal CT thoroughly preoperatively with a clear plan for dehiscence or another abnormality. Any bleeding during surgery in the sphenoid sinus should be treated as injury to ICA and the sinus should be packed immediately. An autologous muscle patch is to be kept ready. After carefully removing the sinus pack, if the bleeding still persists, the muscle patch should be kept over the leak site and the sinus cavity is repacked. The anesthesiologist should be informed to facilitate adequate cerebral blood prefusion (Halderman, et al 2015). Adequate blood transfusion should be arranged. Role of an interventional radiologist is crucial at this stage to identify the leak site by doing angiogram, and balloon occlusion in case of adequate cross-circulation and stenting, if cross-circulation is not adequate (Solarace et al. 2010). Inspite of best possible management, mortality still remains a concern. Anterior ethmoidal artery injury commonly occurs during anterior ethmoidectomy and frontal sinustomy can be controlled with bipolar cautery. If the artery is injured closed to lamina papyracea, it gets retracted into the orbit causing retrobulbar haematoma as described later.

Major bleeding points are anterior ethmoidal, posterior septal artery and the traumatized turbinate.

Packing usually controls bleeding. Cautery may be used judiciously.

Always terminate the surgery, if the bleeding impairs visualization. Never operate in a bloody field. Pack, wait and then proceed. Postoperative blood-stained discharge is a normal phenomenon. Retained blood clot and secretions can cause postoperative nasal block. Use of alkaline saline irrigation can minimize that. Absorbable packing materials also are helpful to minimize postoperative ooze and enhance patient comfort besides reducing the incidence of adhesion (synechia) formation. Postoperative haemorrhage can have serious implications and should be suspected for arterial bleed. It should be managed in the operative set up. Posterior bleeding can be controlled by passing a Foley's catheter into nasopharynx and inflating it and anterior nasal packing.

Synechiae (Figs 11.1 and 11.2)

Synechia is usually caused because of opposed raw surfaces of the middle turbinate and ethmoid cavity. Figure 11.1 is showing the synechia between inferior turbinate and septum and Fig. 11.2 showing early synechia between middle turbinate and lateral wall that may obstruct middle meatal drainage. Only 20% are symptomatic and requiring revision surgery. Symptoms include nasal obstruction, headaches and smell dysfunction. Nayak, et al. in 1998 classified this adhesive condition, based on their site and clinical presentation, into four different groups and advocated use of splint made up of wax plate to prevent this complication.

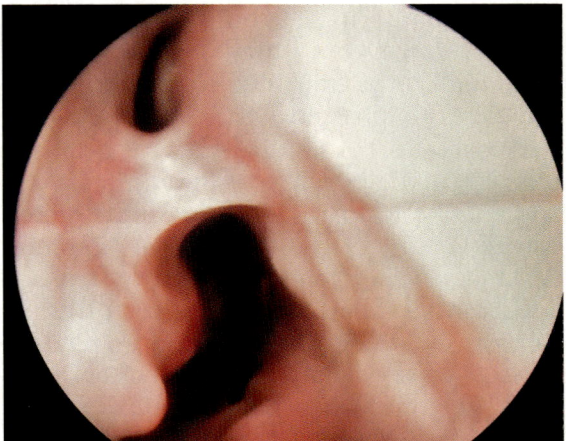

Fig. 11.1: Video endoscopic photograph showing advanced synechia between septum and inferior turbinate

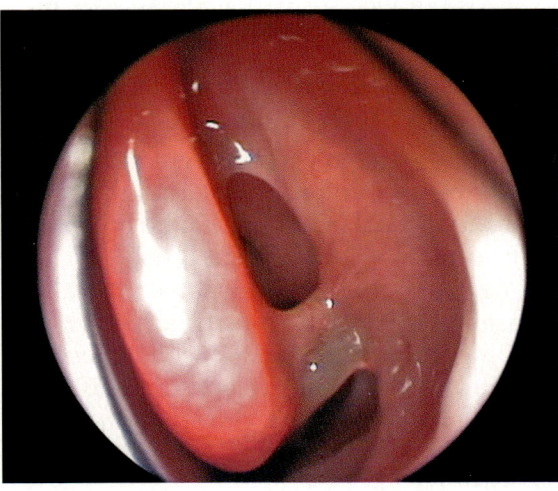

Fig. 11.2: Video endoscopic photograph showing early synechia between middle turbinate and lateral nasal wall

Partial amputation of the middle turbinate anteroinferiorly may prevent synechiae. Gelfoam, MeroGel, etc. have been proposed as spacers. Use of dental wax plate as a spacer in the ethmoid cavity between middle turbinate and lateral wall following endoscopic sinus surgery can prevent synechia formation (Nayak, et al 1998). Most adhesions can be lysed in the early postoperative period during suction and cleaning.

Middle Meatal Antrostomy (MMA) Closure

This occurs in about 2% of cases. A circumferential removal of tissue during antrostomy will contribute to scarring and subsequent closure. However, a 3 mm diameter opening is thought to be adequate for physiological drainage (Hollmstead 1982).

Preservation of natural mucosal drainage pathway at the maxillary ostium is the key to prevent stenosis of middle meatal antrostomy Nayak (2015). Extensive mucosal trimming arround maxillary ostium can lead to shrinkage and fibrosis during healing, resulting in stenosis of MMA, that can be prevented by mucosal conservation, meticulous cleaning of crust and granulations (Kim, et al 2020).

Recent use of steroid-eluting stent is effective in improving wound healing by preserving sinus patency, reducing inflammation, and minimizing adhesions via controlled local steroid delivery without measurable systemic exposure (Murr, et al. 2011).

Nasolacrimal Duct Injury

This occurs due to excessive enlargement of the antrostomy anteriorly. Normally, there is injury to the lacrimal bone found superiorly in the middle meatus (Bolger 1992).

Preventive recommendations include enlarging the maxillary ostium posteriorly and inferiorly. Anterior dissection should be limited to the level of the anterior end of the middle turbinate.

Periorbital Emphysema

Lid oedema, ecchymosis and emphysema all indicate disruption of the lamina papyracea (Fig 11.3). Even in experienced hands, the incidence of orbital complications is at 0.5–1.5%.

These findings usually will resolve spontaneously in 1–2 weeks. Close observation of visual acuity and pressure is necessary.

The presence of yellow orbital fat prolapsing into the operative field along with transmitted movements on movement of the eyeball is almost pathognomonic. All tissues removed during the surgery should be placed in water. Floating tissues normally indicate presence of fat.

Retrobulbar Haematoma

This is characterized by ecchymosis, proptosis, orbital pain, conjunctival haemorrhage. This is caused often due to injury to the anterior ethmoidal artery which retracts into the orbit and continues bleeding. An immediate lateral canthotomy is helpful (Dallan et al, 2009). A lateral canthotomy is done to immediately release intraorbital pressure on operation table and if detected later can aso be performed at the bedside. This should be followed by cantholysis (release inferior orbital septum) to achieve further increase in orbital volume. These procedures are emergency procedures to save vision. Then endoscopic orbital decompression can be done if identified while performing endoscopic sinus surgery or as an emergency adjunctive procedure (Tyler, et al. 2017). Endoscopic orbital decompression is described in Chapter 22 (endoscopic endonasal approach to orbit).

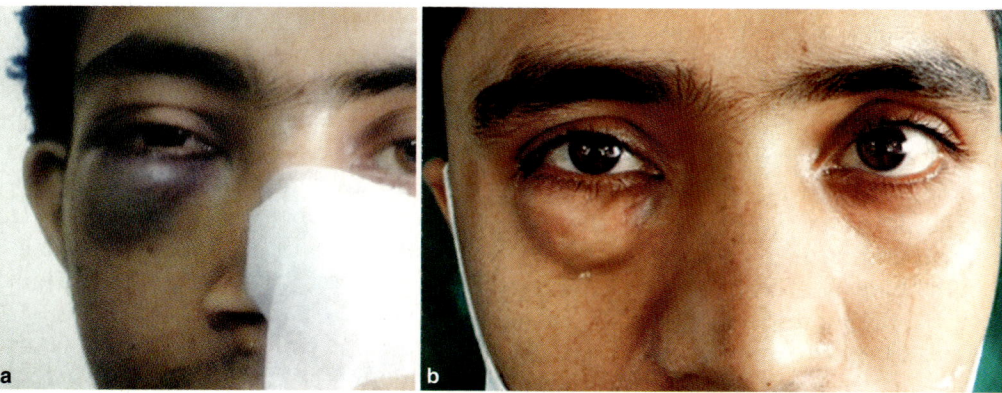

Fig. 11.3: a. Mild proptosis, periorbital ecchymosis, and **b.** Infraorbital emphysema due to breach in lamina papyracea following FESS

Optic Nerve Injury

Direct injury to the optic nerve, in some cases bilaterally, has been reported in literature.

Direct optic nerve injury should be suspected, if the pupil dilates rapidly during surgery (Rene, et al 2001). Probable factors involved are inadequate visualization, poor understanding of anatomy and disorientation secondary to bleeding. 14% of patients have posterior ethmoid cells which extend over the sphenoid (Onodi cells). 88% of sphenoid sinuses juxtaposed the optic nerve and 23% of these had a significant bulge to the sphenoid. Knowledge, therefore, of the sphenoid and the posterior ethmoids is mandatory.

Prevention of orbital complications is possible, if the following guidelines are followed (Flowchart 11.1):

- Preoperative evaluation with regard to history of bleeding diathesis, aspirin use, hypertension, prolonged steroid use, glaucoma, visual acquity, previous nasal surgery are extremely important.

- Preoperative CT is important especially in patients with nasal polyposis and previous nasal surgery. Check for anatomical landmarks prior to surgery.
- Keep the eyes uncovered after draping. Ask the patient to alert you in case of eye pain during the procedure, if under local anaesthesia.
- All tissues removed during surgery should be examined for orbital fat. Orbital ballotment may be necessary during the procedure to check for injury to the orbital periosteum.
- Recognition of orbital haematoma is critical. Intranasal packs should be removed. Eye massage should be started immediately to redistribute the retro-orbital blood into the surrounding fat, thereby decreasing the orbital pressure.
- Diuretics are given to decrease intraocular volume. Mannitol IV 20% over 20 minutes to reduce intraocular pressure, acetazolamide 500 mg IV reduces production of aqueous humor, dexamethasone 10 mg IV bolus.

Flowchart 11.1: Orbital bleed/visual change algorithm

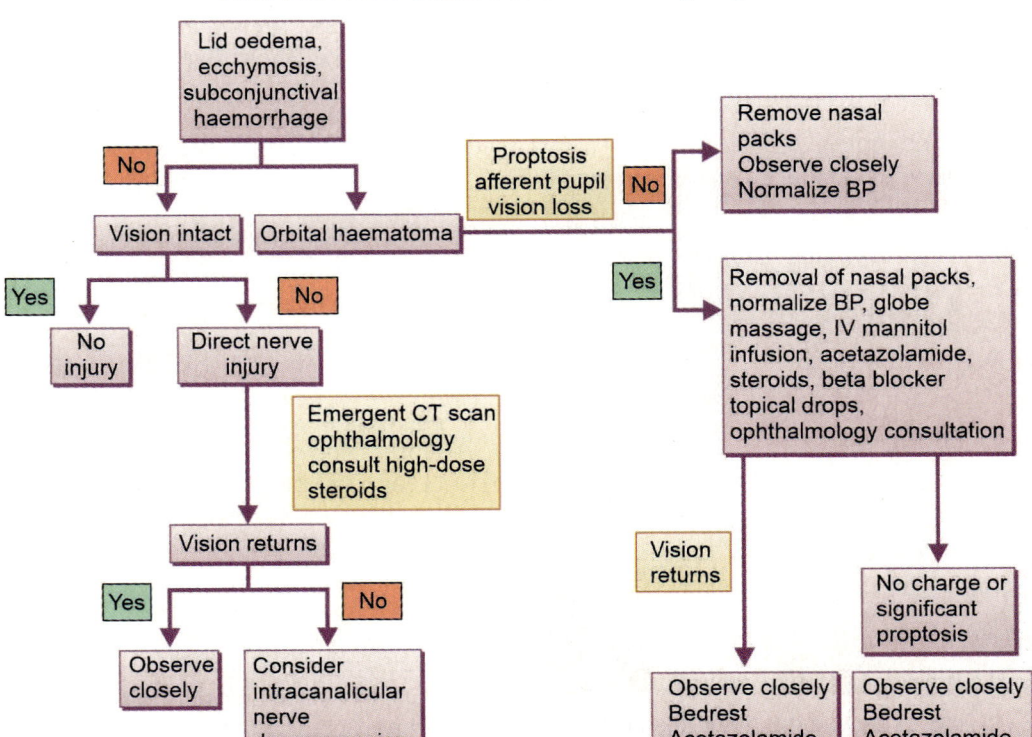

- If conservative management fails, then a lateral canthotomy with superior and inferior cantholysis will allow the orbit to expand.
- A Lynch-Howarth approach with external ethmoidectomy and ligation of anterior and posterior ethmoid arteries will allow the periorbita to expand and help in the control of ocular pressure.
- The intraocular pressure must be normalized within 98 minutes to prevent irreversible damage to the eye.

Cerebrospinal Fluid Leak

The incidence of CSF leak during FESS is reported at 0.05–0.9%. Leaks occur most often from the lateral lamella of cribriform plate, from the roof of the sphenoid or fovea ethmoidalis. Improper visualization, poor orientation, poor knowledge of anatomy, extensive polyposis and anatomical aberrations may cause these accidents. Keros' classification of olfactory fossa is a helpful guideline for the surgeon while dealing with the ethmoidal roof. Keros' type-3 has the highest risk for intracranial entry (Fig. 11.4).

Prevention of this complication is the best arrangement. Intraoperatively, the leak can be plugged with temporalis fascia, fat or muscle. Postoperative leaks usually close spon-

taneously—advise the patient to avoid nose blowing, keep the head elevated, no lifting, bending or straining and absolute bedrest for 48 hours. A lumbar CSF drain may be required in some persistent leaks. If the leak persists in spite of a drain, then an endoscopic repair is advisable as described in Chapter 17. Larger defect requires anterior craniotomy for repair with 3-layer closure including sealing the bony defect.

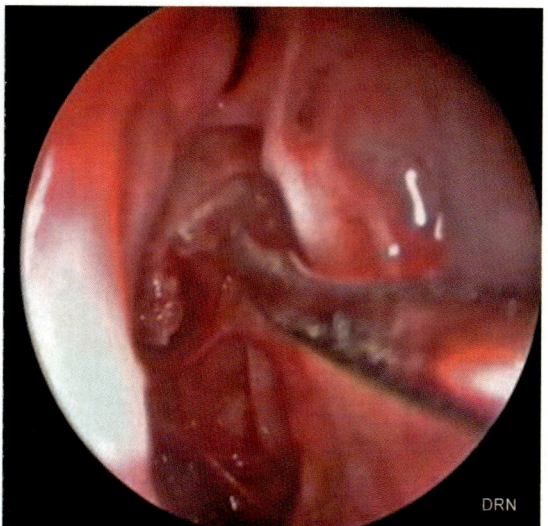

Fig. 11.4: Post sinus surgery dural herniation with CSF leak as pointed with sickle knife

BIBLIOGRAPHY

1. Abridged from Nueman, Turner, Davidson. Complications of Endoscopic Surgery. ENT Journal 1994;73(8): 585–90.
2. Bhatti MT, et al. Ocular motility complications after endoscopic sinus surgery with powered cutting instruments. Otolaryngol Head Neck Surg 2001 Nov; 125 (5): 501.
3. Dallan, et al. Management of severely bleeding ethmoidal arteries. J Craniofacial Surgery 2009, March, 20(2):450–54.
4. Halderman AA, Sindwani R, Woodard TD. Hemorrhagic complications of endoscopic sinus surgery. Otolaryngol Clin N Am 2015; 48:783–93.
5. Hayreh SS, Weingeist TA. Experimental occlusion of the central artery of the retina: Retinal tolerance time to acute ischemia. British Jour Ophthalmol 1980, 64: 818–25.
6. Hollmstead, WH. Anatomy for Surgeons: The Head and Neck. JB Lippincott, Philadelphia. 1982, 93–158.
7. Keros PJ, et al. Laryngology Rhino 1962, 41:809–13.
8. Khanna A, Sama A. Managing complications and revisions in sinus surgery. Current Otorhinolaryngology Reports 2019;7:79–86.
10. Kim HJ, Choi JH, Lee JY. Evaluation of recurrent maxillary sinusitis due to middle meatal antrostomy site stenosis. Ann Otol Rhinol Laryngol 2020;129(10):964–68.
11. Levine HL, et al. Complications of endoscopic sinus surgery: analysis of 2108 patients-incidence and prevention. Laryngoscope 1994 Sep;104 (9):1080–83.
12. Lynch RC. The technique of radical frontal sinus operation which has given the best results. Laryngoscope 1921;31:1–5.
13. Manlglla AJ. Fatal and other major complications of endoscopic sinus surgery. Laryngoscope 1991;101:349–54.

14. Murr AH, et al. Safety and efficacy of a novel bioabsorbable, steroid-eluting sinus stent; Int. Forum Allergy Rhinology 2011 Jan–Feb;1(1):23–32.

15. Nayak DR, Balakrishna R, Hazarika P. Prevention and management of synechia in pediatric endoscopic sinus surgery using dental wax plates. Int J Pediatr Otorhinolaryngol 1998 Dec 15;46(3):171–78.

16. Nayak DR. A tailor made approach to endoscopic sinus surgery for chronic rhinosinusitis. Ojolhns 2015; 9(2):6–8.

17. Rene C, Rose GE, Lenthal R, et al. Major orbital complications of endoscopic sinus surgery. Br J Ophthalmol 2001;85:598–603.

18. Solares CA, Ong YK, Carrau RL, et al. Prevention and management of vascular injuries in endoscopic surgery of the sinonasal tract and skull base. Otolaryngol Clin North Am 2010; 43(4):817–25.

19. Stankiewicz J. Complications in endoscopic intranasal ethmoidectomy: An update. Laryngoscope 1989: 99: 686–90.

20. Stankiewicz JA, Lal D, Connor M, et al. Complications in endoscopic sinus surgery for chronic rhinosinusitis: A 25-year experience. Laryngoscope 2011;121:2684–701.

21. Stankiewicz JA. Blindness and intranasal endoscopic ethmoidectomy: Prevention and management. Otolaryngol Head Neck Surg 1989;101:320–29.

21. Stankiewicz JA. Complications of endoscopic sinus surgery. Otolaryngol Clin North Am 1989;22(4):749–58.

22. Thomas Neuman, Turner WJ, Davldson TM. Complications of endoscopic surgery. ENT Journal 1994;73 (8):585–90.

23. Tyler MA, Citardi MJ, Yao WC. Management of retrobulbar hematoma. Operative Techniques Otol Head and Neck Surg 2017; 28:208–12.

24. VJ Lund, A Wright, J Yiotakis J. Complications and medicolegal aspects of endoscopic sinus surgery. R Soc Med 1997 August; 90(8): 422–28.

25. WE Bolger, Parsons DS, Mair TEA, et al. Lacrimal drainage system injury in endoscopic sinus surgery. Incidence, analysis and prevention. Arch Otolaryngol 1992; 118(11): 1179–84.

Management of Chronic Rhinosinusitis—An Overview

R Singh, DR Nayak, P Hazarika

Definition

Acute rhinosinusitis (ARS): Acute inflammation of mucosal lining of nasal cavity and paranasal sinuses, that starts with and attack of viral infection followed by seconadary bacterial infection with *S. pneumoniae, H. Influenzae, M. Catarrhalis,* etc. The disease is characterized by nasal obstruction, purulent nasal and postnasal discharge and headache/ facial pain of less than 12 weeks duration.

Recurrent ARS: There should be complete remission of symptoms and signs between the episodes of acute rhinosinusitis. They should not be confused with acute exacerbation of chronic rhinosinusitis (CRS) which can be associated with biofilm (Foreman et al. 2009).

Chronic rhinosinusitis: Chronic inflammation of the mucosal lining of one or more paranasal sinuses, usually caused by anatomical/ pathological obstruction to its drainage, and is characterized by nasal obstruction, hyposmia chronic postnasal mucopurulent discharge with or without recurrent headache/facial pain usually two or more symptoms for more than 12 weeks duration (Fokken, et al. 2012) (Fig. 12.1).

Types

1. ***Chronic rhinosinusitis with nasal polyps (CRSwNP):*** It is a form of CRS where visualization of polyps in the middle meatus including endoscopic evidence present. Role of localized IgE mediated response to staphylococcal enterotoxin (Van Zele, et al. 2004) and exotoxin (Bernstein, et al. 2011) has been under evaluation. History of asthma, aspirin intollerance and allergic fungal rhinosinusitis can be associated.
2. ***CRS without polyposis (CRSsNP):*** No visible evidence of polyps including endoscopy.
3. ***Eosinophilic CRS:*** A subgroup of CRS with nasal polyps associated with gross eosinophilic infiltration. It is atributed to staphylococcal enterotoxin (Fujieda, et al. 2019).

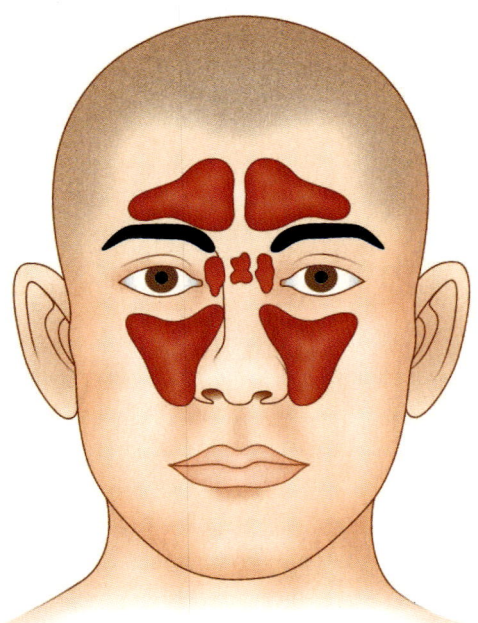

Fig. 12.1: Anatomical position of the anterior group of paranasal sinuses

Flowchart 12.1: Pathogenesis of chronic sinusitis

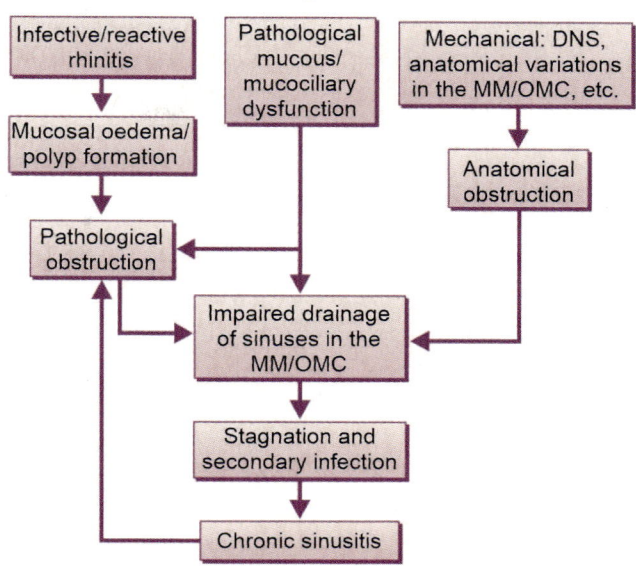

Etiopathogenesis of CRS (Flowchart 12.1)

- Usually rhinogenic. Other routes—rare.
- Unresolved acute sinusitis
- Any form of rhinitis → mucosal oedema in OMC → pathological obstruction
- Any anatomical variation → anatomical obstruction
- Stagnation and secondary chronic sinusitis
- Mucosal oedema
- Mechanical obstruction (anatomical)
- Mucous—thick
- Primary mucociliary dysfunction
- Anterior ethmoid is the key area for causation of chronic anterior group sinusitis because ostiomeatal complex is situated within it, acts as a reservoir of infection.

Bacteriology

- Mixed infection
- *Streptococcus pneumoniae, Streptococcus haemolyticus, Staph. aureus*, gram-negative bacteria, etc.
- Anaerobic infections cause foul smelling discharge.

Pathology

- Mucosal changes
- Hyperemia
- Hypertrophy
- Increased mucosal glands
- Polypoidal changes
- Mucopurulent secretions
- Microabscesses
- Fibrosis, hyalinization
- Atrophy, squamous metaplasia, granulations

Clinical Features

Symptoms

- Mucopurulent/purulent postnasal discharge
- Cachosmia in case of anaerobic infection
- Headache/facial pain—depending on the site and type—usually dull aching.
- Nasal obstruction
- Aural and throat symptoms

Signs

- Discharge in the middle meatus (MM) on anterior rhinoscopy
- Mucosal changes in the MM
- Discharge in MM/superior meatus (SM) on posterior rhinoscopy
- Tenderness in acute exacerbations
- Postural/transillumination tests
- Prominent lateral pharyngeal band

Investigations

- Plain radiographs—Waters view
- Mucosal thickening, haziness, opacity, polyp
- CT scan of OMC/paranasal sinuses (coronal cuts) (Figs 12.2a, b and 12.3)
- X-ray nasopharynx in children to rule out enlarged adenoid
- Diagnostic nasal endoscopy
- Allergic tests, if suspected for nasal allergy
- Proof puncture for maxillary sinus
- Culture and sensitivity—rarely done
- Fungal culture of cheesy discharge, if present.

Treatment

Medical

Mild disease

- Saline irrigation and topical nasal spray
- If improvement—follow same treatment and can add long-term antibiotics

Moderate to severe disease/mild disease not responding to treatment after 3 months:

- Culture and sensitivity. Long-term antibiotics

- Saline irrigation and topical nasal steroids.
- If no improvement—repeat endoscopic evaluation and CT scan to consider for surgery
- Medical treatment to continue even after surgery with saline irrigations and topical steroids

Surgical

- When refractory to medical treatment.
- Surgery for predisposing causes like DNS, polyp, etc.
- Surgical procedure depends on the sinus involved.
- All sinuses may be surgically accessed endoscopically. CT-guided endoscopic surgery helps in identifying various important landmarks like knowing the level of cribriform plate during surgery thus reducing major complications (Fig. 12.4). Knowing this Keros classifications of olfactory fossa is important for a surgeon.

The coronal CT allows to study the level of the cribriform plate and the olfactory fossa as described by Keros. This includes—(a) Keros Type-1: Olfactory fossa 1–3 mm deep, Type-2:

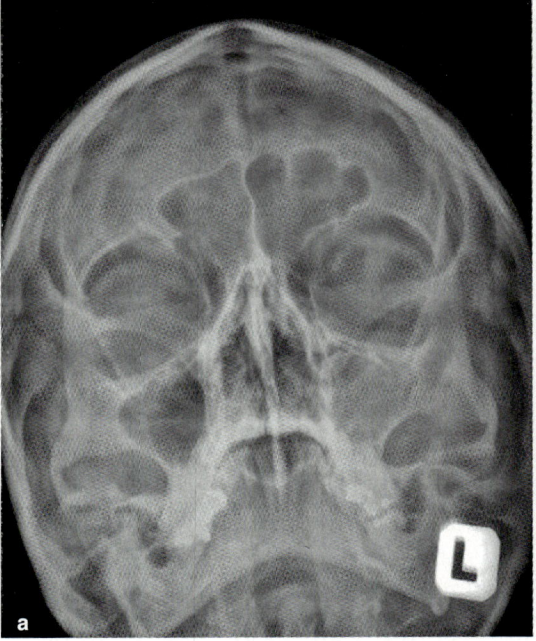 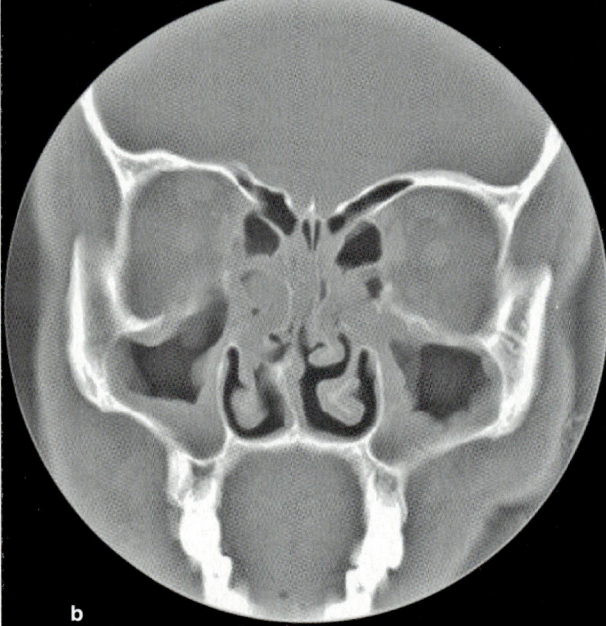

Fig. 12.2: a. X-ray PNS, and **b.** CT OMC coronal cuts suggestive of bilateral OMC disease

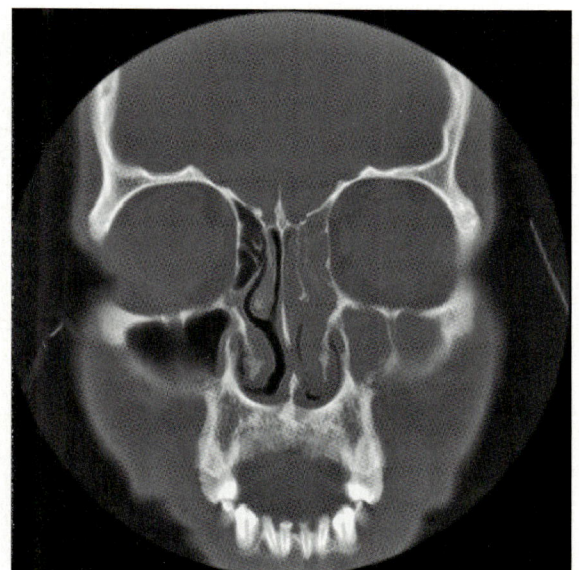

Fig. 12.3: CT OMC coronal cuts left pansinusitis

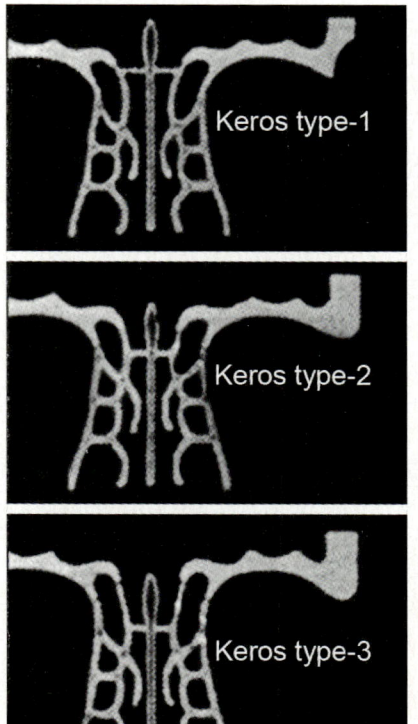

Fig. 12.4: Level of cribriform plate as described by Keros

Olfactory fossa 4–7 mm deep, Type-3: Olfactory fossa 8–16 mm deep.

Surgical Options for Chronic Maxillary Sinusitis

- Antral puncture (rarely being done nowadays)
- Intranasal antrostomy—rarely being done nowadays, only indicated in post-radiation sinusitis, Kartagener's syndrome, etc.
- Endoscopic middle meatal antrostomy (MMA) (Fig. 12.5)
- Endoscopic inferior meatal antrostomy (IMA) as shown in Fig. 12.6 also used as endoscopic access in multiport surgery
- Caldwell-Luc operation (Fig. 12.7)
- Balloon sinuplasty

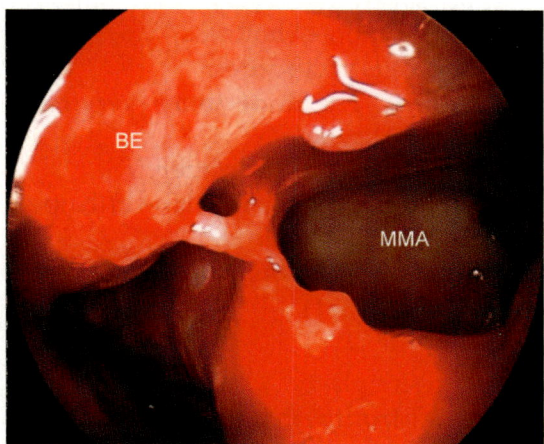

Fig. 12.5: Completed middle meatal antrostomy (MMA) after uncinectomy with intact bulla (BE)

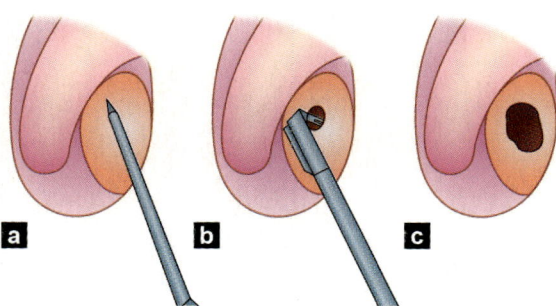

Fig. 12.6: Procedure of endoscopic inferior meatal fenestration (antrostomy)

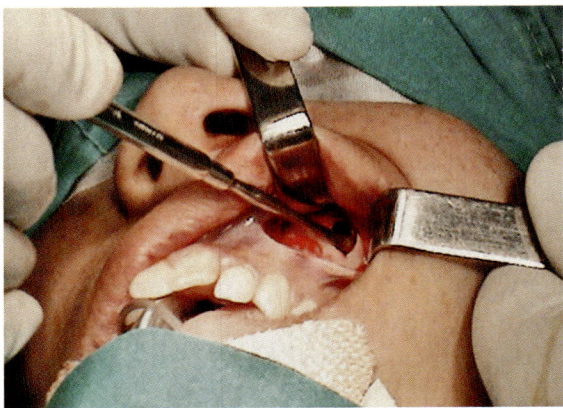

Fig. 12.7: Caldwell-Luc operation in progress

Chronic Ethmoiditis

- **Intranasal ethmoidectomy (abandoned)**
  - Complication—blindness
  - Dangerous procedure
- **Transantral ethmoidectomy (very rarely done)**
  - Via Caldwell-Luc operation
- **External ethmoidectomy** (Howarth operation)
- **Endoscopic ethmoidectomy** (FESS)

Chronic Frontal Sinusitis

- Balloon sinuplasty
- External frontoethmoidectomy (Lynch-Howarth operation rarely being performed nowadays)
- Osteoplastic operation

- Obliteration of frontal sinus
- Endoscopic frontal sinusotomy (Draf I and II): In Draf IIa, frontal ostium is widened medially and laterally between lamina papyracea and middle turbinate, in IIb drainage of frontal sinus between lamina papyracea and nasal septum. Drilling is necessary after identification of 1st olfactory neuron; besides removal of the frontal beak (Nayak 2015).
- Modified Lothrop procedure (Draf III): Involves drilling of the frontal sinus floor and resection of superior nasal septum and inferior interfrontal septum facilitating a common median drainage (Nayak, et al. 2016).

Chronic Sphenoidal Sinusitis

- Intranasal sphenoethmoidectomy (replaced with endoscopic surgery)
- External sphenoethmoidectomy (sometime is done for invasive fungal rhinosinusitis along with medial maxillectomy)
- Endoscopic sphenoidotomy (isolated sinusitis involving sphenoid sinus)
- Endoscopic balloon sinuplasty (for isolated sphenoidal sinusitis)

Steps for Functional Endoscopic Sinus Surgery (Figs 12.8 and 12.9)

- Uncinectomy (infundibulotomy)
- Middle meatal antrostomy
- Frontal recess clearance

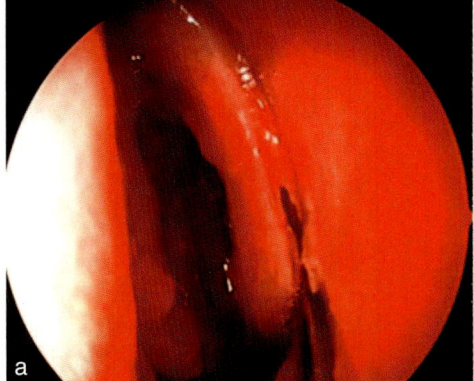
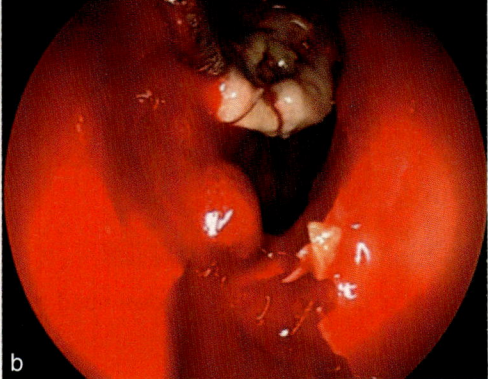

Fig 12.8: Endoscopic sinus surgery in progress: **a.** Uncinectomy, **b.** Bulla is opened, fungal debris can be noted inside bulla

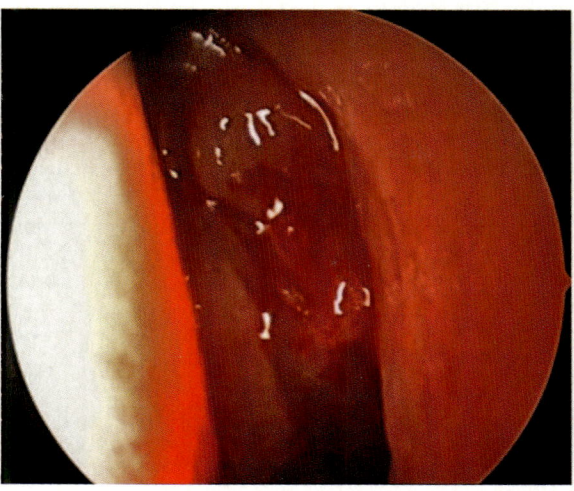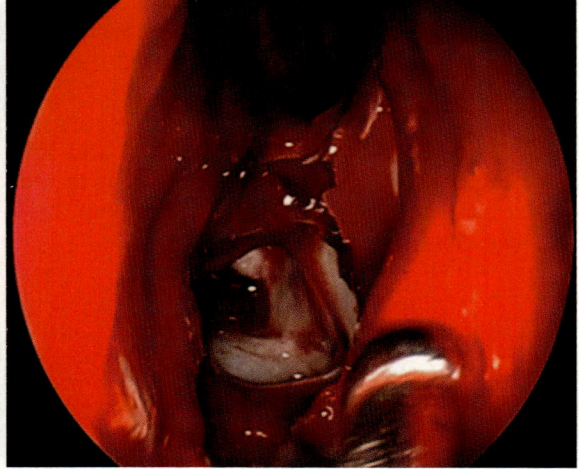

Fig. 12.9: Preoperative ostiomeatal disease and endoscopic sinus surgery in progress, showing ground lamella is opened

- Anterior ethmoidectomy
- Posterior ethmoidectomy
- Sphenoidotomy

Conclusion

- Ostiomeatal complex (OMC) disease is responsible for chronic persistent sinusitis.
- Functional endoscopic sinus surgery (FESS) is the treatment of choice for the management of chronic sinusitis. Use of powered instrument like microdebrider helps in muosal sparing surgery but needs expertise to prevent complications. Navigation can be an important tool in minimizing complications especially in revision cases (Kanai, et al 2017). Microdebrider is a very useful tool to do polypectomy with precision and achieves a relatively bloodless field during endoscopic surgery although the precision depends on the surgeon's anatomical knowledge and operative skills (Singh, et al 2011).
- Meticulous postoperative care is the key to the success of endoscopic sinus surgery.

BIBLIOGRAPHY

1. Kirtane MV. Functional Endoscopic Sinus Surgery, 1993.
2. Head and Neck Surgery—Otolaryngology, Edited by Byron and Bailey (1993).
3. John Groves, Roger F Gray. A synopsis of Otolaryngology, 4th Edition, 1985.
4. Kanai K, Okano M, Haruna T, et al. Evaluation of a new and simple classification for endoscopic sinus surgery. Allergy Rhinol (Province), 2017; 8(3):118–125.
5. Kenedy DW. Functional endoscopic sinus surgery technique. Arch Otolaryngology 1985; 111:634.
6. Nayak DR. A tailor made approach to endoscopic sinus surgery for chronic rhinosinusitis. OJOLHNS 2015;9:2:6–8.
7. Nayak DR, Pai K, Nair S, et al. A short-term subjective and objective analysis of modified endoscopic Lothrop's procedure and its functional outcome: Our experience. Indian J Otolaryngol Head Neck Surg 2016; 68(4): 481–86.
8. Singh R, Hazarika P, Nayak DR, et al. A comparison of microdebrider assisted endoscopic sinus surgery and conventional endoscopic sinus surgery for nasal polypi. Indian J Otolaryngol Head Neck Surg 2013 Jul;65(3): 193–6.
9. Decker BC, Stammberger. Functional Endoscopic Sinus Surgery, Philadelphia; 1991.
10. Stanklewicz JA. Complications in endoscopic ethmoidectomy: An update. Laryngoscope 1989; 99: 686.
11. W Messerklinger. Background and evolution of Endoscopic sinus surgery. ENT Journal 1994; (73) 7: 449–55.
12. Fujeida S, Imoto Y, Kato Y, et al. Eosinophilic chronic rhinosinusitis. Allergology International 2019; 68: 403–12.

13. Fokkens WJ, Lund VJ, Hopkins C, et al. European Position Paper on Rhinosinusitis and Nasal Polyps 2020. Rhinology 2020 Feb 20; 58(Suppl S29):1–464.

14. Zele VT, Gavaert P, Watelet JM, et al. *Staphylococcus aureus* colonization and IgE antibody formation to enterotoxins is increased in nasal polyposis. J Allergy Clin Immunol 2004 Oct;114(4):981–83.

15. Bernstein JM, Allen C, Rich G, et al. Further observations on the role of *Staphylococcus aureus* exotoxins and IgE in the pathogenesis of nasal polyposis. Laryngoscope 121 (2011), pp. 647–55.

16. Foreman A, Psaltis AJ, Tan LW, Wormald PJ. Characterization of bacterial and fungal biofilms in chronic rhinosinusitis. Am J Rhinol Allergy 2009; 23: 556–61.

Endoscopic Septoturbinoplasty

DR Nayak, R Balakrishnan, KD Murty, S Shetty

Decades have passed since septoplasty was first introduced for the management of nasal airway. Numerous medical descriptions are available regarding the pathology and treatment of deviated nasal septum (Freer, 1902; Metzenbaum, 1929; Galloway, 1946; Cottle, et al. 1958; Maran 1974).

The submucus resection was popularized and refined by Killian (1904) and Freer (1902). Due to the increased incidence of complications following such radical surgeries led to more and more conservative septal surgery. Metzenbaum (1929), described the swing-door technique for caudal dislocation and sub-luxation. Galloway (1946) removed the entire septal cartilage and replaced it as a separate autograft. Cottle (1958) described premaxilla-maxilla approach for the correction by making inferior and superior tunnel on concave side and inferior tunnel on convex side to facilitate necessary resection of cartilage and bone to correct the septal deformity. Maran (1974) has described septoplasty, but used a more radical technique in the terms of removal of bony septum. However, none of these descriptions has highlighted a complete surgical management of this condition to improve the nasal airway. Each surgical procedure has its limitations and cannot deal with all the variants of the deformities of the nasal septum. It is essential to know the biomechanical behaviour of the cartilaginous septum (Murakami, et al. 1982). Use of this technique has helped us to refine our technique of endoscopic septal correction. An

ideal surgical correction of the nasal septum should satisfy the following criteria:
1. Should relieve the nasal obstruction.
2. Should be conservative.
3. Should not produce iatrogenic deformity.
4. Should not compromise the ostiomeatal complex.
5. Should relieve all the contact areas.
6. Must have the scope for a revision surgery, if required later.

The traditional surgeries of the nasal septum improve the nasal airway but do not fulfill the above-mentioned criteria in most instances. The reasons outlined for this are poor visualization. Relative inaccessibility, poor illumination, difficulty in evaluation of the exact pathology, need for nasal packing, unnecessary manipulation, resection and over exposure of the septal framework, reducing the scope for a revision surgery (Nayak, et al. 2002). The nasal endoscope allows precise preoperative identification of the septal pathology and its associated lateral nasal wall abnormalities and helps in better planning of endoscope-aided septal surgery (Nayak, et al. 1998). This technique is ultraconservative and fulfills the above mentioned criteria of an ideal septal surgery. As this surgery addresses both the septal and the turbinate pathologies, the term *endoscopic septoturbinoplasty* has been used by Nayak, et al. (2002). In their preliminary study (1998), they demonstrated that endoscopic-aided approach in the management of deviated nasal septum, both subjectively and objectively, is superior to the traditional technique. Simultaneous sinus surgery can be done without the fear of lateralization of the middle turbinate and consequent synechiae formation. Giles et al. (1994) in their series of 38 patients described the use of nasal endoscope in limited septal resection to facilitate endoscopic sinus surgery.

Steps of Endoscopic Septoturbinoplasty (Nayak, et al. 1998, 2001 and 2002)

1. Surface anaesthesia—4% xylocaine with adrenaline 1 in 100,000 for about 10 minutes.
2. Endoscopic infiltration of the nasal septum with 1 in 200,000 xylocaine with adrenaline on the convex side of the cartilaginous septum along the crest and bony septum on both sides including the spur whenever present.
3. Incomplete incision at the caudal end of the septum in its lower half in most cases except when there was a caudal dislocation or anterior buckling (hemitransfixion).
4. Incision is made on the convex side in case with anterior deviation and on the concave side for subluxation, spur or posterior deviation to expose the abnormality at the bony cartilaginous junction. In cases of an isolated spur, incision is made parallel to the floor on the spur itself.
5. Elevation of the initial mucoperichondrial flap using Cottle's elevator and Pilchards nasal speculum. Further elevation is done using 0° Hopkins rod nasal endoscope (4 mm) held in left hand, keeping the tip of the endoscope between the mucoperichondrial flap and the septal cartilage. The right hand is used for instrumentation. Flap elevation in the correct cleavage plane is required to minimize bleeding. The exposure is limited to the target area. The traditional anterior and inferior tunnels described by Cottle et al. (1958) are not followed in the endoscopic method.
6. A subluxated cartilage from the crest is shaved using no. 15-blade Bard-Parker knife to resect the excess cartilage inferiorly, without dislocating the vomerochondral junction. At the anterior nasal spine, the subluxated cartilage was carefully trimmed and repositioned over the crest to prevent a supra-tip deformity (Fig. 13.1a to d).
7. In case of posterior septal deviation or a deviation at the ethmochondral junction, the bony septum is fractured to realign in the midline or a minimum resection of the caudal end of the ethmoidal plate is performed. Dislocation of the ethmochondral junction should be avoided; especially in a child and a deviated septum here is precisely shaved using the Bard-Parker knife. However, a wedge resection can be performed after shaving the thick cartilage at the bony cartilaginous junction in adults (Fig. 13.2a and b).
8. A 'C'-shaped cartilaginous deviation is dealt with by precise multiple wedge resections on the convex side or multiple criss-cross incisions on the concave side aided by the endoscope, placing them on strategic sites and planes (as shown in Fig. 13.1).
9. In cases with caudal dislocation or anterior buckling of the cartilage the correction is done last after correcting the rest of the septum anticipating further increase in the anteroposterior length of the septum.
10. A spur without any other deviation of the septum is resected after incision and exposure made directly over the spur.
11. The gross anterior deviation is dealt with using traditional technique to start with and then treating the posterior deviation and the strategic central portion with the endoscopic approach.
12. A thick septum involving the posterior segment require precise shaving of the cartilage close to the bony cartilage junction and resection of the part of the vomer and perpendicular plate of the ethmoid, if found thick (Fig. 13.2a to d).
13. **Turbinoplasty** (Fig. 13.3): Mucosal preservation is crucial while reducing

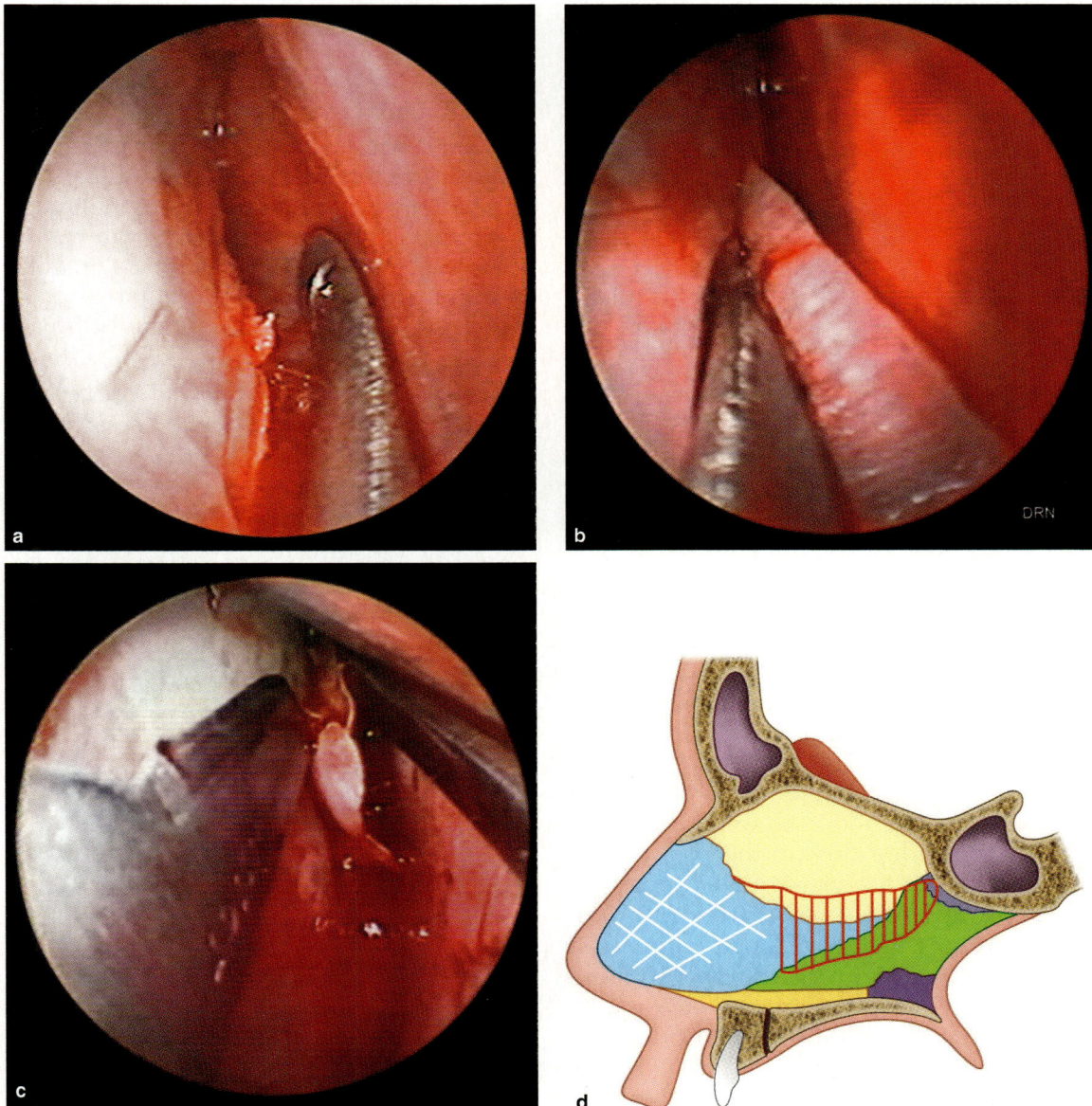

Fig. 13.1: a. Video endoscopic photograph showing elevation of the mucoperichondrial flap, **b.** Resection of excess cartilage of the maxillary crest, **c.** Shaving of thickened cartilage from vomerochondral and ethmoido-chondral junction and resection of the thick portion of the vomer and inferior part of the perpendicular plate of ethmoid, **d.** The area of the cartilage and bone resection and criss-cross incision on the concave side of the cartilage

the hypertrophied turbinates. Micro-debrider and coblator can be used successfully (Fig. 13.3). Alternately an inferolateral partial resection of inferior turbinate can be done while preserving the mucosa on the medial surface. Middle turbinate hypertrophy should be addressed carefully while doing an inferolateral resection by preserving inferior part of ground lamella to prevent middle turbinate instability. A concha bullosa is addressed with lateral partial resection with same principle (Nayak, et al. 2001 and 2002).

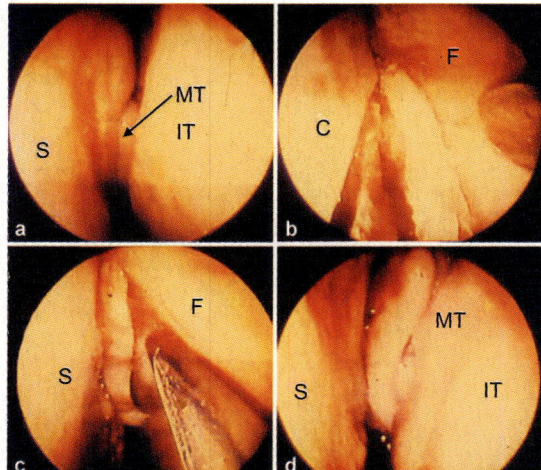

Fig. 13.2: The steps of endoscopic septoplasty: **a.** Gross posterior deviation of septum (S) with septoturbinal compression by middle turbinate (MT) and subluxation of septal cartilage over maxillary crest, **b.** Resection of subluxated cartilage (C) from the crest and elevated septal flap (F), **c.** Shaving of thickened cartilage from vomero-ethmoido-chondral junction with 15-blade Bard-Parker knife, **d.** After correction increase space between septum and middle and inferior turbinate (IT)

14. Splinting is done after a stab incision is made in the inferior aspect of the muco-periosteal flap close to the floor on one side before the closure of the flap, to prevent haematoma formation. The splin-ting is done by using prefashioned dental wax plate (baseplate wax) steri-lized in Cidex solution and anchored by catgut sutures (Nayak, et al. 1995) and can be kept for longer period, if synechiae formation is anticipated after endoscopic sinus surgery, in which case an additional wax plate is kept between middle turbinate and lateral wall.

The advantages of nasal endoscope in septal surgery (Nayak, et al. 1998):

1. Facilitates accurate identification pathology and improved accessibility to remote areas.
2. Better understanding of the lateral wall pathology associated with the septal deformity.
3. Allows limited incision and elevation of the flaps without compromising ade-quate exposure of the pathological site.

4. Allows correct identification of the cleavage planes of flap elevation espe-cially in revision and difficult post-traumatic cases.
5. Elevation of flaps in the correct plane minimizes intraoperative bleeding. Moreover, troublesome bleeding due to removal of bony spurs and from remote areas can be managed better with bipolar cautery using endoscopic aid.
6. Allows realignment by limited and precise resection of the pathological areas and/or by precise repair, by strategically placed wedge resections/shaving of cartilage.
7. Unlike the nasal speculum, the endo-scope does not distort the septal frame-work during its use.
8. Effectively relieve the contact areas and thus contact headaches by allowing accurate intraoperative assessment (Nayak-Balakrishna 2002).
9. Allows ultraconservative as well as effective septal surgery thus not jeopardizing the development of the nose and the midface in children. Ultra-conservation also preserves the support of external framework, thus allowing better concomitant rhinoplasty.
10. With landmarks well preserved, it keeps the option open for revision surgery, if indicated.
11. Helps in accurate nasal splinting thus avoiding the morbidities of nasal packing.
12. Simultaneous sinus surgery can be done without the fear of lateralization of middle turbinate and consequent synechiae formation.
13. Helps in teaching septal anatomy, patho-logy and surgery.
14. Helps in documentation

The limitations of the nasal endoscope use may include loss of binocular vision, need for frequent cleaning of the tip of the endoscope especially when there is more bleeding and that combined traditional and endoscopic methods may be required, if pathology also involves the caudal most part of the septum,

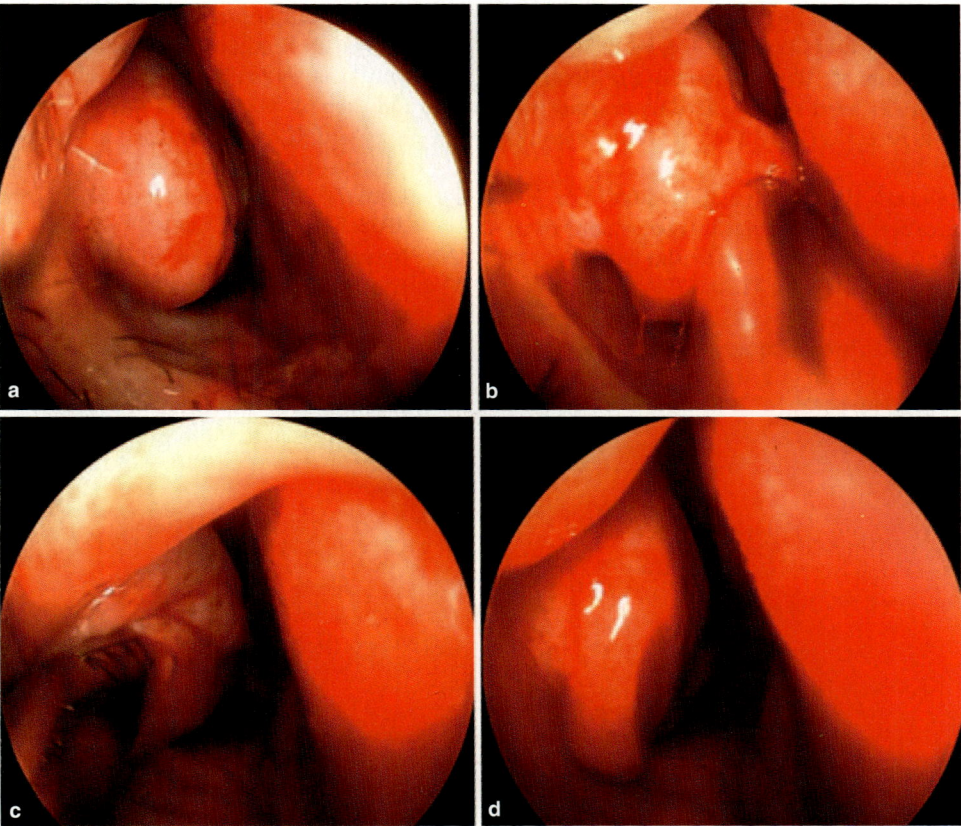

Fig 13.3: a. Hypertrophied inferior turbinate, **b & c.** Subepithelial reduction of turbinate by microdebrider which is withdrawn gradually while preservation of the mucosa, **d.** Post reduction appearance of inferior turbinate with no gross bleeding noted

i.e. anterior buckling and trimming of excess caudal end of the septum.

Endoscopic septoturbinoplasty for a deviated nasal septum is a viable alternative to conventional septal surgery. This is safe, effective and conservative with future scope for revision surgery. The author advocates combination of approaches—endoscopic for the inaccessible middle and posterior part and traditional to accessible anterior most portion of the nasal septum especially caudal dyslocation and anterior buckling. Endoscopic septoplasty can be used as a complimentary procedure to rhinoplasty operation (Nayak, et al 1998, 2002). A preliminary diagnostic nasal endoscopy is crucial for proper evaluation and planning and placement of incision. Incision should be given in the anterior most part, particularly near the

caudal end of the septum. It gives wider exposure to the cartilage and bony cartilaginous junction. If large part of cartilage needs to be resected, incision must preserve Killian's L-strut (Pons, et al 2015).

BIBLIOGRAPHY

1. Cottle MH, et al. The maxilla-premaxilla approach to extensive nasal septum surgery. Archives of Otolaryngology 1958; 68: 301.
2. Freer O. The correction of deflections of the nasal septum with a minimum of traumatism. Journal of American Medical Association 1902; 38: 636.
3. Galloway T. Plastic repair of the deflected nasal septum arch. Otolaryngology 1946;44:141.
4. Giles et al. Endoscopic septoplasty. Laryngoscope 1994; 104:1507–09.
5. Killian G. Die submucöse Fensterresektion der Nasenscheidewand. Archiv fur Laryngologie and Rhinologie 1904;16:362.

6. Maran AGD. Septoplasty. Journal of Laryngology and Otology 1974; 88: 393–402.
7. Metzenbaum M. Replacement of the lower end of the dislocated septal cartilage versus submucous resection. Archives of Otolaryngology 1929;9:282.
8. Murakami WT, Wong LW, Davidso TM. Application of biomechanical behaviour of the cartilage in nasal septoplastic surgery. Laryngoscope (1982); 92,300–309.
9. Nayak DR, Balakrishna R. Endoscopic approach to middle turbinate squeeze syndrome. Indian Journal of Otolaryngol and Head and Neck Surgery 2012; 64(2):167–71.
10. Nayak DR, et al. Endoscopic physiologic approach to allergy-associated chronic rhinosinusitis: A preliminary study. ENT Journal 2001; 80(6): 392–403.
11. Nayak DR, et al. Endoscopic septoturbinoplasty—our update series. Indian Journal of Otolaryngology and Head and Neck Surgery 2002; 54(1): 20–22.
12. Nayak DR, et al. An endoscopic approach to the deviated nasal septum—a preliminary study. Journal of Laryngology and Otology 1998; 112: 934–39.
13. Nayak DR, et al. Septal splints using wax plates. Journal of Postgraduate Medicine 1995;41:70–71.

Endoscopic Dacryocystorhinostomy

DR Nayak, S Pillai, K Pujary, K Devaraja

Obstruction of the lacrimal system, either congenital or acquired, is a common problem. There are multiple causes of the nasolacrimal duct obstruction, the most common of which is recurrent dacryocystitis. The contributing factors include nasal allergy, septal deviation and sinusitis. The nasolacrimal duct obstruction can be corrected with dacryocystorhinostomy (DCR) by creating a fistula between lacrimal sac and nasal cavity. The most common indication for DCR is stenosis of nasolacrimal duct causing annoying epiphora or repeated infection. External DCR was first introduced by Toti in 1904 and transnasal procedure was described by Caldwell in 1893 which was subsequently modified by West in 1911. The transnasal approach did not become popular because of the relative inaccessibility and poor visibility and problem of bleeding during surgery.

These limitations are overcome by the use of nasal endoscope for dacryocystorhinostomy, as popularized by McDonough and Meiring 1989. Endoscopic endonasal dacryocystorhinostomy (EDCR) is considered to be superior alternative technique to conventional external DCR and is quite successful in failed cases of external DCR.

Tests to Find Nasolacrimal Obstruction

- The Jones test is a test of the patency of the nasolacrimal system. The test is performed by placing fluorescein in the conjunctival sac and seeing whether or not this fluorescein can be visualized in the nose. If after a period of five minutes there is impaired outflow, it is likely that there is an obstruction somewhere in the duct or somewhere in the system. If dye is not seen in the nose after five minutes, then a secondary test can be performed by irrigating the duct. If after irrigating the duct no dye is found in the nose, the dye has never really reached the lacrimal sac to begin with. The obstruction is likely proximal. If dye is seen in irrigate, then dye did reach the nasolacrimal sac, and it is likely that the obstruction is distal.

- Dacryocystogram
- Dacryoscintigraphy with radio labelled materials
- CT scan

Operative Technique of Endoscopic DCR

This surgery can be done both under local and general anaesthesias. The local anaesthetic technique is similar to that described under the Chapter Endoscopic Sinus Surgery. Topical 2% xylocaine should also be instilled into the conjunctival sac. The lateral wall anterior to the attachment of the middle turbinate was infiltrated submucosally with 2% xylocaine with 1 in 2 lakh dilution of adrenaline using 0 to 30° nasal endoscope in all the cases (including cases under GA). A, U, C shaped mucoperiosteal flap is created in the lateral wall which is superiorly or posteriorly based 1 square cm size anterior to the attachment of

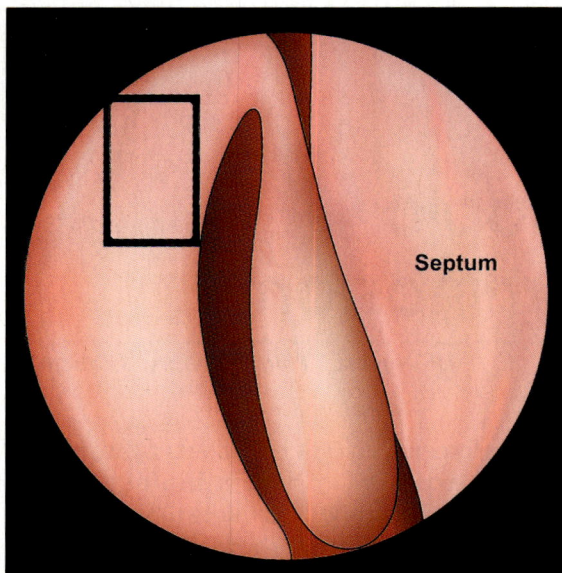

Fig. 14.1: The black square area just anterior to the attachment of middle turbinate (MT) where a raw area has to be created to expose the lacrimal bone

middle turbinate to expose the lacrimal bones or 1 square cm of raw area can be created over the lateral wall at the same site by using diathermy/bipolar cautery or laser (shown as black square area in Fig. 14.1).

The lacrimal bone thus exposed was drilled initially using a cutting burr and later a diamond burr to expose the sac. The sac can easily be identified from the surrounding periosteum. At this stage, saline infiltration can be done through the lacrimal punctum, which will allow the sac to expand and thus can be identified easily (Fig. 14.2).

The bone can also be removed by using a Kerrison rongeur/DCR punch after initial exposure with a drill. Chisel or gouge should be avoided to prevent penetrating of small bony spicule into the soft tissue and can cause secondary infection and closure of fistula site. After the complete exposure of the sac, the trained assisting surgeon or ophthalmologist is asked to pass a lacrimal probe. The lacrimal sac can also be inflated with normal saline by using syringe for irrigation of lacrimal sac. Irrigation is important, if KTP laser is to be used to prevent damage to the mucosa within the sac. KTP-532 laser is applied over the

exposed and inflated sac, till free flow of saline comes out through the fistula thus created (Fig. 14.3).

The sac can also be opened by tenting the lacrimal sac as described above and opening it with a sickle knife. A portion of the medial sac mucosa should be everted, to prevent closure (Fig. 14.2a to h). No stenting with silastic tube is required. However, for revision, DCR silastic tube stenting is required after creation of the opening in the lacrimal sac.

A jelco cannula no. 20 is used along with the lacrimal probe like a trocar. Once jelco is inserted into the nasal cavity through the lower punctum, the lacrimal probe is removed keeping the cannula in place. Then a silastic cannula of appropriate size is passed through the jelco and brought out through the nasal cavity. Keeping it *in situ*, the jelco cannula is removed. The silastic cannula can be removed after 3–6 weeks.

Postoperative Care

1. The nasal cavity should be cleaned.
2. Granulation tissue, if any, should be removed and cauterized. Silastic cannula is one of the causes for granulation, and should be removed immediately, if granulation appears. The nose should be irrigated in every alternate day for a period of 7–10 days.
3. Irrigation should be started from the 1st postoperative day in case of primary DCR without cannulation and should be continued weekly intervals till the healing is complete (Fig. 14.4).

Causes for Failure

The most common cause of a surgical failure in endoscopic DCR is obstruction of the neo-ostium by granulation tissue or synechia that forms postoperatively. Inadequate exposure of the lacrimal sac, due to limited resection of bone and excessive and unnecessary removal or injury of surrounding nasal and lacrimal sac mucosa, and, hence, exposure of bone around a small neo-ostium, appear to contribute to obstruction of the neo-ostium by granulation tissue (Jin, et al. 2006). DNS should be corrected prior to endoscopic DCR.

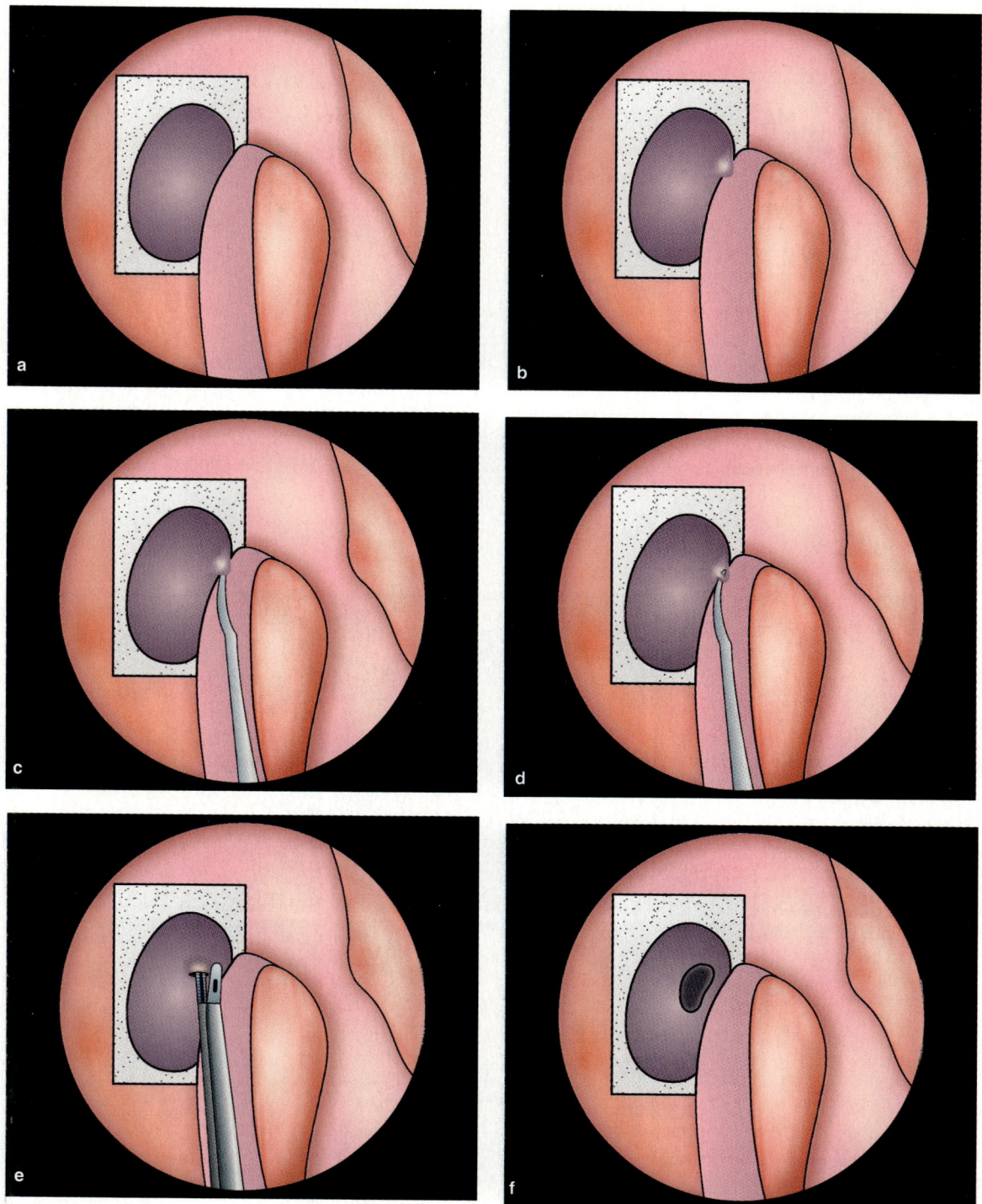

Fig. 14.2: Steps of endoscopic dacryocystorhinostomy: **a.** Exposure of the sac, **b.** Tenting of the sac by passing a lacrimal probe through lower punctum into the sac, **c** and **d.** Opening of the sac with sickle knife, **e.** Enlargement of the opening in the sac with the help of through cutting forceps, **f.** Completion of dacryocystorhinostomy

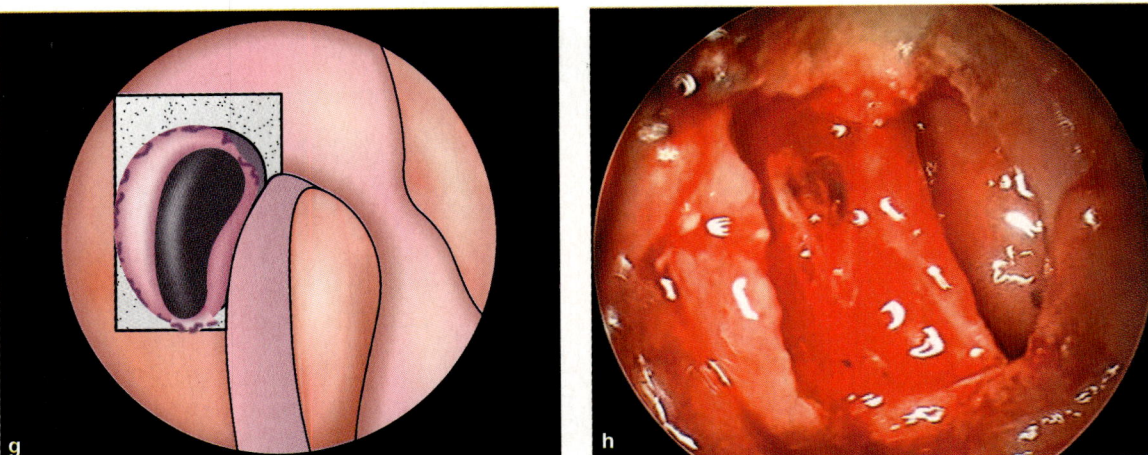

Fig. 14.2: Steps of endoscopic dacryocystorhinostomy: **g.** The mucosal flap is everted and reflected into the nasal cavity to complete the endoscopic dacryocystorhinostomy. This prevents closure of rhinostomy site, **h.** Endoscopic picture showing sac being opened and the mucosal margin has been everted

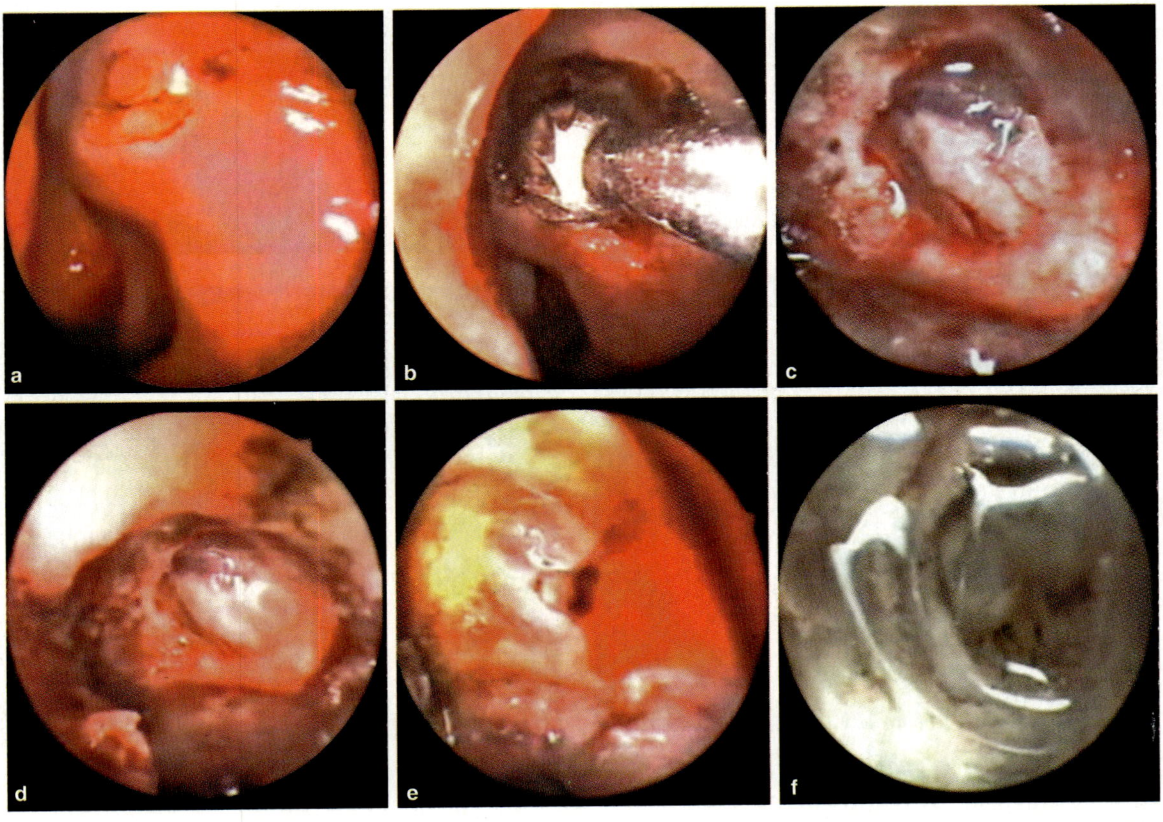

Fig. 14.3: **a.** Mucosa is vaporized with KTP532 laser to expose the lacrimal bone, **b.** Lacrimal bone is drilled to expose the sac, **c.** Lacrimal sac is exposed, **d.** Sac is inflated with saline, **e.** Inflated sac is opened with KTP532 laser, **f.** Free flow of saline is noted after creation of an adequate size opening in the sac

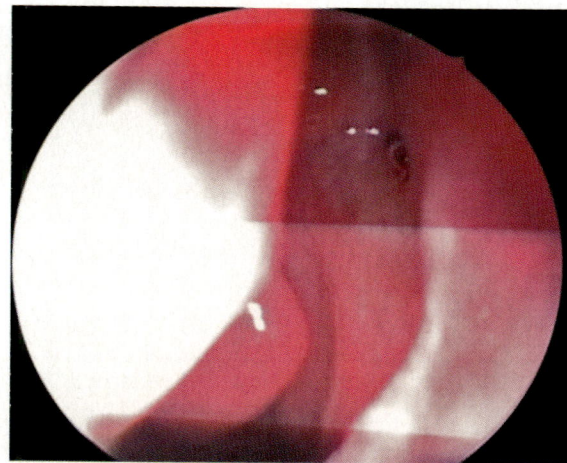

Fig. 14.4: Postoperative endoscopic DCR site which is well epithelialized and healed with patent DCR opening

Sinusitis should be treated with functional endoscopic sinus surgery. Silastic cannulation, if used, should not be kept for a longer period as it can produce granulation and subsequent closure after tube is removed.

It is important to note that, septoplasty and co-existing sinonasal diseases can be managed simultaneously while performing endoscopic DCR by the same surgeon (Deviprasad, et al. 2009).

Complications

- Haemorrhage during surgery
- CSF rhinorrhoea due to fracture of the ethmoid
- Corneal injury
- Orbital cellulitis
- Granulations
- Synechia
- Lacrimal sump syndrome and reinfection.

BIBLIOGRAPHY

1. Caldwell. Two new operation for obstruction of the nasal duct. New York Medical Journal 1893; 57:581–82.

2. Deviprasad D, Mahesh SG, Pujay K, et al. Endonasal endoscopic dacryocystorhinostomy: our experience. Indian J Otolaryngol Head Neck Surg 2009 Sep;61(3): 223–6. doi: 10.1007/s12070-009-0071-z. Epub 2009 Sep 27.

3. Jin HR, et al. Endoscopic dacryocystorhino-stomy: Creation of a large marsupialized lacrimal sac. J Korean Med Sci 2006 August; 21(4):719–23.

4. Nayak DR, Hazarika P, Rodrigues R AW, Pillai S, Balakrishnan R. Endoscopic dacryocystorhino-stomy vs KTP 532 laser-assisted endoscopic dacryocystorhinostomy. Indian Journal of Otolaryngology and Head and Neck Surgery 2005; 57 (4), 278–82.

5. Nayak DR, Satish R, Shah Parul, Poojary K, Balakrishnan R. Endoscopic dacryocystorhino-stomy and retrograde nasolacrimal duct dilatation with cannulation—our experience. Indian Journal of Otolaryngology and Head and Neck Surgery 1999–2000: 52(1): 23–27, ISSN 0019–5421.

6. Rice DN. Endoscopic dacryocystorhinostomy: A cadaveric study. Ann of Rhinol 1998; 2,127–28.

7. Toti A. Nuovo metodo conservatore di eura radicale delle suporazioni chroniche del sacco lacrimale (dacriocistorhinostomia). Clin Mod Firenze 1904;10:385–89.

8. Weston JM. A window resection of nasal duct in case of stenosis. Transaction of Am Oph Society 1910;12(Pt2) 654–58.

9. McDonough M, Meiring JH. Endoscopic transnasal DCR. JLO 1989;103(6):585–87.

Management of Nasal Allergy

D Rao, DR Nayak, A Menon, P Rao

Nasal allergy is a very common condition and frequently acts as a triggering factor for both acute and chronic rhinosinusitis. Nasal inflammation associated with allergic rhinitis can cause obstruction in the area of ostio-meatal complex, thereby predisposing to bacterial infection of the sinuses. This process accounts for many cases of acute and chronic bacterial sinusitis. The term allergic rhino-sinusitis is the most appropriate terminology when nasal allergy is associated with sinusitis. Patients with perennial allergic rhinitis—especially those with significant sensitivity to moulds and/or house dust mites—are parti-cularly susceptible to acute sinusitis and many patients with chronic sinusitis also have nasal allergy. Thus, failing in the management of nasal allergy can lead to treatment failure in sinusitis. Therefore, it is essential to include nasal allergy management in the treatment strategy for chronic sinusitis.

ALLERGIC RHINITIS

History

- First described by John Bostock in 1819 as seasonal catarrah
- 1873, Blackley observed the first reaction by applying pollen to excoriated skin
- 1911, treatment began by Leonard Noon on the assumption of antitoxins.

Definition

Allergic rhinitis is an acute IgE mediated, type-1 hypersensitivity reaction of nasal mucosa in response to antigenic substance (allergen) associated with episodic attacks of sneezing, watery rhinorrhoea, watering of the eyes. Patient may also present with tightness of chest due to subclinical bronchospasm.

Types

- Seasonal (or intermittent) allergic rhinitis (most often referred to as hay fever) is triggered by air-borne pollen most comm-only from grasses, weeds and sometimes trees.
- Perennial (or persistent) allergic rhinitis occurs throughout the year and is most commonly triggered by exposure to house dust mites.
- Mixed when both seasonal and perennial types coexist. As per ARIA (Allergic Rhinitis and Its Impact on Asthma) guideline, seasonal and perennial allergic rhinitis have been replaced with intermittent and persistent, respectively.

ARIA classification (Flowchart 15.1): Allergic rhinitis is a chronic disease where causation is multifactorial and manifestation is multifocal. It is very important to obtain a proper history with respect to various predisposing factors and possible causative agent (allergen), the pathophysiological mechanism and progress of nasal allergy. The symptom of the patient and the type of allergy depend on a number of factors.

Flowchart 15.1: ARIA classification of allergic rhinitis (Small, et al. 2007)

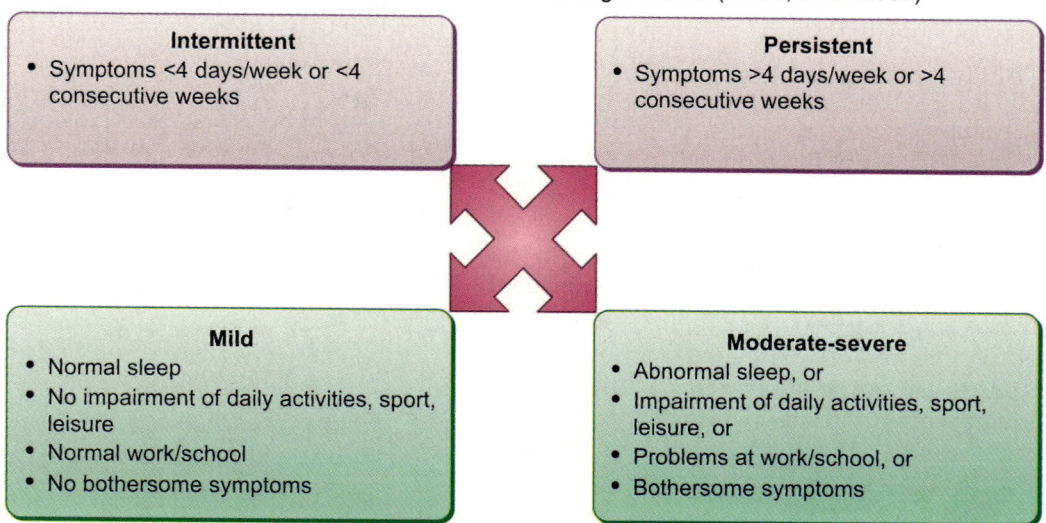

Precipitating Factors

Aerobiological Flora

This is determined by the allergens present in that environment of which inhalant allergen is more common.

Common Allergens (Min 2010)

I. *Inhalant:* Commonest cause
- Pollen and dust including house dust mite—75%
- Fungus
- Animal danders
- Miscellaneous.

House dust mite species are the most common. The fecal matter of house dust mite is highly allergenic and is associated with allergic rhinitis. These mites feed on organic material in households, particularly the skin that is shed from humans and pets. They can be found in carpets, upholstered furniture, pillows, mattresses, comforters, and stuffed toys. While they thrive in warmer temperatures and high humidity, they can be found year-round in many households. On the other hand, dust mites are rare in arid climates.

II. *Food allergy:* Certain food like milk, wheat, eggs, nuts, etc. can have immunologic response causing allergic rhinitis. This chapter will discuss only about inhalant allergy.

Predisposing Factors

a. *Age:* Patients with any age are susceptible to allergy. However, young patients are more affected. About 70% of the cases present with symptoms of nasal allergy before 30 years of age (Yadav *et al.* 2003).

b. *Sex:* Males are more commonly affected with male to female ratio of about 3:2. Some report equal predilection.

c. *Industrialization and urbanization:* Incidence of allergic rhinitis is ever increasing because of industrialization and urbanization responsible for environment pollution. Reported incidence of allergic rhinitis is 1.4–39.7% of population in the Western countries. In UK, there is fourfold increase in incidence of allergic rhinitis in last 30 years.

d. *Genetic predisposition:* Atopy refers to the genetic tendency to develop allergic diseases such as allergic rhinitis, asthma and atopic dermatitis. Atopic march refers to the natural history or typical progression of allergic diseases that begins early in life as atopic dermatitis (skin) and may progress to food allergy, allergic rhinitis and finally to asthma.

e. Focal sensitivity of nasal mucosa can trigger the allergic reaction.

f. IgA deficiency state makes the patient more prone for allergy.

g. Psychology

h. ***Living conditions:*** Residential and workplace conditions play a significant role in the etiology. Crowding, dusty environment, air-conditioned rooms may predispose. Dust may accumulate in the carpets, curtains, bed sheets, bookshelves, store shelves, etc. and its exposure may precipitate the allergic response in genetically predisposed individuals. Allergy may be an occupational hazard also wherein the individual is exposed to allergen in his workplace, e.g. librarian, store-keeper, factory worker, etc.

i. ***Environment:*** Depends on the aerobiological flora of the particular environment. Climatic conditions including season, altitude can affect the manifestation of the symptoms. Based on this, the allergic manifestations may be classified into seasonal and perennial allergic rhinitis. In seasonal allergic rhinitis, the symptoms are more in a particular season, e.g. pollens in spring, fungus in rainy season, etc. In perennial, the symptoms are present throughout the year. Common examples are house dust mite, pets, etc. (Fig. 15.1).

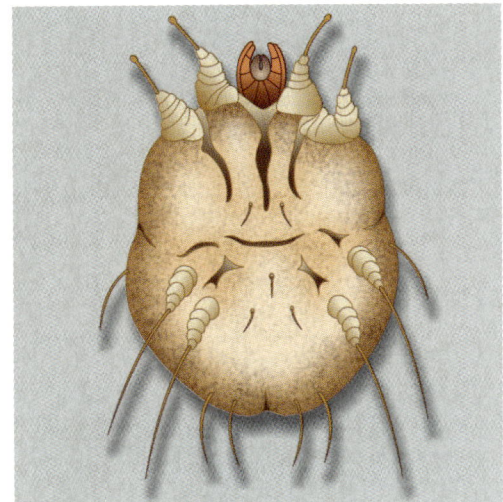

Fig. 15.1: House dust mite

Pathophysiology (Min, 2010)

Primary Response or Sensitization

This is also called priming. After initial exposure to the allergen (antigen), in genetically predisposed individual. The sensitization process begins in the nasal tissues when antigen presenting cells phagocytose and process the inhaled allergen and, subsequently, present the processed antigen to CD4 T cells in local lymph nodes. The allergen stimulated T cells proliferate in a T-helper type 2 (Th2) pathway and release cytokines, including interleukin (IL) 3, IL-4, IL-5, IL-13, among others. These cytokines lead to local and systemic production of IgE antibodies by plasma cells. These antibodies bind to the high-affinity receptor (FcRI) on mast cells and basophils. This process is referred to as sensitization (Fig. 15.2).

Early phase response: On allergen reexposure, cross-linking of IgE-FcRI complexes facilitates degranulation of mast cells and basophils, which release preformed mediators, including histamine and enzymes (e.g. tryptase). There also is rapid de novo synthesis of other mediators, such as cysteinyl-leukotrienes (leukotriene C4, leukotriene D4, leukotriene E4) and prostaglandin D2 (PGD2). Histamine produces pruritus, rhinorrhoea, and sneezing, whereas leukotrienes and PGD2 are associated more with the development of nasal congestion. This process comprises the early or **immediate-phase response**.

Late phase response: Cytokines released during the immediate phase response mediate a cascade of events over the next 4–8 hours, referred to as the late-phase response.

Clinical symptoms in early and late responses are similar, but nasal congestion predominates in the late phase response (Fig. 15.2).

Mechanism (Fig. 15.2)

Clinical Features

Symptoms: The symptoms may be seasonal or perennial. All symptoms are simply a manifestation of the body's defense mechanism to the allergen.

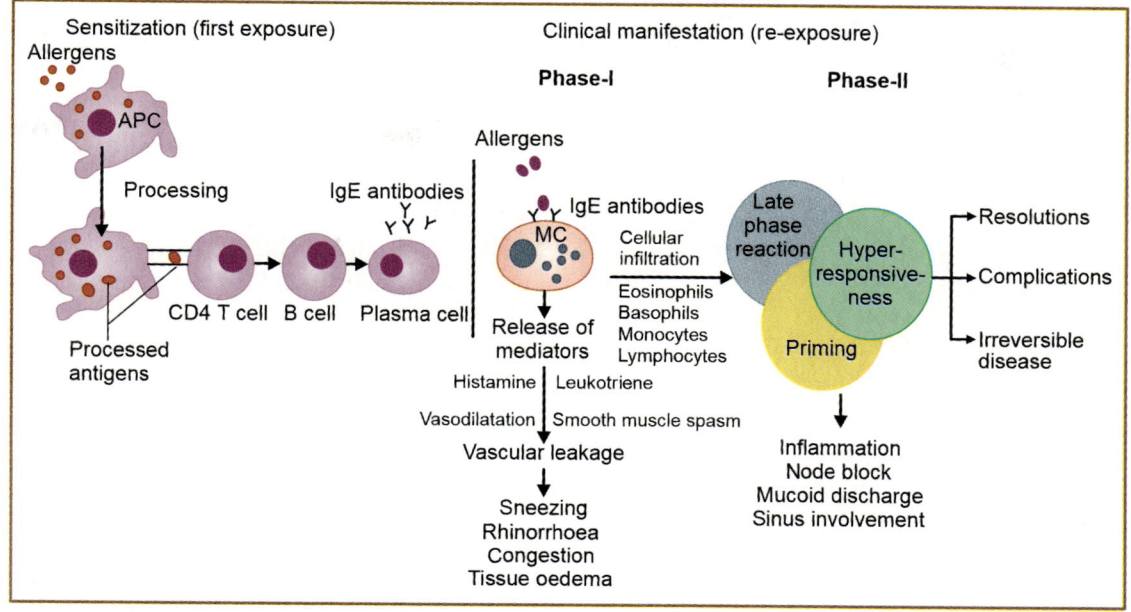

Fig. 15.2: Mechanism of allergic rhinitis, allergen sensitization (priming), APC (allergen presenting cell), MC (mast cell degranulation)

Classical: Mainly seen in seasonal allergic rhinitis. This includes paroxysmal bouts of sneezing, watery rhinorrhoea and nasal obstruction with itching of the nose on exposure to known or unknown allergen. This may be associated with non-nasal manifestations like watering and itching of the eyes, itching of the palate and skin and in some it may be associated with bronchospasm, which may be sub-clinical. Patient may complain of hyposmia or anosmia depending on the severity of the disease.

In perennial allergy, the symptoms are usually less severe and may present as recurrent cold or nasal stuffiness with sneezing and watery rhinorrhoea.

Signs
- Pale bluish oedematous nasal mucosa (Fig. 15.3)
- Bulky oedematous turbinates with bluish/purplish tinge of the mucosa
- Mucosa coated with clear/mucoid secretions
- In advanced cases, the mucosa of the middle turbinate may be polypoidal and

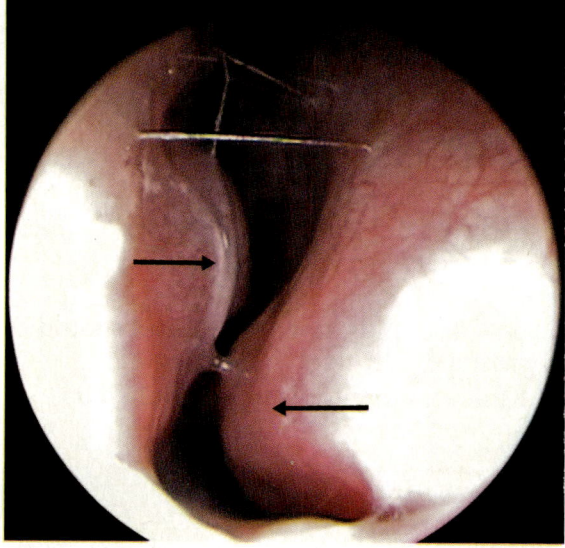

Fig. 15.3: Endoscopic picture showing the pale oedematous turbinates with septal spur coated with clear mucoid secretions [Turbinate (→), septal spur (←)]

frank polyposis may be seen in the middle meatus (Fig. 15.4).
- Septum may be thickened due to mucosal swelling.

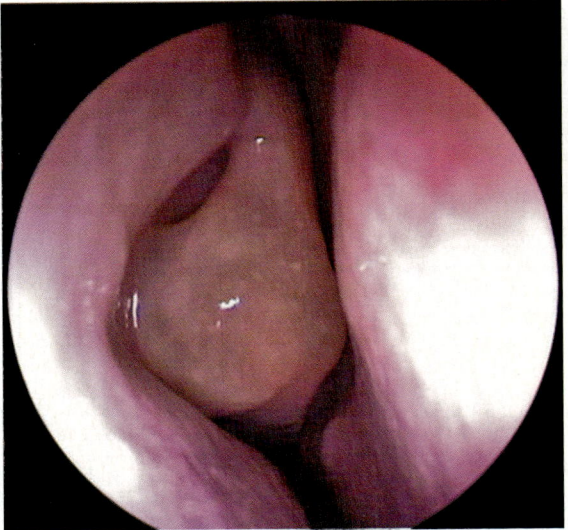

Fig. 15.4: Polypoidal changes of middle turbinate

Classical signs associated with allergic rhinitis
- Overriding maxillary incisors
- High arched palate
- Allergic shiners (Fig. 15.5)
- Allergic salute
- Transverse crease above the tip of nose and lower eyelids (Fig. 15.6).
- Conjunctival congestion
- Periorbital swelling.

Diagnosis

Patient with the following features should be considered allergic rhinitis.
- Recurrent upper respiratory infections

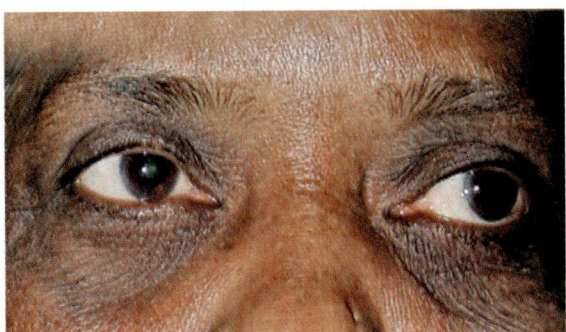

Fig. 15.5: Dark circle around the eyes (allergic shiners)

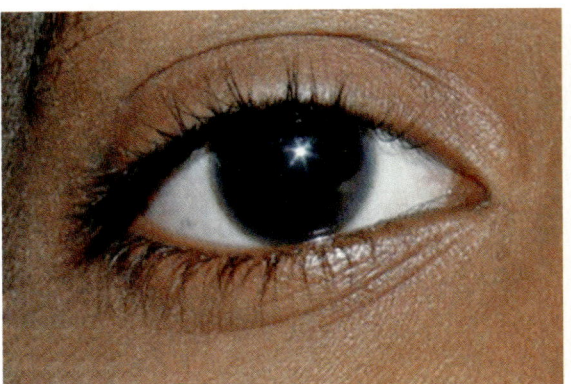

Fig. 15.6: Transverse crease below the lower eyelid

If a patient has the following features, he may be considered as having allergic rhinitis:
1. History of allergy in the family—atopy
2. Recurrent episodes of sneezing.
3. Throat irritation and dryness
4. Ear itching

Differential Diagnosis

1. Common cold
2. Vasomotor rhinitis
3. Chronic sinusitis
4. Rhinitis medicamentosa
5. Occupational rhinitis

Investigations

Nonspecific

Nasal smear for eosinophils
- Total WBC count and differential count
- Absolute eosinophil count
- Histamine test

Specific (Qualitative and quantitative tests)

1. *In vivo* tests (Smart, 1999)
- *Skin tests*
  - i. *Subcuticular test—prick/scratch test:* Skin prick test detects sensitization and indicates the presence of specific IgE antibodies on the surface of sensitized mast cells. This is the most popular, practical and safe test. It may be used as a screening test (Bernstein, et al. 2008). This test is more readily reproducible, has lower incidence of

false positive results, is more accurate and has less risk of anaphylaxis. In this test, a drop of test extract solution (with histamine and saline as control) is placed on the unprepared skin of the medial aspect of forearm. Using a lancet at about 45° to the skin through the drop, the epidermis is pricked with a lifting motion. Care is taken not to penetrate the dermis. The area is examined after 10 minutes for histamine control and after 20 minutes for the allergen. Wheal response around the prick is measured in mm. A reaction is considered positive, if the wheal size is 3 mm more than the negative control (saline). A positive reaction indicated sensitization to that particular allergen. A patient can be sensitized while not being allergic. Hence, to determine if an individual is truly allergic to a particular allergen, the skin prick test results must be co-related with history. Anaphylactic reaction can occur while doing allergy test and it is necessary to have the emergency kit while doing allergy test (Fig. 15.7). The patient must be observed for swelling of lips, tongue, oropharynx, larynx, rashes over the entire body. The most important drug in the emergency kit is Inj. adrenaline, given as 1:1000 dilution 0.3 mg IM, and repeated after 5 min, in case of severe anaphylaxis. This can be life saving.

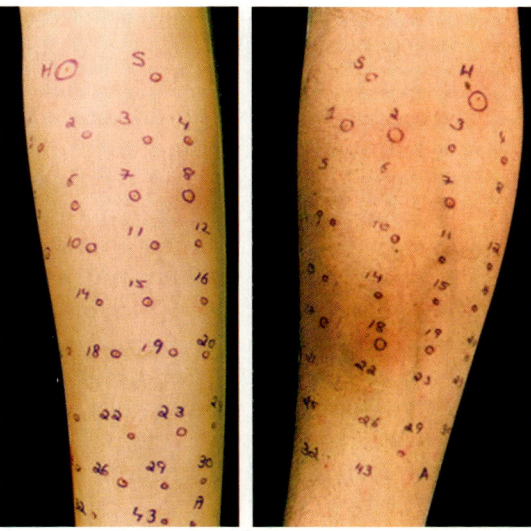

Fig. 15.8: Skin prick test: **a.** Wheal formation for histamine (H) of 8 mm and control saline (S) of 2 mm. Wheal formation is also seen in number 8—pollen ricinus communis, **b.** Wheal formation in number 2—house dust mite and number 18—Dog epithelia

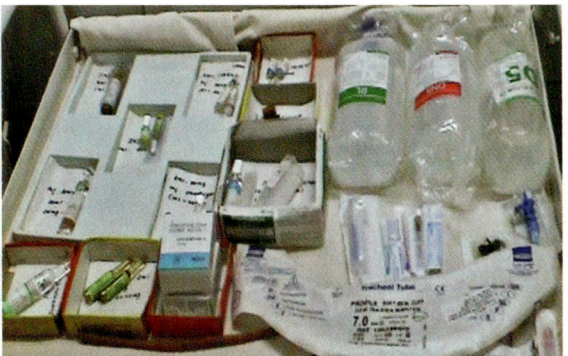

Fig. 15.7: Emergency kit consisting of injectable antihistamines like avil, Inj. adrenaline, endotracheal tube, saline infusion, etc.

The kit should also contain antihistamines, oral steroids, injectable steroids, intubation kit and a tracheostomy set. Prick test is contraindicated in cases with dermographism, patients on antihistamine and NSAID medications (Fig. 15.8).

ii. *Intradermal skin test:* This has higher chances of anaphylaxis and has to be done only with resuscitation drugs and equipment ready.

iii. *Serial skin end-point titration test:* This is a quantitative intradermal skin test for specific allergen. This test is done using a dilute and known concentration of an allergen, which is injected intradermally, and the response is noted. The dose is increased gradually intradermal skin test technique using 1:5 serial dilutions of allergenic extract. This technique is safe, reliable and is well standardized intradermal injections of 0.01 ml allergenic extract applied to the upper lateral arm. Wheal and flare beyond 5 mm suggest positive response. Maximal whealing occurs at

15 minutes. The end-point is defined as the antigen dilution which yields a wheal at least 2 mm larger than the preceding negative wheal, and which is followed by a wheal at the next stronger dilution. The confirming wheal is important for determining the true end-point. This test is not very popular due to its unreliability and is less sensitive than skin prick test.

iv. *Nasal challenge (nasal provocation) test:* Not a very popular test due to potential risks of anaphylaxis and has limited clinical applications. The test dose is delivered in a nebulizer using a specific allergen.

v. *Nasal cytology:* It can be done using a dry wipe technique without surface anaesthesia. The specimen is applied to the slide with a firm rolling action. The smear is fixed immediately with 95% alcohol and is stained with Wright-Giemsa stain. Following cell types are noted.
- Eosinophils
- Mast cells/basophils/both
- Epithelial cells
- Lymphocytes
- Neutrophils
- Goblet cells

In allergy, patients have increased eosinophils of more than 10%.

2. *In vitro* tests (Smart, 1999)

i. *Radioallergosorbent test (RAST):* This is very useful test especially in case with dermographism. This is less sensitive than skin prick test but is more expensive. While skin prick test detects specific IgE bound to mast cell, RAST detects free IgE in the blood. The amount of specific IgE produced to a particular allergen approximately correlates with the allergic sensitivity to that substance. These tests allow determination of specific IgE to a number of different allergens from one blood sample, but the sensitivity and specificity are not always as good as accurate skin testing (depending on the laboratory and assay used for the RAST). As with skin testing, virtually all of the allergens that cause allergic rhinitis can be determined using the RAST, although testing for some allergens is less well established compared to others.

ii. *Fluoroallergosorbent test (FAST):* The fluoroallergosorbent test (FAST) is similar to the ELISA, except for the use of a fluorogenic substrate which produces fluorescence that can be read with a fluorometer. The test procedure can be completed in 6 hours. There is good correlation with skin prick test and RAST against aeroallergens. An automated version of the FAST, the CAP system is now available. It is claimed that its sensitivity and specificity are better than RAST. Being automated, it has a faster turnaround time and is less demanding on human resources. Results are expressed in kilo units per liter which is advantageous for comparison with other techniques (Seltzer, et al, 1989).

iii. *MAST CLA:* The multiple allergosorbent test chemiluminescent assays (MAST CLA) have shown good correlation with skin prick test and RAST against several aeroallergens. In this assay, allergens are coated onto threads. It performs simultaneous determination of total IgE and 35 allergen specific IgE in serum (Scolozzi, 1998).

iv. Paper immunoallegrosorbant test (PRIST) is a recognized effective test for the determination of serum concentration of IgE antibody.

Other Tests

These are done to rule out associated sinus pathology and polyposis.
a. X-ray PNS
b. CT OMC
c. Diagnostic nasal endoscopy

TREATMENT OF ALLERGIC RHINITIS

The goals of treatment for allergic rhinitis are to provide a complete symptomatic relief to the patient with improved quality of life while minimizing the adverse effects (Panigrahi & Acharya 2016).

Therapeutic Goals

These include medical line of management with short-, medium- and long-term goals.

1. Short-term relief that usually helps within days (medication).
2. Medium-term measures to reduce reliance on medication (allergen avoidance, if possible).
3. Long-term options including immuno-therapy, particularly if medication is poorly tolerated or ineffective and allergen avoidance is difficult.

Medical

Avoidance of Allergen

This is ideal but is not always possible. Some of the known allergens can be avoided, like paper dust, house dust, animal dander, etc. by avoiding pets, washing curtains regularly, keeping less articles in the living room, changing bed sheets and pillow covers frequently, use of ironed bed sheets, pillow covers before use and washing it in hot water, drying it in the sun (kills dust mite). Use of mask/nasal filters air purifier with HEPA filter (high efficiency particulate air) while cleaning the house, prefer vacuum cleaning or wet mopping to dry mopping, avoidance of carpets, etc. will also control most of the aeroallergens effectively. Seasonal and environmental allergen can be avoided to certain extent by knowing and avoiding the aerobiological flora of that particular environment. Allergy skin tests may be useful in identifying the allergens.

Pharmacotherapy

a. *Antihistamines:* This is the mainstay of treatment for allergic rhinitis, when avoidance of allergens is not possible. It is most preferred during the acute attack. These are basically H-1 receptor antagonists and block the effect of histamine on the receptors. Various antihistamines are available and the recent ones like fexo-fenadine, loratidine, rupatidine levo-cetrizine, etc., have faster onset of action, longer duration and with less side effects like sedation and cardiovascular changes and anticholinergic effects. Antihistamine nasal sprays and eye drop—antihistamines like azelastine (Azep) can be used as a nasal spray with no long-term side effects. It acts rapidly (within minutes) to relieve sneezing or itching and are generally well tolerated. In general, they are less effective at relieving severe nasal congestion.

TAK-427 is a long-acting antihistamine in Guinea pigs, which suppresses acute phase of allergic reactions and may have a long-lasting antihistamine activity with minimum sedative side effect (Fukuda, et al. 2003).

b. *Steroids:* Intransal corticosteroids act by inhibiting the inflammatory reaction. Steroid nasal sprays like beclomethasone, budesonide, fluticasone, mometasone, etc. are particularly useful as they have lesser side effects and may be used for longer period. Reduction in middle meatal oedema may facilitate drainage of the sinus secretions.

c. *Anticholinergic sprays:* Ipratopium bromide nasal spray is very effective in reducing watery rhinorrhoea.

d. *Sodium chromoglycate:* Mast cell stabilizing nasal sprays or eye drops (e.g. Ifiral/Fintal) reduce inflammation by stabilizing the mast cells and preventing its degranulation. It is available as nasal drops or nasal spray for allergic rhinitis/eye drops for allergic conjunctivitis. This is mainly used for prophylaxis and, therefore, should be used regularly and before the attack.

e. *Decongestants:* They are useful to reduce nasal obstruction and mucosal oedema and rhinorrhoea. Oral preparations are available with antihistamines. Long-term use of topical decongestants is best avoided as they can cause rhinitis medicamentosa and should not be given for more than 4–5 days. Oral preparations include pseudo-ephedrine hydrochloride, phenylephrine hydrochloride, etc. Topical decongestants include oxymetazoline, xylometazoline, ephedrine in saline, etc.

f. *Saline irrigation of the nasal cavities:* Help in removing secretions and prevent secondary infection.

g. *Antileukotrienes:* They include montelukast, zafirlukast—leukotriene receptor antagonists and zileuton—leukotriene synthesis inhibitor. They are viable alternative to antihistamine in treating seasonal allergic rhinitis but less than intranasal corticosteroids (Lagos & Marshall 2007). Nasal obstruction is currently thought to be closely related to the presence and abundance of lipid mediators, such as leukotriene and thromboxane (TX) A2. The novel drug **ramatroban**, a TXA2 receptor antagonist, has been demonstrated, in clinical trials, to improve nasal obstruction in the treatment of patients with allergic rhinitis and it has recently become commercially available. **Ramatroban** suppresses the secretion of chemical mediators in nasal mucosa that are thought to be involved in the allergic reaction in patients with perennial allergic rhinitis (Ohkubo, 2003).

Immunotherapy (Desensitization)

Allergen immunotherapy (AIT) is the only disease-modifying treatment option besides allergen avoidance (Klimek, et al. 2017). It is the closest thing to a cure for allergic rhinitis. The role of immunotherapy is limited especially in case of multiple allergens. However, people with allergy to limited number of allergens may find it useful. The unique aspect of allergy immunotherapy is the capacity to modify the natural course of disease by inducing long-term immunological tolerance (Larcen, et al 2016). Immunotherapy is often recommended for treatment of allergic rhinitis (and sometimes asthma) when:

- Symptoms are severe.
- The cause is difficult to avoid (e.g. grass pollen).
- Medications are unhelpful or cause adverse side effects; and patients need medication most days.

It is effective only in about 40% of cases and involves the administration of gradually increasing amounts of allergic material, usually given to patients by injection or sublingually over a period of years. It is administered by giving subcutaneous injections in diluted form at weekly intervals. The dose is gradually increased. RAST/skin end-point titration based immunotherapy is more effective since the quantitative analysis can be done and the patient can receive higher dose without the fear of anaphylaxis. Hence, they get an early response. Immunotherapy helps in reducing the specific serum IgE level and a decrease in basophil sensitivity and increase in IgG blocking antibody level which helps in preventing the allergen from reaching the mast cells and thus preventing their degranulation. The proper selection of allergen extracts is important in maintaining an efficient allergy practice. The selection of tree, grass, and weed pollen extracts depends very much on where the clinician's practice is located (aerobiological flora).

Sublingual immunotherapy is gaining popularity in recent days and has the distinct advantages over subcutaneous immunotherapy. It can be administered safely with less risk of anaphylaxis than subcutaneous immunotherapy (Calderon, et al 2011).

Allergen extracts given sublingually are primarily taken up by the dendritic cells in the mucosa and are presented to T cells in the draining lymph nodes. Likely mechanisms of action include activation of T regulatory cells and down regulation of mucosal mast cells. Allergenic proteins that reach the small intestine are processed through columnar mucosal cells and are presented to T lymphocytes within Peer's patches. Changes in the humoral responses to allergens are seen with this technique are 'increased allergen specific IgG4' production under the control of IL-10. There is blunting of seasonal increases in allergen specific IgE. The CD8+ T cells are increased and there is a decrease in the CD4:CD8 T cell ratio. In contrast to the subcutaneous immunotherapy, the IgG level decreases in sublingual immunotherapy and is safer and comfortable for patient. It can be taken by the patient himself at home after proper advice. The initial administration needs to be supervised as there is possibility of anaphylactic reaction (Bufe, et al. 2009, de Goot and Bijl, 2009).

Local nasal immunotherapy is an alternative form of mucosal immunotherapy and its ability to reduce rhinitis symptoms and medication usage, as well as to decrease nasal reactivity towards offending allergen has been well established (Meheta and Smith 1975, Motta, et al. 2000). Nasal immunotherapy with single allergen (aqueous mixed weed) extract administered with cromolyn sodium pre-treatment for 17 to 21 weeks was effective in reducing both nasal and ocular symptoms of weed pollen-induced allergic rhinitis (Gaglani, et al. 1997).

Role of omalizumab: Omalizumab is a molecularly cloned humanized monoclonal antibody inhibiting human IgE. It binds specifically to the region of the IgE molecule that binds to the IgE receptor on the mast cell or basophils. Studies have shown that omalizumab is effective in the treatment of seasonal allergic rhinitis (Casale, et al. 2001). The anti-inflammatory effects of omalizumab at different sites of allergic inflammation and the clinical benefits of anti-IgE therapy in patients with allergic asthma and allergic

rhinitis emphasize the fundamental importance of IgE in allergic inflammation (Holgate & Casale, et al. 2005).

ARIA guidelines for management of nasal allergy (Flowchart 15.2): Appropriate selection of pharmacotherapy is most essential for treating allergic rhinitis to control disease while considering various factors to manage. Grading of Recommendations Assessment, Development and Evaluation (GRADE) guidelines have considerably improved the treatment of allergic rhinitis. The revised ARIA guideline has been proposed with an algorithm for allergic rhinitis by an expert group to classify allergic rhinitis treatments (Courbis 2018) is depicted in Table 15.1.

ARIA in 2016 recomended a revised guideline for management of allergic rhinitis which includes (Brozek et al 2017):

1. In patients with seasonal allergic rhinitis, either a combination of intranasal cortico-steroids (INCS) + Oral antihistamine (OAH) or INCS alone, can be given

2. In patients with perennial allergic rhinitis, INCSs alone are recommended rather than a combination of an INCS + an OAH.

3. In patients with seasonal allergic rhinitis, either a combination of an intranasal corticosteroids + an intranasal antihistamine or an intranasal corticosteroid alone

Flowchart 15.2: ARIA guidelines for alleric rhinitis management (Todorova, et al 2014)

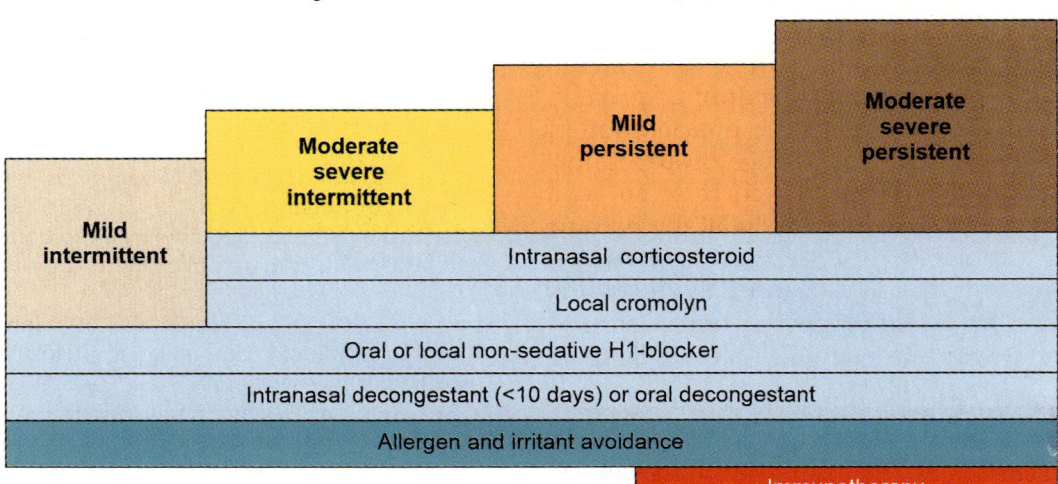

Table 15.1: Classification of treatment used in allergic rhinitis

T1	Nonsedating H1-antihistamine (oral, intranasal, and ocular), leukotriene receptor antagonists, or cromones (intranasal and ocular)
T2	Intranasal corticosteroids (INCSs)
T3	INCSs + intranasal azelastine
T4	Oral corticosteroid as a short course and an add-on treatment
T5	Consider referral to a specialist and allergen immunotherapy

may be given, based on patient's preference. At initiation of treatment (first 2 weeks), a combination of an INCS + an INAH might act faster than an INCS alone and might, therefore, be preferred by some patients. In settings in which the additional cost of combination therapy is not large, a combination therapy might be a reasonable choice.

4. In patients with Perennial allergic rhinitis, either a combination of an INCS + an INAH or an INCS alone can be given.

Surgical Management

Role of surgery is limited to reduction of the size of the turbinate, correction of septal deviation and limited endoscopic sinus surgery, if sinuses are involved. The inferior and the middle turbinate are trimmed by inferolateral partial resection using microdebrider or turbinectomy scissors or microdebrider assisted turbinoplasty. Septal deviation should ideally be dealt with limited ultraconservative endoscopic approach. Limited sinus surgery with preservation of uncinate process may reduce postoperative postnasal discharge, which is often seen following traditional functional endoscopic sinus surgery (FESS) for allergy associated chronic sinusitis (Nayak, et al. 2001) including polyposis. Antiallergy treatment should continue even after surgical intervention.

BIBLIOGRAPHY

1. Bernstein IL, Li JT, Bernstein DI, Hamilton R, Spector SL, Tan R, et al. Allergy diagnostic testing: An updated practice parameter. Ann Allergy Asthma Immunol 2008; 100:S1–148.
2. Bousquet J, Khaltaev N, Cruz AA, et al. Allergic rhinitis and its impact on asthma (ARIA) 2008 update (in collaboration with the World Health Organization, GA(2)LEN and AllerGen). Allergy. 2008;63 (Suppl 86):8–160.
3. Brozek JL, Bousquet J, Agache I, et al. Allergic Rhinitis and its Impact on Asthma (ARIA) guidelines—2016 revision. J Allergy Clin Immunol 2017;140:pp. 950–58.
4. Bufe, et al. Safety and efficacy in children of an SQ-standardized grass allergen tablet for sublingual immunotherapy. J Allergy Clin Immunology 2009, 123(1):167.
5. Calderon MA, et al. Allergen-specific immunotherapy for respiratory allergies: From meta-analysis to registration and beyond. J Allergy Clin Immunol 2011 Jan;127(1):30–38.
6. Casale T. Anti-IgE (omalizuman) therapy in seasonal allergic rhinitis. Am J Resp Crit Care Med 2001; 164:1821.
7. Courbis AL, Murray RB, Arnavielhe SD, et al. Electronic Clinical Decision Support System for allergic rhinitis management: MASK e-CDSS. Clin Exp Allergy, 48 (2018), pp. 1640–53.
8. Crimi E, Brusasco V, Crimi P, Brancatisano M, Bregante A. The fluoro-allergosorbent test: A comparison with RAST and skin test in respiratory allergy. Ann Allergy 1988;61:371–4.
9. de Groot H, Bijl A. Anaphylactic reaction after 1st dose of sublingual immunotherapy tablet. Allergy 2009; 64(6):963.
10. Dzul AI. Selecting allergenic extracts for inhalant allergy testing and immunotherapy. Otolaryngol Clin North Am 1998; Feb; 31(1):11–25.
11. Fukuda S. et al. Characteristics of the antihistamine effect of TAK-427, a novel imidazopyridazine derivative. Inflm Res 2003; May; 52(5):206–14.

12. Gaglani B, et al. Nasal immunotherapy in weed-induced allergic rhinitis. Ann Allergy Asthma Immunol 1997 Sep; 79(3):259–65.

13. Holgate S, Casale T, et al. The antihistaminic effect of Omalizumab confirm the central role in allergic rhinitis, J Allerg Clin Immunology 2005; March: 115(3):459–65.

14. Klimek L, et al. Allergen immunotherapy in allergic rhinitis: current use and future trends. Expert Rev Clin Immunol 2017 Sep;13(9):897–906.

15. Lagos JA, Marshall GD. Montelukast in the management of allergic rhinitis. Ther Clin Risk Manag 2007 Jun; 3(2): 327–32.

16. Larcen JN,Broge L, Jacobi H. Allergy immunotherapy-the future of allergy treatment. Drug Discovery Today, 2016;21(1):26–37.

17. Min YG. The Pathophysiology, diagnosis and treatment of allergic rhinitis. Allergy Asthma Immunol Res 2010 Apr; 2(2): 65–76.

18. Meheta SB, Smith JM. Nasal hyposensitization and hay fever. Clin and Experimental Allergy 1975; 5:279–86.

19. Motta G, et al. A multicenter trial of specific local nasal immunotherapy. Laryngoscope 2000 Jan; 110(1):132–39.

20. Nayak DR, Balakrishnan R, Murty KD. Endoscopic physiologic approach to allergy associated chronic rhinosinusitis: A Preliminary study. ENT Journal 2001 June; 80(6): 392–403.

21. Nayak DR, Balakrishnan R, Murty KD. Functional anatomy of the uncinate process and its role in endoscopic sinus surgery. Indian Journal of Otolaryngology and Head and Neck Surgery 2001; Jan, 53(1): 27–31.

22. Ohkubo K, Gotoh M. Effect of ramatroban, a thromboxane A2 antagonist, in the treatment of perennial allergic rhinitis. Allergology International (2003)52:131–138.

23. Panigrahi R, Acharya SK. Recent trends in the management of allergic rhinitis. Clinical Rhinology 2016; 9(3):130–36.

24. Scolozzi R, Boccafogh A, Vicentini L, Baraldi A, Bagni B. Correlation of MAST Chemiluminescent assay (CLA) with RAST and skin prick tests for diagnosis of inhalent allergic disease. Ann Allergy 1998; 62: 193 a–b.

25. Seltzer JM, Georges M, Halpern M, Tasy YG. Correlation of allergy test results obtained by IgE FAST, RAST and prick-puncture method. Ann Allergy 1989; 1985; 54: 25–30.

26. Small P, Frenkiel S, Becker A, et al. The Canadian Rhinitis Working Group. Rhinitis: a practical and comprehensive approach to assessment and therapy. J Otolaryngol 2007; 36(Suppl 1):S5–27.

27. Smart BA. Allergy testing using in vivo and in vitro techniques. Immunol Allerg Clin North Am 1999; 19(1): 35–45.

28. Todorova A, Tsvetkova A, Dimitrov D, et al. Script Scientfic a Pharmaceutica, 2014. DOI:10. 14748/ssp.v1i2.779

29. Varghese B, Murthy PSN, Rajan R, Nayak DR, Hazarika P, Murty KD, Mathew KJ. "Nasobronchial relationship: a controversial entity?". Kerala Journal of ENT, 1995; 3(3); 6–12. 18.

30. Yadav A, Verma J. Singh Study on Nasal Mucous Clearance in Patients of Perennial Allergic Rhinitis. Indian J Allergy Asthma Immunol 2003; 17(2):89–91.

16

Transnasal Endoscopic Balloon Sinuplasty

DR Nayak

Inflammatory disease of the paranasal sinuses is a common problem that affects millions of people. Functional endoscopic sinus surgery is one of the most accepted modalities of surgical treatment for patients who have failed to respond to medical therapy. Over the past 20 years, many patients have benefited from endoscopic sinus surgery.[2] The objective of the functional endoscopic surgery (FES), although it has been discussed by some authors, is to increase the ventilation and draining of the paranasal sinuses involved and allow the return of adequate functioning of the muco-ciliary movements of the nasal mucosa. Many of these patients treated surgically respond poorly to extensive endoscopic surgery and could be benefited with less invasive methods, with major preservation of the nasal mucosa.[1,2] Nayak and collaborators proposed the physiological endoscopic approach, with conservation of the nasal mucosa and the uncinate process in the surgical management of patients with chronic rhinosinusitis associated with allergic symptoms.[1]

Balloon sinuplasty is a new medical procedure which uses a balloon catheter system to dilate ostium of various major paranasal sinuses, similar to the technique used in angioplasty instead of instruments such as microdebriders and forceps. It is currently used in the maxillary, frontal and sphenoid sinuses.[3] Balloon sinuplasty technology was developed by Acclarent, Inc., and was brought to the market in 2005, after FDA approval. This procedure involves the dilation of the desired region, which may lead to 16 atmospheres pressure in the balloon, producing local microfractures that end up remodelling the anatomy, dilates the ostia and allows a PNS normal aeration without, however, the removal of the tissues and damage to the nasal mucosa. This makes the procedure less invasive than a classical functional endoscopic sinus surgery.[3,4] Excellent results were seen on long-term follow-up following balloon sinuplasty.[9]

BALLOON SINUPLASTY TECHNIQUE

Using a sinus guide catheter and an ultra-flexible guidewire the targeted sinus is entered (Fig. 16.1). After confirming with C-arm/Relieva Luma system, the sinus balloon catheter is advanced over the sinus guidewire (Fig. 16.2). The balloon is placed at the site of obstruction/stenosed ostium.

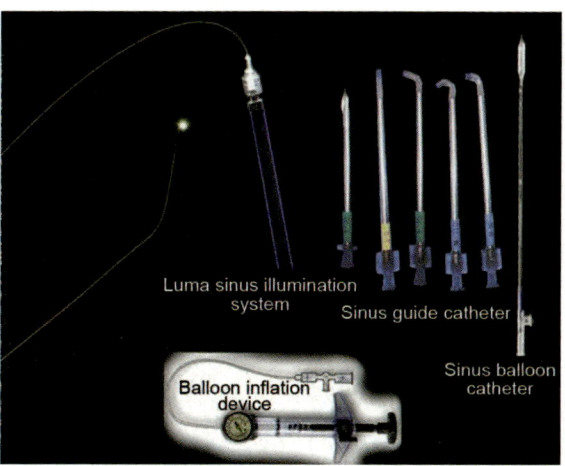

Fig. 16.1: Acclarent balloon sinuplasty system

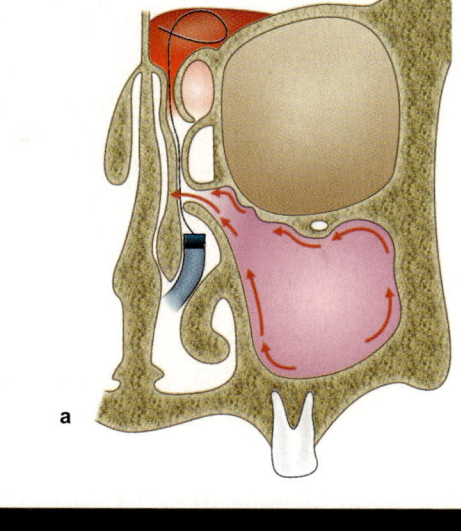

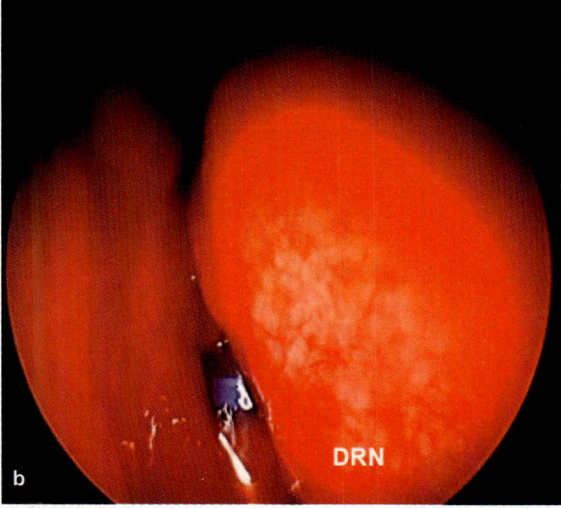

Fig. 16.2: a. Frontal sinus guidewire being passed into the frontal sinus, **b.** After confirmation of guidewire being passed into the frontal sinus by Relieva Luma system, sinus balloon catheter is advanced over the guidewire

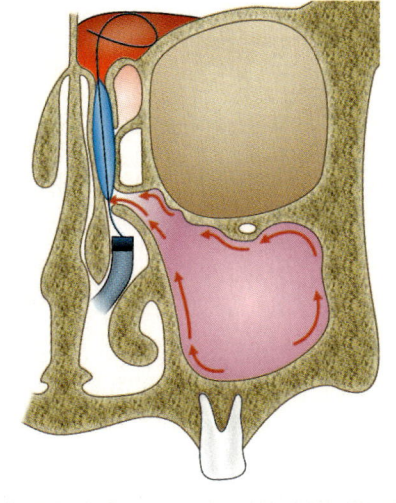

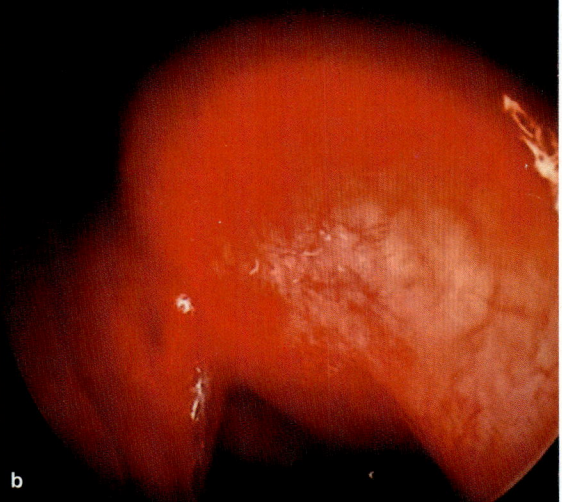

Fig. 16.3: a. Balloon catheter is dilated after placing at the site of narrow frontal recess and ostium, **b.** The inflated balloon after dilatation of the frontal recess

Balloon sinuplasty for frontal sinus: A 70° sinus guide catheter is used for frontal sinus. The passage of Relieva sinus guidewire is confirmed by the glow seen over the frontal sinus. Then the sinus balloon catheter is advanced gently.

Once the position of the sinus balloon catheter is confirmed, the balloon is gradually inflated with saline (8–10 atmospheres) to open and remodel the narrowed or blocked ostium (Fig. 16.3). The balloon catheter is then deflated and withdrawn (Fig. 16.4) and instead an irrigation catheter is advanced over the guidewire into the affected sinus to irrigate and flush out the tenacious sinus secretions accumulated within. Irrigation catheter is then removed from the targeted sinus (Fig. 16.5). The first author of this book (DRN) prefers to place a small elongated piece of NasoPore (bio-degradable synthetic polyurethane foam) soaked with povidone-iodine solution along with triamcinolone which does not require

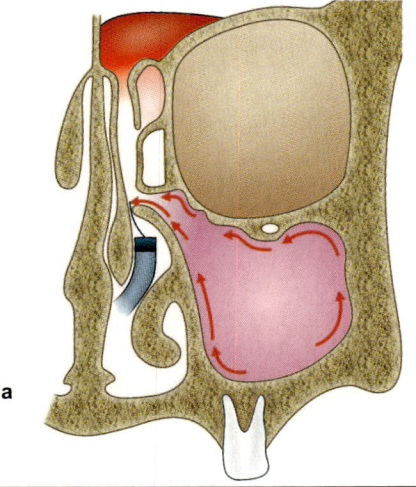

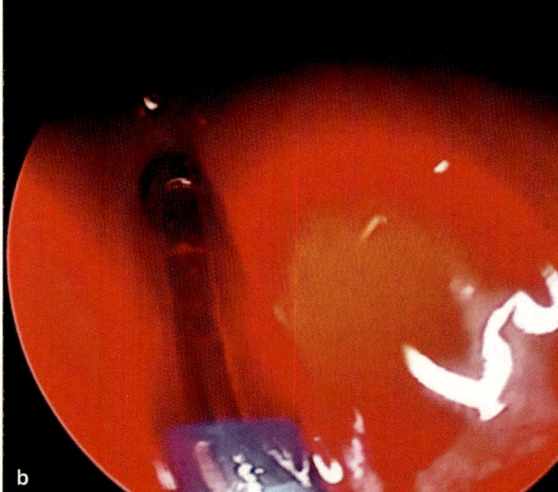

Fig. 16.4: a. Balloon catheter being withdrawn after dilatation, **b.** The cannula being passed to irrigate the frontal sinus after dilatation

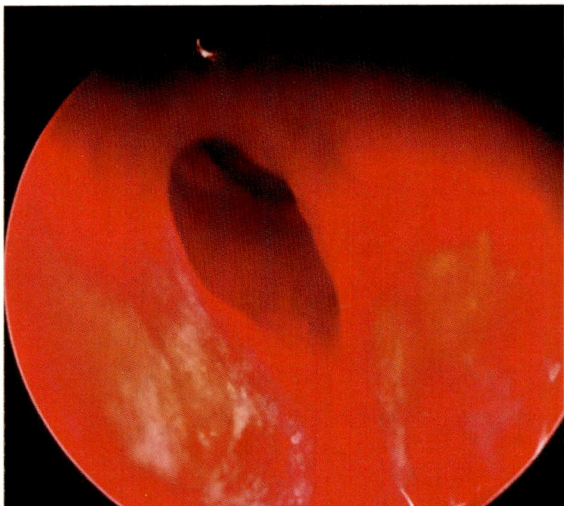

Fig. 16.5: The frontal recess and frontal sinus ostium after balloon dilatation

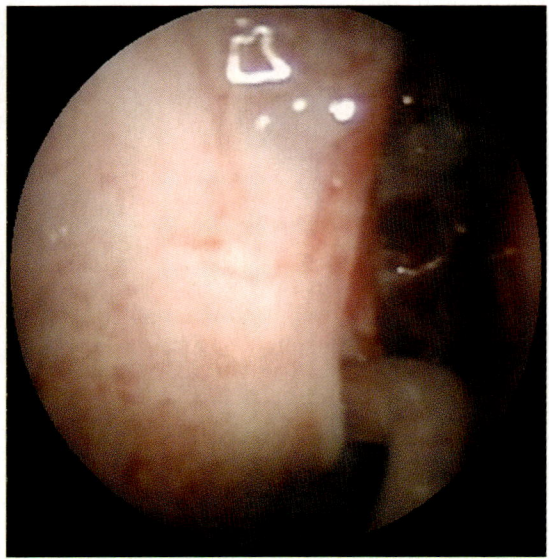

Fig. 16.6: 110° guide catheter being kept near inferior part of hiatus semilunaris close to maxillary ostium

removal and gets absorbed with the course of time. It provides excellent anti-inflammatory action and relieves oedema around the ostium.

Balloon sinuplasty of maxillary sinus: The initial procedure is same as described under frontal sinusitis. A 110° guide catheter is passed instead of 70° used for frontal sinus (Fig. 16.7) and the tip of is directed inferiorly and laterally towards the hiatus semilunaris.

Through this, Luma guidewire is passed gently into the maxillary sinus through the maxillary ostium without resistance. Repeated attempt is made to pass, if there is resistance. If one faces difficulties in passing, a partial uncinectomy can be done to facilitate smooth passage of guidewire (Nishioka 2018). Once Luma guidewire is passed successfully confirmed by glow over canine fossa/check, the balloon catheter is passed gently till it is in the midway of maxillary ostium (Fig. 16.7) and is dilated with saline till 10.0 atmospheric pressure. As the balloon is dilated, the uncinate process is bulged out (Fig. 16.7).

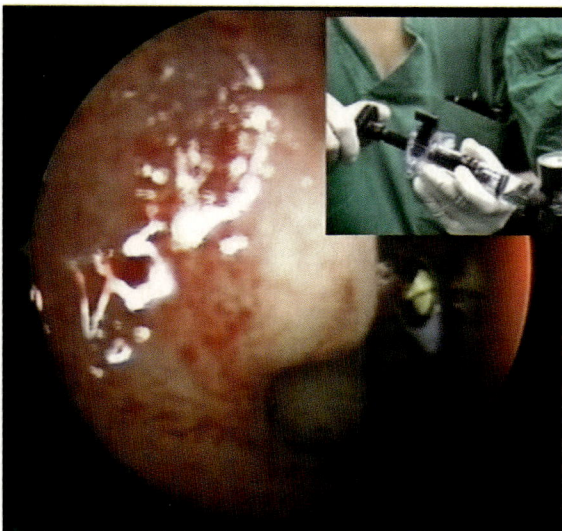

Fig. 16.7: Balloon is dilated at the maxillary ostium using inflation device. Note the bulging of the inferior part of the uncinate process, confirming the correct position

The balloon catheter is withdrawn sently followed by the guide wire and the sinus catheter. The sinus cavity is then inspected and any secretions present can be sent for culture and then can be irrigated (Fig. 16.8).

Balloon sinuplasty for sphenoid sinus: The procedure is similar except the use of a 0° guide catheter (*see* Fig. 4.4d).

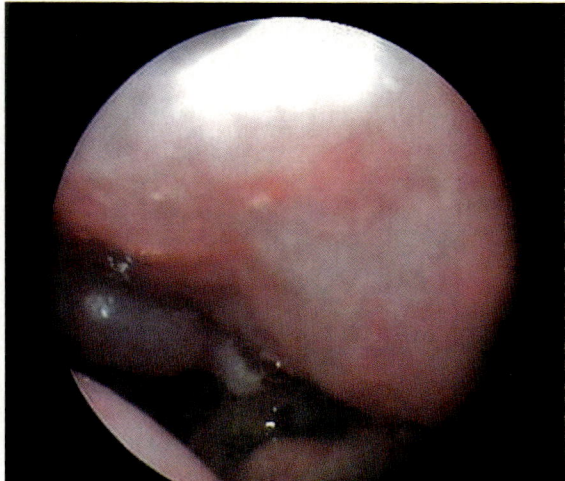

Fig. 16.8: Dilated maxillary ostium, through which secretions can be seen in the maxillary sinus cavity being sucked out.

Advantages

- Safe and effective
- Less invasive
- Minimal bleeding
- Early recovery
- Revision possible
- Short hospital stay/office based procedure.

Disadvantages

- Disposable catheter and balloon
- Expensive
- Long-term results have yet to be ascertained
- Not effective in cases of extensive polyposis/allergic fungal sinusitis.

Complications

The potential complications include CSF leak, orbital injury, turbinate lateralization.[7,8,10] Levine and Rabago on an examination of adverse events during a post-marketing assessment of balloon sinuplasty identified a total of 3 major complications among 28,500 patients, with a total of >85000 treated sinuses.[8] Balloon sinuplasty although is considered to be a safe technique, in an inexperienced hands or wrongly applied, complications may occur, as with any surgical tool rigid enough to breach through skull base.[7] No serious adverse events or complications were reported between one year and two years in the 65 study patients.[9] If fluoroscopy is used, the risk of radiation exposure should be kept in mind, especially to the lens leading to lenticular opacity (Chandra 2007).

BIBLIOGRAPHY

1. Brown CL, Bolger WC. Safety and feasibility of balloon catheter dilation of paranasal sinus ostia: A preliminary investigation. Ann Otol Rhino Laryngol 2006;115:293–99.
2. Bolger WE, Brown CL, Church CA, Goldberg AN, Karanfilov B, Kuhn FA, et al. Safety and outcomes of balloon catheter sinusotomy: A multicenter 24-week analysis in 115 patients. Otolaryngol Head Neck Surg 2007, 137:10–20.
3. Chandra RK. Estimate of radiation dose to the lens in balloon sinuplasty. Otolaryngol Head Neck Surg 2007; 137(6):953–55.

4. Howard Levine, David Rabago. Postgraduate Medicine 2011; 123(2):112–18.

5. Joao Flavio Nogueira Junior, Maria Laura Solferini Silva, Fabio Pires Santos, Aldo Cassol Stamm. Balloon sinuplasty: A new concept in the endoscopic nasal surgery. Intl Arch Otorhinolaryngol São Paulo 2008; v.12, n.4, pp 538–45.

6. Levine HL, Sertich AP 2nd, Hoisington DR, Weiss RL, Pritikin J. Multicenter registry of balloon catheter sinusotomy outcomes for 1,036 patients. Ann Otol Rhinol Laryngol 2008, 117(4):263–70.

7. Nayak DR, Balakrishnan R, Murty KD. Endoscopic physiologic approach to allergy-associated chronic rhinosinusitis: A preliminary study. Ear Nose Throat J 2001, 80:390–403.

8. Nishioka GJ. Modified in-office maxillary balloon sinus dilation for post-procedure sinus monitoring and access. Int Arch Otorhinolaryngol 2018 Jan;22(1):68–72.

9. Raymond L Weiss, Christopher A. Church Frederick A. Kuhn, Howard L. Levine, Michael J. Sillers, and Winston C Vaughan. Long-term outcome analysis of balloon catheter sinusotomy: Two-year follow-up. Otolaryngology—Head and Neck Surgery 2008; 139, S38–S46.

10. Tomazic PV, Stammberger H, Koele W, Gerstnberer C. Ethmoid roof CSF leak following frontal sinus balloon plasty Rhinology. 2010 June; 48(2):247–50.

Chapter 17

Transnasal Endoscopic Repair of the CSF Rhinorrhoea

DR Nayak, P Hazarika

Definition: Leakage of cerebrospinal fluid (CSF) from a fistula between the dura and the skull base leading to discharge of CSF from the nose. Dandy in 1926 was the first person to perform a surgical repair of CSF leak by a frontal craniotomy. Wigand in 1981 used the endoscope to assist the repair of a skull base defect with CSF rhinorrhoea. In the last three decades, endoscopic repair has become the preferred method to deal with CSF rhinorrhoea.

ANATOMICAL CLASSIFICATION

- Frontal sinus
- Ethmoid sinus
- Cribriform plate
- Sphenoid sinus
- Paradoxical (eustachian tube)

Etiology

Can be classified as traumatic or non-traumatic.

Traumatic

Majority of the cases of CSF rhinorrhoea occur as a result of trauma and the incidence can vary from 80–90%. The commonest sites of CSF leak following trauma are anterior cranial fossa floor (cribriform plate and fovea ethmoidalis) and the posterior wall of the frontal sinus (Iffenecker, et al. 1999).

- **Non-surgical:** This is the most common cause of CSF rhinorrhoea and is usually associated with closed head trauma that may present with an immediate or delayed onset.

- *Surgical:* CSF leak commonly occurs following endoscopic surgery of the nose and paranasal sinus or major skull base surgery involving anterior cranial fossa for tumour removal or inflammatory disease. Although the incidence of CSF leak following endoscopic sinus surgery is less than 2%, it is still one of the most common causes of CSF leak (Brodie 1997). This can be present with immediate or delayed onset. The common sites being fovea ethmoidalis and lateral cribriform lamella.

Non-Traumatic

A. **High pressure:** Conditions that increase the ventricular pressure can cause CSF rhinorrhoea.
  - **Tumour**
    - Direct infiltration of dura
    - Indirectly due to raised intracranial tension
  - **Hydrocephalus**

B. *Normal pressure*
  - **Congenital:** Spontaneous CSF leak can be associated with congenital bony dehiscence with prolapse of arachnoid granulations. This can be associated with meningoceles or meningoencephaloceles.
  - **Focal atrophy of the dura** at the cranial defect may lead to CSF leak.
  - **Osteomyelitic erosion**
  - **Idiopathic:** This occurs due to **spontaneous rupture** of the meningeal dura and fistula formation due to pre-existing

intracranial problem. The term idiopathic although used for unexplained CSF leak, in reality are secondary to raised CSF pressure of varied intracranial causes. Rarely arachnoid granulations along the cribriform plate can cause spontaneous leak.

CLINICAL FEATURES

Recurrent clear and nonsticky watery fluid draining from nose, often unilateral is the frequent presenting symptom. Any such case of unilateral watery rhinorrhoea should be investigated thoroughly and should be suspected for CSF leak and should never be treated with steroid nasal spray till the diagnosis is established. Hyposmia/anosmia are associated with 60–80% of cases. Headache is seen in 20% of cases and associated meningitis or raised intracranial pressure should be ruled out. Recurrent meningitis may be associated with CSF leak and will always present with classical features including fever. Wet handkerchief from nasal secretions that fails to dry without stiffening should be suspected for CSF leak (Handkerchief test).

INVESTIGATIONS

1. *Testing of nasal secretions:*
   a. Beta 2 transferrin assay: It is a highly sensitive test as beta 2 transferrin is only found in CSF, perilymph and the aqueous humour.
   b. Glucose protein determination is a highly unreliable but rapid test.
   c. Beta-trace protein is not a very specific test

2. *Diagnostic nasal endoscopy:* It is one of the useful investigations that may help in identifying the site of the leak in certain cases, and particularly post-surgical cases but in general, has a very limited role in diagnosis of the majority of the cases. Injection of intrathecal fluorescein has been used to diagnose and localize the site(s) of CSF rhinorrhoea during nasal endoscopy usually 30 minutes after injection at a dose of 0.1 ml of 10% non-ophthalmic solution is

diluted in 10 ml of CSF and reinjected into the subarachnoid space over a period of 10 minutes. This test can also be done at the time of surgery to facilitate immediate repair.

3. *Imaging studies:*
   a. *HRCT paranasal sinus and the skull base* is the imaging of choice to identify the defect in the skull base with CSF rhinorrhoea (Fig. 17.1).
   b. *CT cisternography:* CT scans with or without intrathecal contrast and preoperative nasal endoscopy are the most frequently used investigation to preoperatively localize the site of the leak. Intrathecal contrast injection before the CT scan can provide more accurate information about the leakage (Jones, et al. 2000).
   c. *Metrizamide CT cisternography:* It is the best tool in establishing the diag-nosis and to locate the site of leak.
   d. *MRI and MRI cisternography:* Non-invasive images to locate leak site (Fig. 17.2).

MANAGEMENT

Most of CSF leaks can close spontaneously within 7 to 10 days with conservative management. The risk of meningitis and other intracranial complications should be kept in mind in post-traumatic cases and surgical

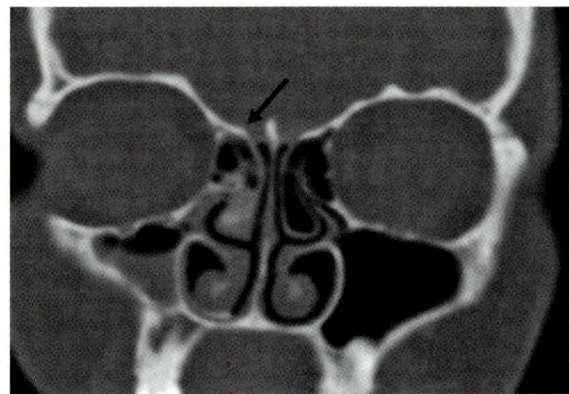

Fig. 17.1: CT scan showing the leak site at the attachment of the middle turbinate to fovea ethmoidalis. Also note associated maxillary sinusitis

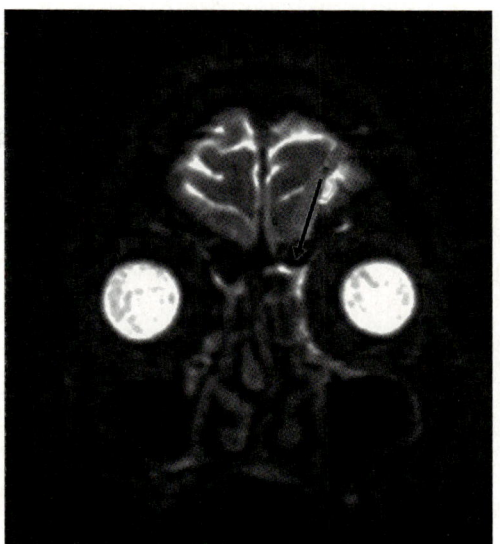

Fig. 17.2: MRI showing the leak site in the fovea ethmoidalis (black arrow)

intervention should be the preferred modality apart from antibiotics and other medical treatment.

Medical Treatment

1. Prophylactic antibiotic.
2. Bed rest in head up position (head of bed position at 15–30°)
3. Coughing, sneezing, and blowing of nose, weight lifting needs to be avoided and should be adequately treated whenever present.
4. Mild laxative to prevent increase in CSF pressure.
5. Repeated or continuous lumbar puncture may be requiring in certain cases. The timing for surgery and CSF drainage procedures must be decided with great care and with a clear strategy.
6. Diuretics like acetazolamide can be given.
7. Mannitol can be started preoperatively.

Surgical Treatment

Basic Principles of Surgery

- Positive identification of leak site
- Meticulous preparation of recipient bed
- Accurate placement of an appropriate graft material

This includes two approaches:

1. *Intracranial:* This approach was frequently being used by a frontal craniotomy approach and still a preferred approach for selected cases by the neurosurgeon. Repair includes the use of pedicled pericranial or dural flap. Some surgeons prefer fascia lata graft for repair.

2. *Extracranial:*

    a. *External or combined endoscopic approach:* Commonly approached with a bicoronal incision and osteoplastic flap to expose the posterior table of the frontal bone to locate the defect in that area. This approach is particularly suitable for defect above the floor. Graft material like fascia lata and bone/cartilage can be used to seal the defect.

    A combined approach also can be advocated by using a small incision in the eyebrow and frontal sinus trephination for endoscopic visualization and instrument manipulation along with endoscopic frontal sinusotomy.

    b. *Endoscopic approach:*

        i. *Overlay technique*
            1. Localize the skull base defect.
            2. Surrounding mucosa is elevated at least 3–5 mm in all directions to prevent mucosa from interfering with graft adhesion.
            3. Place the free graft, which is glued over the underlying structure.

        ii. *Underlay technique*
            1. Localize the site of the defect.
            2. Elevate the dura of the skull base for 2–3 mm, thus creating the epidural space.
            3. Connective tissue graft is placed in this pocket.
            4. Then proceed to remove the mucosa as in overlay technique.
            5. Placing the overlay graft.
            6. Thus triple layer seal is achieved.
            7. Useful for large defect.

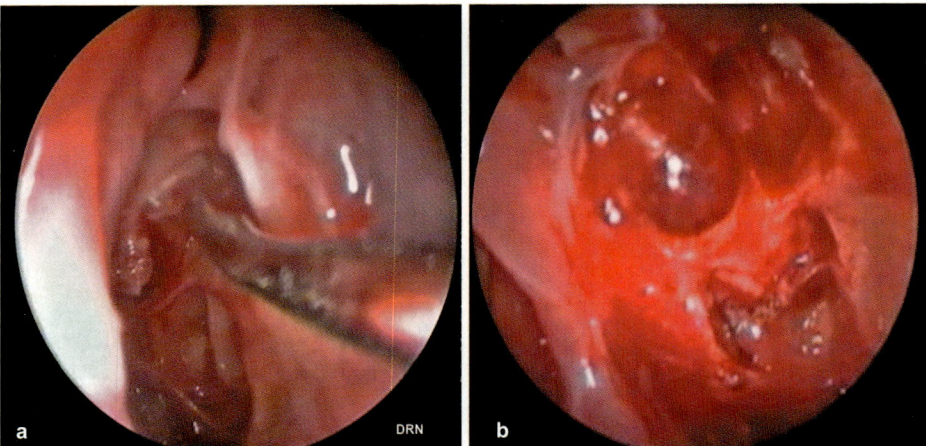

Fig. 17.3: a. The leak site being expose by removing mucosa over the small area of herniated brain tissue, **b.** Striping of the mucosa to create a raw bony surface around for graft placement

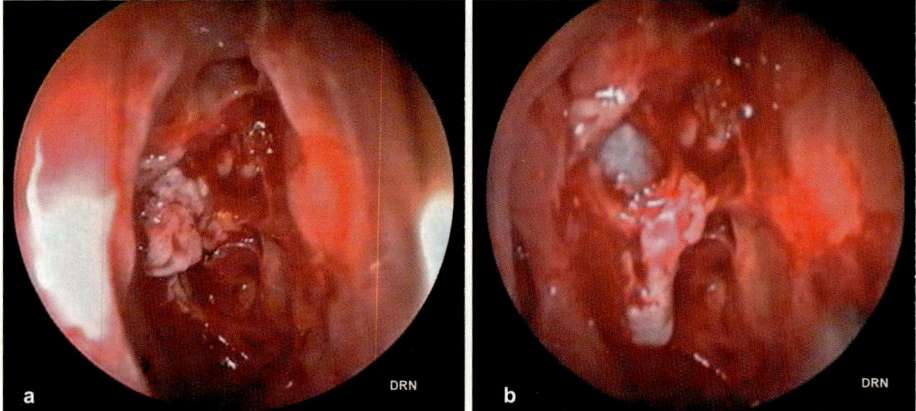

Fig. 17.4: a. Placement of an underlay fascia lata graft followed by placement of a cartilage. **b.** Note part of the fascia has been outside to prevent migration of the cartilage

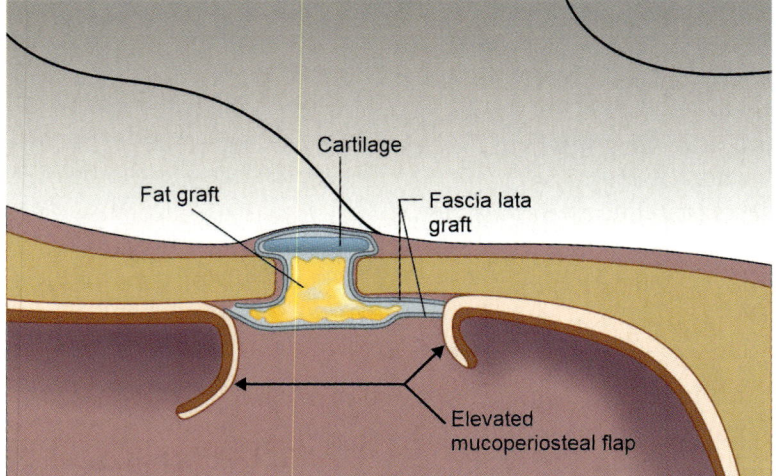

Fig. 17.4c: Underlay fascia lata and cartilage graft for sealing large bony defect in CSF leak

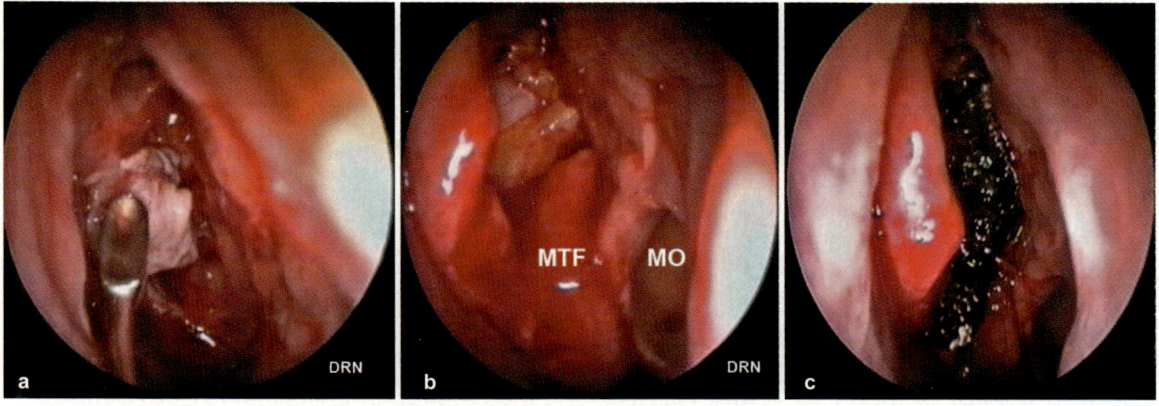

Fig. 17.5: a. Placement of an additional fascia lata, **b.** Middle turbinate being partially resected as a pedicled flap (MTF) and placed over graft for early epithelialization, maxillary ostium (MO) can be seen, and **c.** Surgicel is placed over the flap to keep it in place

Indications and Surgical Details
(Figs 17.3 to 17.6)

It is one of the most preferred approaches at present with a success rate of more than 90–95% in an experienced hand. Some surgeons prefer to put a lumbar drain prior to surgery to inject intrathecal fluorescein. The key to endoscopic repair is the accurate identification of the site of the leak as well as the relevant anatomy of the area so as to make proper surgical planning. Depending on the site of the leak (cribriform plate, fovea ethmoidalis or sphenoid sinus), exposure is done. A complete ethmoidectomy, maxillary and frontal sinusotomy, sphenoidotomy, middle and superior turbinectomies may be required. After identifying the leak, the graft bed is prepared by striping/elevating the surrounding mucosa from the bone (Fig. 17.3a and b). For a small defect, fat graft is preferred to give a dumbbell-shaped seal followed by an additional layer of fascia lata as onlay graft. In case of a larger leak with bony defect of more than 1 cm, an underlay bone or cartilage gafting is done in addition to fascial graft placement to prevent prolapse of brain or meningeal tissue and also to hold the graft in place (Fig. 17.4a to c). If the mucosa is elevated as a flap instead of being striped, it can be reapplied over the graft to facilitate early epithelilization (Fig. 17.5a and b). Alter-natively, part of the middle turbinate can be used as a pedicled flap. Application of Surgicel® helps in stabilizing the graft in place followed by Merocel (Fig. 17.5c). The author (DRN) prefers NasoPore® soaked with antibiotic solution for the same as it does not prevent early epithelialization. Immediately after surgery, the surgeon should request the anaesthesiologist for removal of the swallowed blood clot from the stomach. Antiemetic is given immediately after surgery before patient is recovered from anaesthesia to prevent postoperative nausea and vomiting.

Postoperative Treatment
  i. Placement of a lumbar drainage
 ii. Head end of the bed is elevated to 15–30°
iii. Bed rest
 iv. Stool softener
  v. Diuretics
 vi. Pack removal on 10th day
vii. Light activity after 6 weeks of surgery.

Postoperative follow-up: This is absolutely essential as recurrent CSF leak at an alternate site after recent repair is common. Regular endoscopic inspection with minimal debridement of the surgical site should be performed over the long term to identify recurrence of disease.

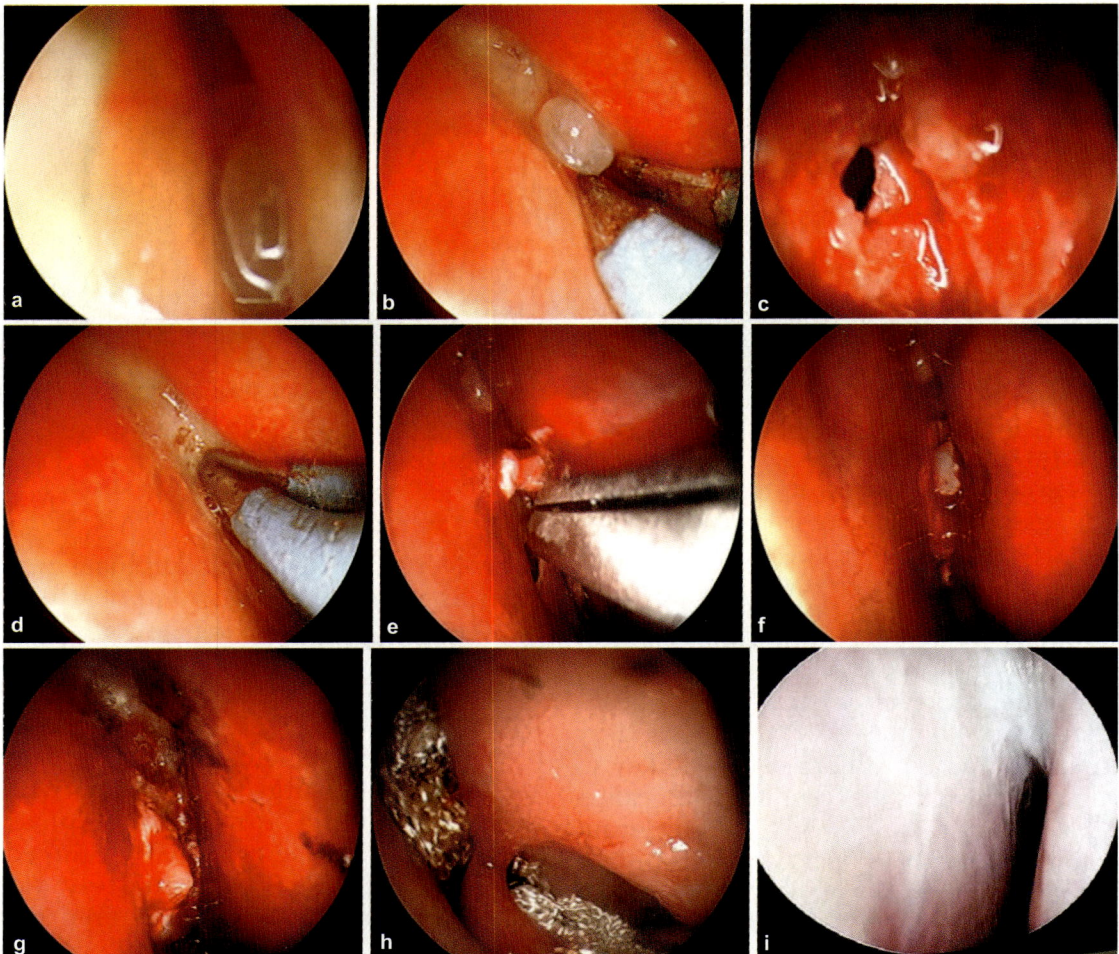

Fig 17.6: a. CSF leak associated with meningocele, **b.** Resection of meningocele with bipolar cautery, **c.** Defect site for CSF leak after removal of meningocele, **d.** Cauterization of the adjacent mucosa to create raw area, **e.** Creation of septal and adjacent turbinate mucosal flap, **f.** Showing after placing fascia lata, a small piece of septal cartilage inserted to snuggly to fit the defect, **g.** Additional layer of fascia lata was placed to cover the inserted layer of cartilage as shown in Fig 17.4c and septal and middle turbinate mucosal flap was placed over the graft for epithelialization, **h.** Surgicel® was placed over the repaired area and middle meatus to prevent displacement of graft, **i.** Healing of the defect after two months

BIBLIOGRAPHY

1. Brodie H. Prophylactic antibiotics for post-traumatic cerebrospinal fluid fistulae: A meta-analysis. Archives of Oto: 1997 July;123(7):749–752.
2. Dandy WD. Pneumocephalus. Arch Surg 1926; 12:949–82.
3. Iffenecker C, Benoudiba F, Parker F, Fuerxer F, David P, Tadie M, et al. The place of MRI in the study of cerebrospinal fluid fistulas. J Radiol 1999; 80:37–43.
4. Jones ME, Reino T, Gnoy A, Guillory S, Wackym P, Lawson W. Identification of intranasal cerebrospinal fluid leaks by topical application with fluorescein dye. Am J Rhinol 2000; 14:93–96.
5. Wigand ME. Transnasal ethmoidectomy under endoscopic control. Rhinology 1981;19:7–15.

18

The Role of Nasal Endoscopy in the Management of Nasopharyngeal Cancer

JS Sahota, A Kumar

INTRODUCTION

The rigid nasal endoscope, now used by nearly all ENT surgeons, was developed in the 1970s and was instrumental in changing the diagnostic and therapeutic modalities for treatment of sinonasal pathology, especially chronic sinusitis. As surgeons became more experienced in nasal endoscopy, its use expanded to include the diagnosis and treatment of various nasal masses and nasopharyngeal pathology. The use of the nasal endoscope not only permits close, accurate, and magnified views of the nasal cavities and the nasopharynx but also proves immensely useful in diagnosing small submucosal lesions which, otherwise, would be missed by conventional techniques. Traditionally, the nasopharynx is difficult to visualize using speculums since the view is often limited by anatomic and pathologic variations like deviated septum, hypertrophied turbinate, or concha bullosa. Postnasal examinations using mirrors are also complicated by a limited view and the gag reflex which precludes a thorough examination. The use of the nasal endoscope to evaluate the nasopharynx is, therefore, particularly useful.

ANATOMY OF THE NASOPHARYNX

The nasopharynx measures about 4 cm high, 4 cm wide, and 3 cm anteroposteriorly. The posterior wall is located about 8 cm from the pyriform aperture. Endoscopic assessment of the nasopharynx is usually done with the 0° rigid endoscope. The most important region of the nasopharynx with respect to nasopharyngeal cancer is the fossa of Rosenmüller. This recess/region measures up to 2.5 cm in depth and is located between the lateral and posterior walls, just behind the torus. The eustachian tube orifice lies on the lateral wall about 1.5 cm from the roof, posterior wall, choana, and floor.

Endoscopic Diagnosis of Nasopharyngeal Cancer

Typically, patients with suspected nasopharyngeal cancer (NPC) usually present with hard lymph node swelling just below the angle of the mandible. These patients may also have nasal symptoms and some will have a unilateral hearing loss caused by the obstruction of the eustachian tube either by tumour, oedema, or lymphoid enlargement around the tubal orifice. Consequently, the endoscope is used to visualize the region around the fossa of Rosenmuller and the eustachian tube. A suspected lesion may appear as a submucosal bulge, a frank growth, or an infiltrating lesion (Fig. 18.1). There may be oedema around the orifice of the eustachian tube endoscopic photograph showing a large tumour arising from the left fossa of Rosenmüller (Fig. 18.2). The eustachian tube opening is seen just anteriorly. Indeed, the endoscope has revolutionized the diagnosis of such lesions by enabling the surgeon to take focused, targeted biopsies from this region. Before the development of endoscopes, one had to rely

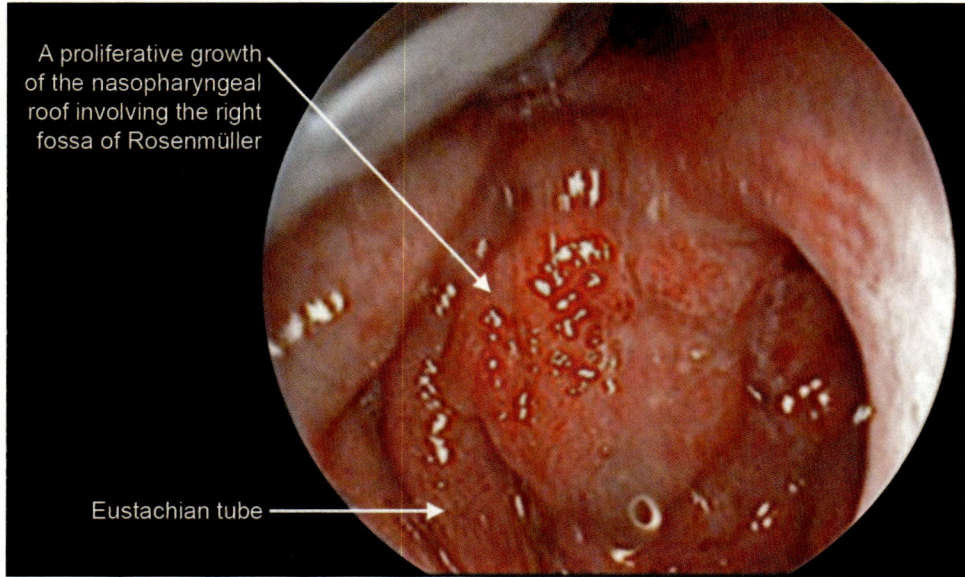

A proliferative growth of the nasopharyngeal roof involving the right fossa of Rosenmüller

Eustachian tube

Fig. 18.1: Proliferative growth of the nasopharynx

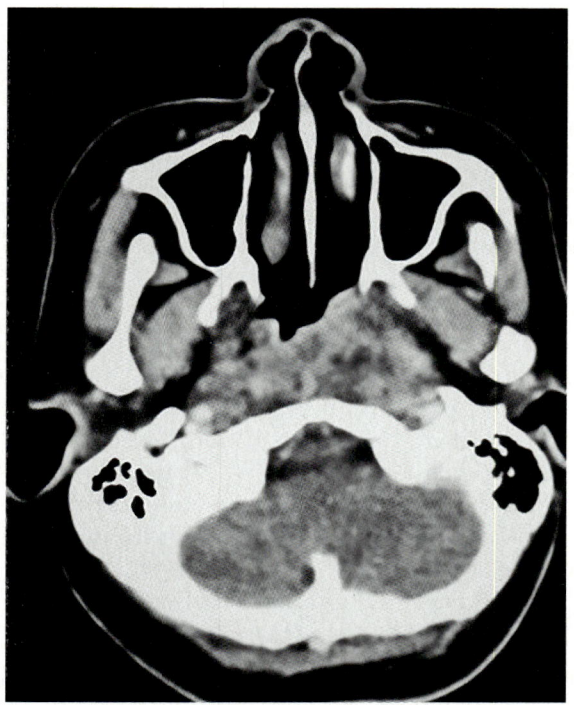

Fig. 18.2: Involvement of left fossa of Rosenmüller

on "blind" punch biopsies from the nasopharynx, which did not always detect small malignant lesions. Now, such biopsies can be taken in the outpatient department and at the same time the rest of the nose and sinuses can be examined.

Role of Preoperative CT Scan

CT evaluation is very important to detect tumour extension, especially erosion of the bone: Contrast CT can show enhancement of the tumour and helps in evaluation of the neck node. Besides nasopharynx, CT of brain and CT neck should be done to rule out intracranial involvement and involvement of neck node (Figs 18.3a,b and 18.4). MRI is important in planning for intracranial extension and soft tissue involvement and has become the integral part of the management. Recently FDG PET and FDG PET/CT have a growing role in the diagnosis and management of NPC especially when patient presents with unkown primary neck metastases (Mohandas, et al. 2014).

Newer Modalities for Diagnosis of NPC

Narrow band imaging is fast emerging as an efficient diagnostic and screening modality for early NPC. Wang et al. report that narrow band imaging when used with nasal endoscopy is a rapid and effective screening

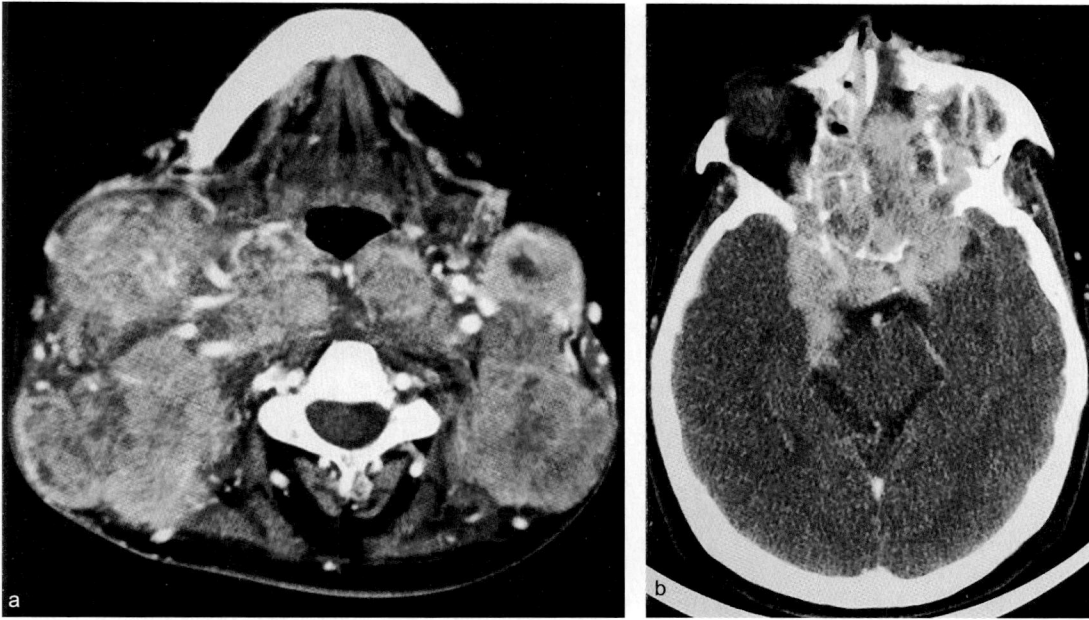

Fig. 18.3: a. Infiltration into parapharyngeal space infratemporal fossa with fungating neck nodes, **b.** Intracranial extension

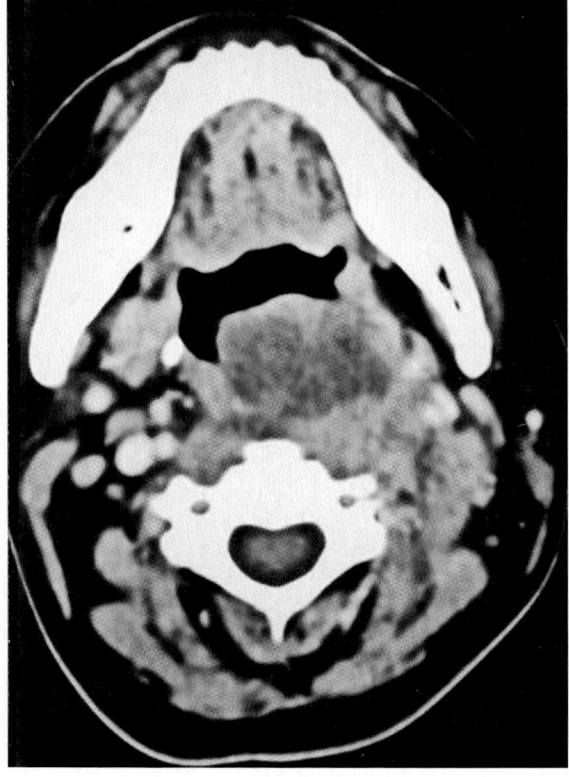

Fig. 18.4: Involvement of prevertebral fascia

tool for nasopharyngeal cancers. Contact endoscopy using methylene blue to stain for malignant epithelium was evaluated by Pak et al. 1991. In this method, the suspicious areas are stained with methylene blue and viewed with an endoscope. The malignant epithelium shows distinct patterns when compared with normal epithelium of the nasopharynx. Presently Ebstein-Barr virus-specific antibodies were found to be useful for early detection of NPC and can help in mass screening programs to identify patients with early-stage NPC (Young and Dawson, 2014).

Role of Endoscopes in Treatment of NPC

Although most patients will undergo external beam radiotherapy as the standard treatment for their disease, some patients will require salvage therapy in the form of a localized nasopharyngectomy and/or neck dissection. Accurate mapping of the tumour and its anatomical localization is essential in planning precise radiotherapy because radiotherapy can cause complications like choanal atresia or stenosis. Chronic sinusitis occurs due to blockage of sinus ostia by radiation-induced oedema. Endoscopic techniques prove to be useful in the aforesaid conditions. Endoscopic nasopharyngectomy for locally recurrent nasopharyngeal carcinoma has been performed with encouraging results (Rohaizam 2009). Role of immunotherapy has been evaluated in clinical trials with some success but is still in experimental stage (Peri, et al. 2019).

SURGICAL TECHNIQUE OF ENDOSCOPIC NASOPHARYNGECTOMY

1. After creation of a posteriorly and inferiorly based septal flap (Hadad-Bassagasteguy flap) in the healthy side the posterior half of the bony nasal septum is removed to gain access to the contralateral Rosenmüller fossa.
2. Resection of the posterior half of the nasal septum increases the maneuverability of endoscopes and instruments to facilitate the access.
3. Resection of inferior turbinate is warranted to provide better access.
4. The curved-blade harmonic scalpel/ KTP532 laser is utilized to achieve a bloodless mucosal incision on the nasopharynx, and for a wide resection of tumour.
5. Margins should be taken for histopathological confirmation.
6. First, superior mucosal incision is given followed by the lateral wall, including the cartilaginous portion of the eustachian

tube, the roof of the nasopharynx and the inferior margins are resected depending on the extent (Fig. 18.5).
7. Difficulties are usually encountered in peeling the mucosa and periosteum from the bony nasopharynx.
8. The exposed bony surface with flaps is compulsory to prevent infection or osteoradionecrosis in irradiated patients.
9. Hadad rotational flap is used from septum and alternately an inferior turbinate flap can be used and can be glued and packed. Packs are removed after 24–48 hours.
10. Patients can be discharged home within two to three days after the surgery.

CONCLUSION

Endoscopic evaluation of the nasopharynx is an indispensable tool in the diagnosis and treatment of tumours of the nasopharynx. It permits accurate localization and evaluation and allows targeted biopsies, resulting in improved diagnostic yield. Further advances such as contact endoscopy and narrow band imaging will help in early diagnosis and greatly aid in screening as well.

Endoscopic nasopharyngectomy is considered mostly for rT1 or rT2 tumours and selected rT3 nasopharyngeal cancer. The surgical techniques varies, although certain key elements common in most approaches. With proper case selection and appropriate

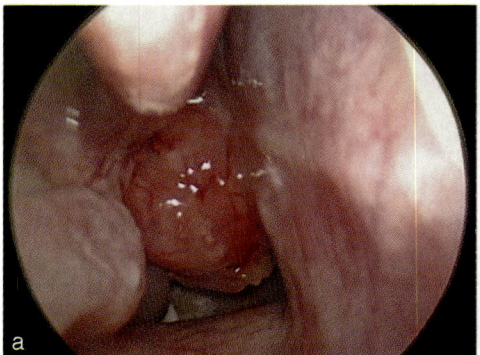 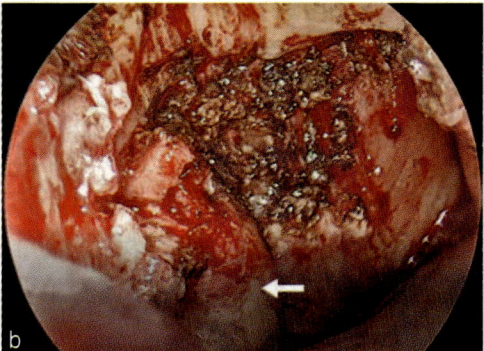

Fig. 18.5: a. Preoperative endoscopic picture showing right nasopharyngeal carcinoma (poorly differentiated non-keratinized squamous cell carcinoma) arising from the fossa of Rosenmüller extending to the roof of nasopharynx, **b.** Endoscopic picture showing area of resection after partial nasopharyngectomy. Note the white arrow showing the right eustachian tubal orifice

surgical execution, patients with recurrent nasopharyngeal carcinoma can be successfully managed endoscopically (Monteiro and Witterick, 2014).

BIBLIOGRAPHY

1. Rohaizam J. Endoscopic nasopharyngectomy: The Sarawak experience. Med J Malaysia Vol-64 No 3 September 2009.
2. Mohandas A, et al. FDG PET/CT in the management of nasopharyngeal carcinoma. Am J Roentgenol 2014 Aug;203(2):W146–57.
3. Monteiro E, Witterick I. Endoscopic nasopharyngectomy: Patient selection and surgical execution. Operative Techniques in Otolaryngology—Head and Neck Surgery 2014; 25,3:284–88.
4. Pak, et al. In vivo diagnosis of nasopharyngeal carcinoma using contact rhinoscopy. Laryngoscope. 2001 Aug; 111(8):1453–58.
5. Peri F, Scarpati GDV, Caponigro F, et al. Management of recurrent nasopharyngeal carcinoma: Current perspectives. Onco Targets Ther. 2019; 12: 1583–91.
6. Wang, et al. Nasopharyngeal carcinoma detected by narrow-band imaging endoscopy. Oral Oncol 2011 Aug; 47(8):736–41. Epub 2011 Mar 9.
7. Young LS, Dawson CW. Epstein-Barr virus and nasopharyngeal carcinoma. Chin J Cancer 2014 Dec; 33(12): 581–90.

Allergic Fungal Rhinosinusitis Including Other Forms—An Overview

DR Nayak, S Pillai, A Dora, P Sharma, T Karanth

Allergic fungal sinusitis (AFS) is a non-invasive form of highly recurrent chronic allergic hypertrophic rhinosinusitis that can be distinguished clinically, histopathologically and prognostically from other forms of chronic fungal rhinosinusitis. It is a form of noninvasive fungal rhinosinusitis and is associated with a hypertrophic sinus disease (HSD). It has clinicopathological features that make it similar, but not identical, to allergic bronchopulmonary aspergillosis (ABPA).

The classification of fungal sinusitis described by deShazo et al. (1997), Ferguson (2000) and Adelson et al. (2005) into different invasive and non-invasive types. However, consensus on terminology, pathogenesis, and optimal management is lacking. The International Society for Human and Animal Mycology convened a working group to attempt consensus on the terminology and disease classification has led to the following conclusion (Chakarbati A; Denning D; Fergusson B; Ponikau J, et al. 2009).

Fungal Rhinosinusitis (FRS)

It is a distinct clinical entity characterized by inflammation of the sinus mucosa due to a fungal infection, and may be seen in immunocompetent or immunocompromised hosts. A consensus panel led by Chakravarti, et al (2009) classified the fungal sinus disease based on tissue invasion into two types—invasive and non-invasive.

Classification

1. Invasive
   - Acute fulminant
   - Chronic invasive
   - Chronic granulomatous
2. Non-invasive
   - Saprophytic fungal infestation
   - Fungal ball
   - Fungal related eosinophilic sinus disease (allergic fungal sinusitis)

AFS is a recently described clinical entity that has gained increased attention as a cause of chronic sinusitis. Allergic aspergillosis was first recognized by Lamb and Miller 1982 (ABPA). Allergic fungal sinusitis (AFS) was first described by Katzenstein et al. (1983), when histopathological similarities were noted between the surgically removed sinus debris of some patients with sinusitis and the bronchial mucus plugs of patients with allergic bronchopulmonary aspergillosis.

The term allergic fungal sinusitis was first coined by Robson et al. in 1989. It is the most common type of fungal rhinosinusitis. Allergic bronchopulmonary aspergillosis, a disorder analogous to AFS, was recently reported to have HLA-MHC class II associations.

Pathogenesis

Allergic fungal sinusitis is mediated by both Type-I (IgE) and Type-III (IgG antigen immune complexes) Gell and Coomb reactions. Patients with allergic fungal sinusitis and hypertrophic sinus disease have HLA-DQB1 03 alleles as a

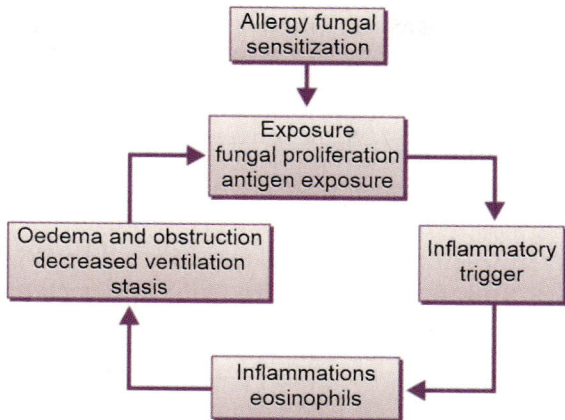

Fig. 19.1: The events associated following exposure to fungal antigen

risk factor for disease, with AFS having the highest association. The association of ABPA, AFS, and HSD with class II genes of the major histocompatibility complex places the initiation of these inflammatory diseases within the context of antigen presentation and the acquired immune response.

It is a benign non-invasive sinus disease related to a hypersensitivity reaction to fungal antigens that triggers inflammatory response leading to oedema and obstruction of the affected sinus ostium and forms a vicious cycle (Fig. 19.1). It should be suspected in any atopic patient with refractory nasal polyps.

Commom Fungi Involved

- *Aspergillus fumigatus*
- *Bipolaris*
- *Drechslera*
- *Alternaria*
- *Curvularia*
- *Exserohilum*

Diagnostic Criteria

Bent and Kuhn (1996) proposed diagnostic criteria for allergic fungal sinusitis. This has been divided further into two groups, i.e. major and minor.

Major Criteria

- Type-I hypersensitivity
- Nasal polyposis

- Characteristic CT findings
- Positive fungal smear
- Allergic mucin with fungal elements and no tissue invasion

Minor Criteria

- Asthma
- Unilateral predominance
- Radiographic bone erosion
- Positive fungal culture
- Charcot-Leyden crystals
- Serum eosinophil

Diagnosis of Allergic Fungal Sinusitis

Significant overlap exists between the clinical, radiological, and immunological features of AFS, invasive fungal disease, and ethmoidal polyposis. A definitive preoperative differentiation of these entities is desirable for diagnosis as it influences the choice of surgical procedure and the perioperative adjunctive medical treatments (Diwakar, et al. 2003).

- *History:* A history of sinus disease strongly recalcitrant to traditional medical and even surgical therapy aimed largely at bacterial rhinosinusitis. A detail history should be elicited for the following complaints:
  - Sneezing and a runny nose as seen classically in allergic rhinitis
  - Nasal obstruction
  - Thick and mucopurulent viscid nasal discharge.
  - Headache
  - Postnasal drip
  - Occasional facial pain
  - Cough seen more at night
- *Objective findings:*
  - **Allergic mucin** (Fig. 19.2): Extramucosal allergic mucin (that is also seen grossly at surgery as a characteristic 'peanut-buttery' material)
  - Fungal specific IgE
  - No evidence of invasion
- *Endoscopic mucosal staging system* (Kupferberg, et al. 1996):
  - Stage 0: No mucosal oedema or allergic mucin

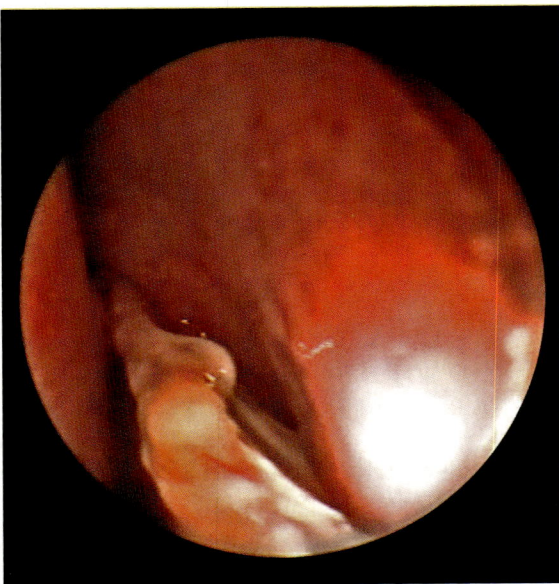

Fig. 19.2: Endoscopic picture showing allergic mucin suctioned out from the frontal sinus

– Stage I: Mucosal oedema
– Stage II: Polypoid oedema
– Stage III: Sinus polyps

Radiological findings (Fig. 19.3): Sinus computed tomography scans showing chronic rhino-sinusitis (often with the presence of hyper-attenuating sinus contents). Schubert (2000, 2009) noted that computed tomography (CT) scans are always associated with the abnormal findings in the paranasal sinuses. The characteristic findings that can be noted are:

• Central areas of increased contrast (hyper-attenuation) within abnormal paranasal sinuses.
• Marked soft tissue sinus mucosal hyperplasia evident in multiple sinuses.
• Areas of increased density attributed to the presence of fungal-containing allergic mucin.
• Extrasinus extension of the disease is common in the form of expansion.

Histopathology: Histopathology shows the presence of eosinophilic-lymphocytic sinus mucosal inflammation and scattered silver stain positive fungal hyphae within the allergic mucin but not in the mucosa. Based on histopathological criteria, Kathleen, et al. (2013) classified **fungal sinusitis** into following types:

• *Non-invasive FRS*
  – Fungus ball (FB)
  – Allergic fungal rhinosinusitis (AFRS)
  – Mixed FB/AFRS
• *Invasive FRS*
  – Acute (AIFRS)

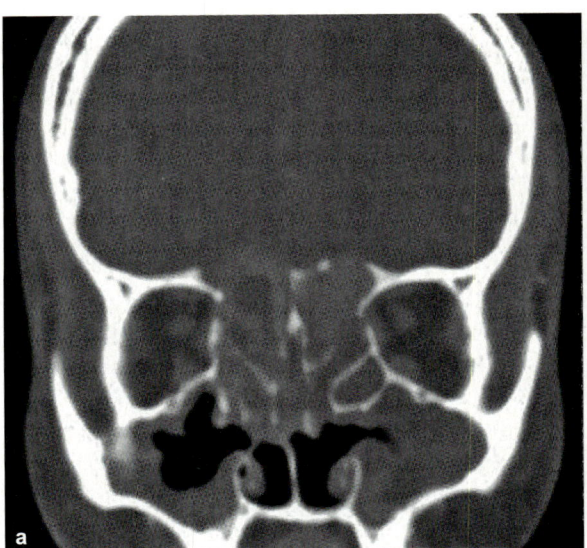
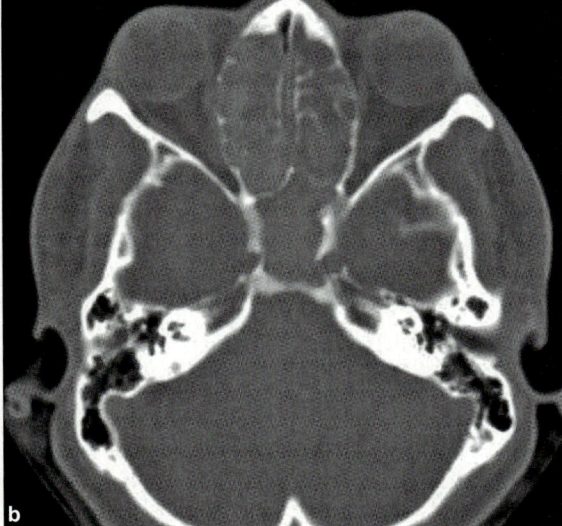

Fig. 19.3: a. Coronal CT, **b.** Axial CT, showing hypertrophic sinus diseases associated with areas of hyper-attenuation due to fungal containing allergic mucin. Also note expansion of sinus wall

- Chronic (CIFRS)
- Chronic granulomatous (CGFRS)
- *Mixed non-invasive/invasive*
- *Fungal culture:* Fungal cultures should be interpreted with caution. They are best used as supportive evidence because of their variable yield.
- *Lab studies:*
  - Elevated total serum IgE
  - Positive inhalant allergy skin tests
  - Microscopically, the mucin often takes on a chondroid appearance with sheets of eosinophils, frequently with the presence of eosinophilic breakdown products or Charcot-Leyden crystals.

Treatment

Extensive surgical debridement followed by the use of systemic antifungal agents was initially common place for all forms of fungal sinusitis. Eventually this notion was challenged by the theory that AFRS represented an immunologic response to presentation of a fungal antigen within a susceptible host (Gungor, et al. 1998) and is only adopted for invasive fungal sinusitis. The initial treatment of extensive allergic fungal sinusitis is surgery to confirm the diagnosis and remove the diseased mucosa (Schubert 1998, 2000).

Incomplete surgical removal of the involved hypertrophic sinus tissue may render the patient vulnerable to relapse of allergic fungal sinusitis. Oral corticosteroid therapy post surgery can prevent relapses and potential of corticosteroid side effects needs to be balanced against the risk of recurrent disease.

Surgical treatment involves aggressive sinus surgery followed by aggressive post-operative medical management of allergic inflammatory disease includes allergen immunotherapy, topical and systemic corti-costeroids, antihistamines and antileuko-trienes (Fig. 19.4). Radical endoscopic surgical debridement of nose and PNS is being adopted for invasive fungal infection like **mucormycosis** with complete removal of dead tissue and anti-fungal treatment with Amphotericin-B, Isavuconazole and Posaconazole. Treatment of AFS is directed at endoscopic removal of the inciting antigenic material via complete surgical removal of allergic mucin and debris while also amelio-rating the underlying inflammatory process through the use of limited systemic and topical steroid preparations (Mabry 2000).

All patients with AFS should undergo surgical debridement of the respective sinuses. Extensive disease of the frontal sinus may require a **Draf II** (Fig. 19.5a) or a modified

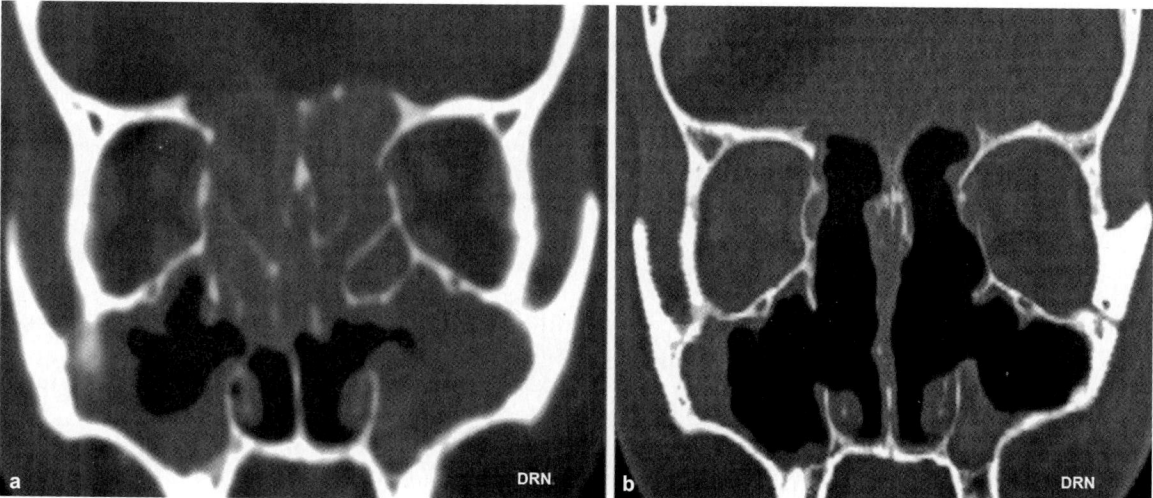

Fig. 19.4: a. Preoperative CT showing allergic fungal sinusitis, **b.** Postoperative CT of the same patient showing good clearance of disease

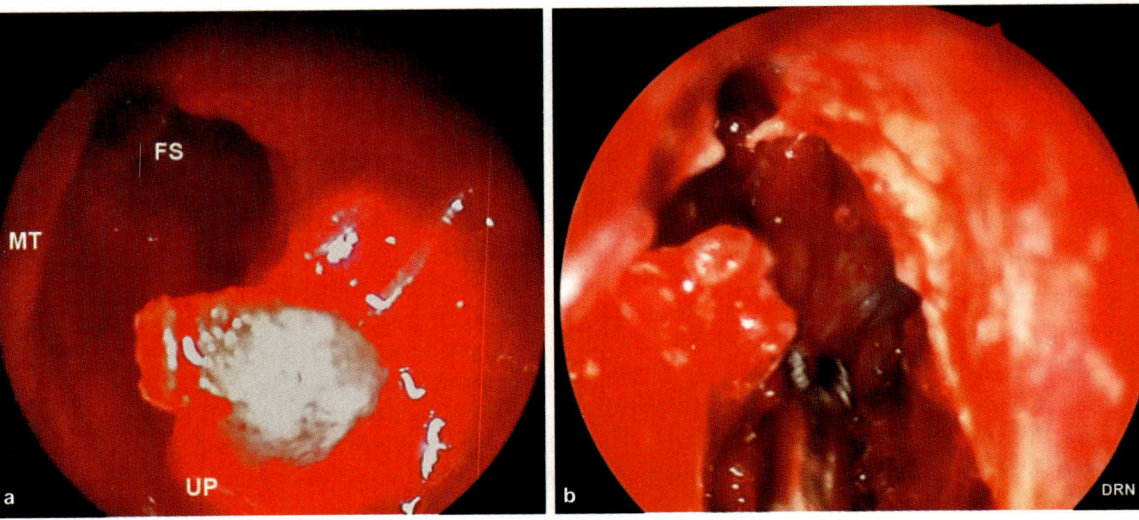

Fig. 19.5: a. Draf II procedure in progress for a case of allergic fungal sinusitis of left frontal sinus, **b.** Modified Lothrop procedure for bilateral frontal sinus disease in progress—microdebrider is used to clear the polypoidal tissue

Lothrop procedure (Fig. 19.5b) also refer Chapter-22 for surgical technique. Immunotherapy may be beneficial, rather than harmful, as a component of treatment for AFS. Antifungal therapy often was used in an attempt to provide some degree of control over recurrence of AFS. Data on the effects of this form of therapy for AFS have been limited. Topical application of antifungal agents may hold some benefit in the control of postoperative recurrence. Total serum IgE levels should be followed postoperatively as they can be prognostic for recurrent disease.

Prognosis is good with integrated medical-surgical follow-up, but recurrence remains problematic (Schubert 2006).

BIBLIOGRAPHY

1. Bent JP 3rd, Kuhn FA. Antifungal activity against allergic fungal sinusitis organisms. Laryngoscope 1996 Nov; 106 (11):1331–4.
2. Bozeman S, deShazo RD, Stringer S, et al. Complications of Allergic Fungal Sinusitis. Am J Med 2016; 124,4:359–368.
3. Chakravarthi, et al. Fungal rhinosinusitis: A categorization and definitional schema addressing current controversies. Laryngoscope 2009 Sep; 119(9): 1809–1818. doi: 10.1002/ lary.20520
4. deShazo, et al. A new classification and diagnostic criteria for invasive fungal sinusitis. Arch Otolaryngol Head Neck Surg 1997 Nov; 123(11):1181–88.
5. deShaz RD, et al. Criteria for diagnosing sinus myotome. J Allergy Clin Immunol 1997;99:475–55.
6. Dhiwakar, et al. Preoperative diagnosis of allergic fungal sinusitis. Laryngoscope 2003; 113:688–694.
7. Gungor, et al. Fungal sinusitis: Progression of disease in immunosuppression a case report. Ear, Nose and Throat J 1998; 77: 207–15.
8. Katzenstein A, Sale S, Greenberger P. Pathologic findings in allergic aspergillus sinusitis. J Allergy Clin Immunol 1983; 72:89–93.
9. Lamb D, Millar J, Johnston A. Allergic aspergillosis of the paranasal sinuses. J Pathol 1982;137:56.
10. Mabry RL, Otolaryngol Head Neck Surg. Jan 2000; 122(1):104–6.
11. Robson M, et al. Aust. NZJ Med. 1989; 19:351–353.
12. Schubert and Goetz. J Allergy Clin Immunol 1998; 102:395–402.
13. Schubert M. Ann Allergy Asthma Immunol (2000) Aug; 85:90–101.
14. Schubert, et al. Clin Rev Allergy Immunol 2006 Jun; 30(3):205–16.
15. Schubert M. Med Mycol 2009; 47 Suppl 1:S324–30.

Endoscopic Pituitary Surgery

R Govindaraju, TI Ping, VW Mathaneswaran, P Narayanan

Introduction

Pituitary surgery has seen a remarkable shift from transcranial approaches to pituitary tumours (lateral pterional and subfrontal midline) to microscopic surgery (endonasal or sublabial approach) performed by neuro-surgeons to a currently minimally invasive fully endoscopic surgery performed in collaboration between the neurosurgeon and the rhinologist.[1] The rhinologist's role here is mainly to provide an access for the neurosurgeon to remove the tumour and subsequently assist to provide the endoscopic view and an extra hand for instrumentation while the neurosurgeons are free to use both hands for instrumentation.

Characteristics of Pituitary Tumours

Pituitary tumours are mostly benign and consist of pituitary adenomas. Based on the size of the tumour, it can be classified into either microadenoma (<10 mm) or macroadenoma (>10 mm). Though benign, pituitary tumours are located in a critical area adjacent to the cavernous sinus, cavernous carotid artery (CCA), optic nerve (ON) and chiasma (Fig. 20.1).

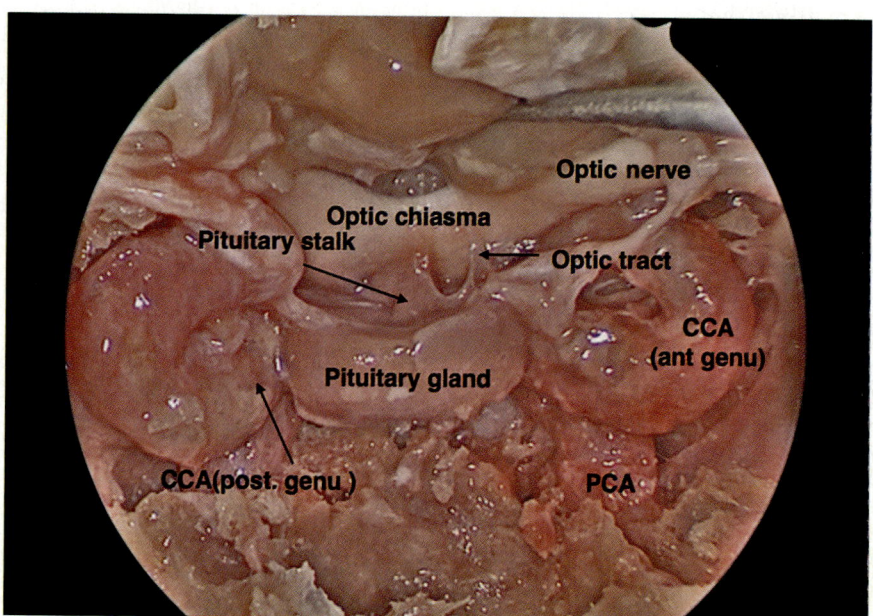

Fig. 20.1: Cadaveric dissection demonstrating the normal pituitary gland and its relation to the cavernous carotid artery and optic nerve and chiasma. CCA–cavernous carotid artery; PCA–paraclival carotid artery; post. genu–posterior genu; ant genu–anterior genu

The tumour may grow out of the **sella turcica** into the suprasellar region superiorly (Fig. 20.2a), and laterally it may encase the cavernous sinus and the cavernous part of the internal carotid artery (ICA) (Fig. 20.2b) and inferiorly extend to the sphenoid sinus and clivus (Fig. 20.2c). Extrasellar extension of pituitary tumour can be categorized using the Wilson's grading system for pituitary adenomas (Table 20.1).[2]

The clinical presentation of pituitary adenoma depends not only on the size of the tumour and compression of adjacent structures (anterior pituitary gland or extrasellar structures) but also on the hormonal status of the tumour, further classifying the tumour as endocrine-active or endocrine-inactive

tumours.[3] Common presenting symptoms in an endocrine-inactive tumour are visual disturbances (diplopia, bitemporal hemianopias), hypopituitarism and headaches.[3]

Table 20.1: Wilson's grading system for extrasellar extension of pituitary adenomas

Stage	Extension
O	No suprasellar extension
A	Extension into suprasellar cistern only
B	Extension into anterior recess of the third ventricle
C	Obliteration of anterior recess and deformation of floor of third ventricle
D	Intradural extension into anterior, middle or posterior fossa
E	Extradural invasion into cavernous sinus

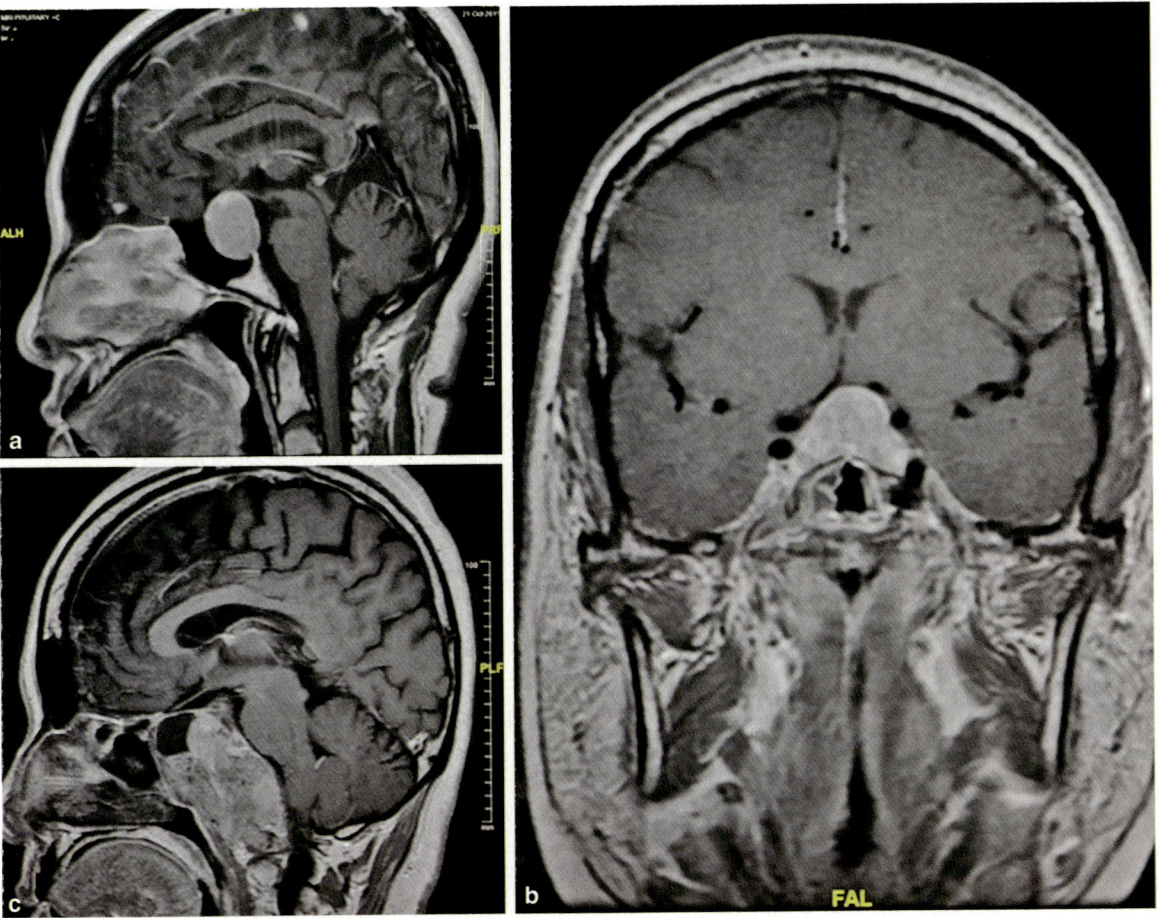

Fig. 20.2: Magnetic resonance images (MRI) showing: **a.** Suprasellar extension of the pituitary tumour in the sagittal plane, **b.** Cavernous sinus extension of the pituitary tumour seen in the coronal plane and **c.** Invasion into the sphenoid sinus and erosion of clivus seen on a sagittal view

Endocrine-active tumours hypersecrete hormone; commonly prolactin and less commonly growth hormone (GH), adeno-corticotrophic hormone (ACTH), follicular-stimulating hormone (FSH), luteinizing hormone (LH) and thyroid-stimulating hormone (TSH) with clinical features accordingly. Hypersecreting tumours are additionally challenging as total tumour removal is critical to achieve normal hormonal levels. In the rare cases of pituitary apoplexy secondary to haemorrhage or necrosis, patients present more acutely with headaches, visual disturbances and ophthalmoplegia.

Endoscopic Approach for Pituitary Tumours

A completely endoscopic surgery of the pituitary tumours though widely practiced is still subject to acceptance by the neuro-surgeons.[4] Institutions already utilizing the technique are expanding its indication as skill improves and better instrumentations allow visualization of previously inaccessible spaces. Endoscopic pituitary surgery has certain advantages over microscopic surgery.

Advantages[5,6]

1. Panoramic view of the sellar floor and the surrounding anatomy of critical importance: The cavernous carotid artery, cavernous sinus, optic nerve and chiasma, planum sphenoidale and clivus.
2. Better illumination and improved view for intrasellar exploration and extrasellar extensions (better visualization of corners not seen with microscope with the use of angled telescopes)
3. Lower nasal morbidity
4. Faster recovery period postoperatively with same endocrinological results as microscope.
5. Concurrent use of image-guided surgery (IGS) system guides the exact site of tumour, depth and limit of surgery and location of critical structures.
6. It also serves as a platform for surgeons to develop their skill for more advanced parasellar and suprasellar tumours.

Disadvantages

The disadvantages from the neurosurgeon's point of view:[5]
1. Technical unfamiliarity
2. Two-dimensional vision, with the lack of accurate depth perception.
3. The need to keep the endoscope and its light path clear and clean.
4. The need to use an assistant or an endoscope holder for the 3-hand technique essential for performing microneurosurgery using the endoscopic approach.

Preoperative Work-Up

Besides the usual blood investigations and preoperative assessment for fitness for surgery, there are some specific preoperative requirements:
1. Ophthalmological assessment (visual acuity, perimetry), neurological assessment and endoscopic examination of the nose by the rhinologist
2. Endocrine blood investigations
3. *Radiology:* HRCT scan of the paranasal sinuses, high resolution MRI brain with IGS protocol

Radiological Imaging

Analysis of the radiology films preoperatively prepares the surgeon for variations in anatomy as well as extension of tumour.

The study of the CT films should be systematic and the below listed anatomical variations must be looked for:
1. Septal deviations and concha bullosa (Fig. 20.3a)
2. *Sphenoid sinus pneumatization in sagittal view:* Conchal, sellar and presellar configuration (Fig. 20.3b).
3. Indentation in the sphenoid sinus caused by ON and ICA and if bony dehiscence over ON and ICA is present.
4. Presence of Onodi cells (sphenoethmoidal cells)
5. Septations on ICA (Fig. 20.3c and d) and ON. See also Fig. 20.4.

MRI films are indispensible to analyze the tumour. Typical imaging protocol includes a

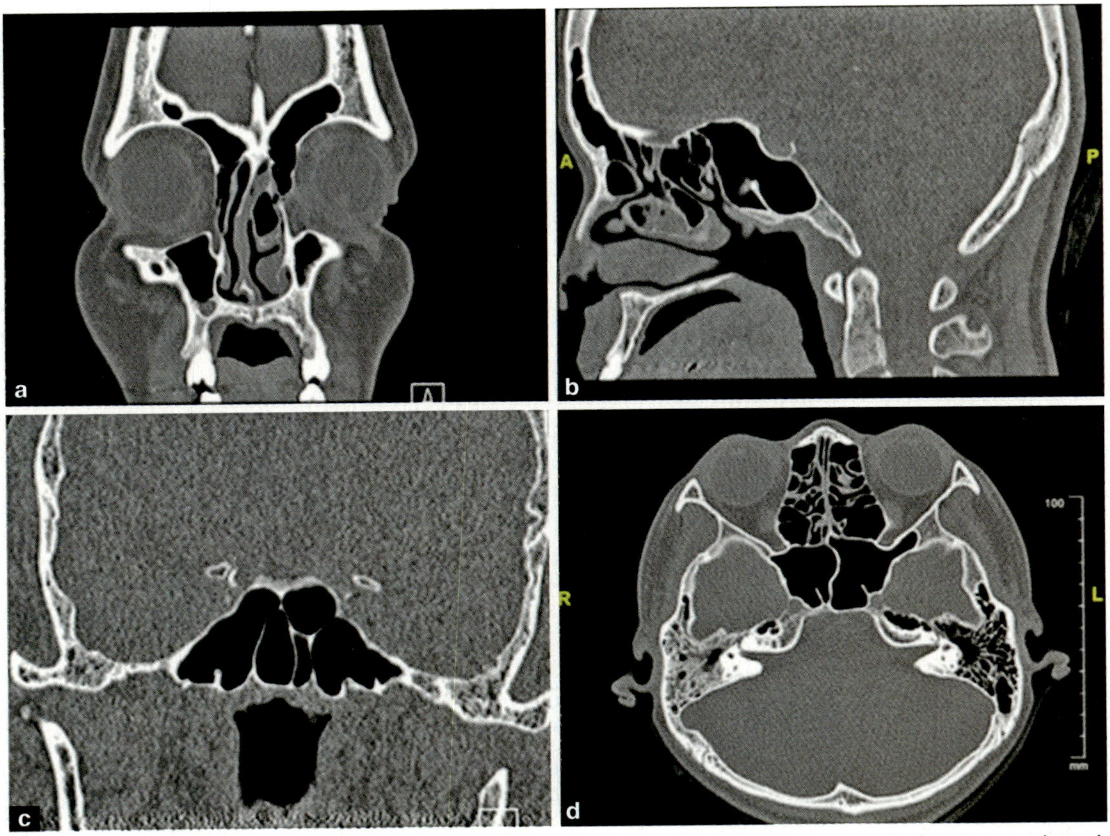

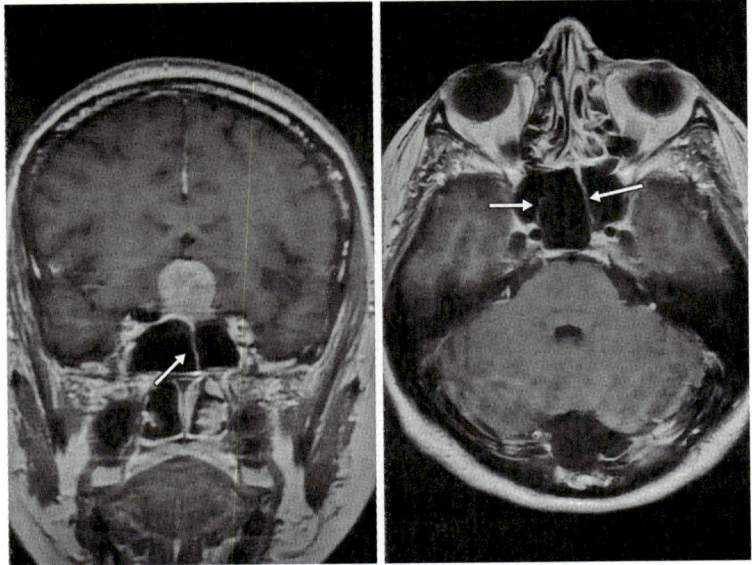

Fig. 20.3: Images of computed tomography (CT) paranasal sinus of importance during transsphenoidal surgery demonstrating: **a.** Deviated nasal septum and left concha bullosa seen on a coronal plane, **b.** Pneumatization of sphenoid sinus—sellar type which is the commonest, **c.** Sphenoidal septations running to ICA seen on (c) coronal image, and **d.** axial plane. ICA–internal carotid artery

Fig. 20.4: Sphenoidal septations (white line with arrowhead) running to ICA may also be seen on high quality images of MRI scan

T1-weighted spin-echo (SE) sequence pre- and post-contrast images in coronal and sagittal plane, whereas T2 images seem to have a limited role in pituitary tumours. Small microadenomas often enhance similar to normal pituitary and present diagnostic challenges and at present dynamic contrast enhanced images are used to identify small microadenomas. Newer methods (Fast SE and a high resolution 3D gradient echo) are also being utilized to overcome the limitations of current methods and improve sensitivity.[7]

Features of Pituitary Adenoma in MRI[7]

a. *T1 pre-contrast:* Isointense to normal pituitary, high signal, if there are areas of focal haemorrhages.
b. *T1 post-contrast:* Adenoma hypoenhancing within a hyperenhancing gland.
c. *T2:* Low signal with calcification and diffuse iron deposition; high signal intensity, if there are areas of cystic change.
d. *T2-weighted gradient echo:* Acute and old haemorrhage appear as areas of low signal intensity.
e. *T2-weighted flow attenuated inversion recovery scan (FLAIR):* Cyst shows higher signal intensity compared to solid tumour.

Other informations to be sought from MRI[7] (Fig. 20.5):

1. Size of tumour
2. Presence of suprasellar extension and the degree of extension
3. Nature of tumour (cystic, solid component) and location of the cystic component with respect to the solid component.
4. Location of normal pituitary and infundibulum.
5. Aberrations in the course of ICA and aneurysms.
6. Extension of tumour into cavernous sinus, encasement of ICA, compression of optic chiasma, erosion of adjacent structures, e.g. clivus, indentation of temporal lobes.

Surgical Procedure

The route to the sphenoid sinus through which the surgery is performed is variable among surgeons according to their personal preferences and includes the transseptal, transnasal and transethmoidal approach.

In our institution, the preferred access for surgery is via transseptal transsphenoidal route. This technique was initially used with the assistance of a modified speculum but

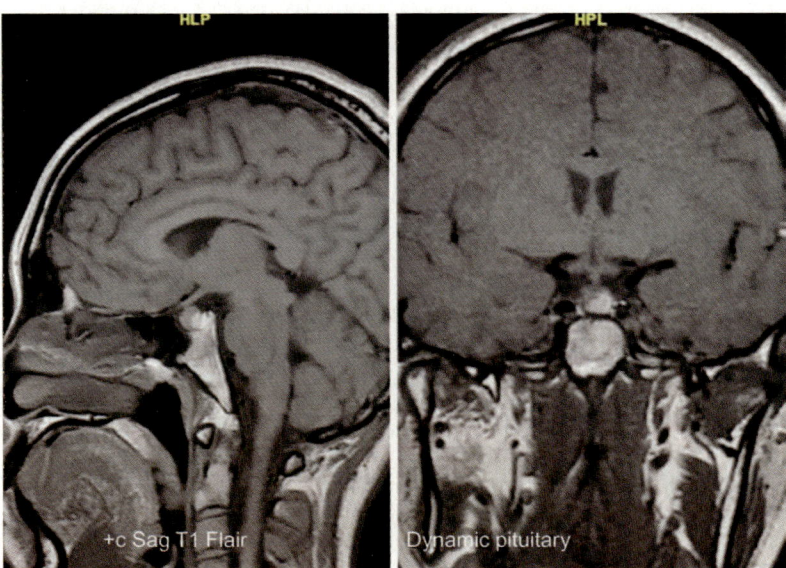

Fig. 20.5a: MRI images of pituitary adenomas: Pituitary microadenoma in a 20-year-old female student; tumour in anterior lobe of pituitary showing delayed enhancement in dynamic pituitary assessment and a normal posterior lobe

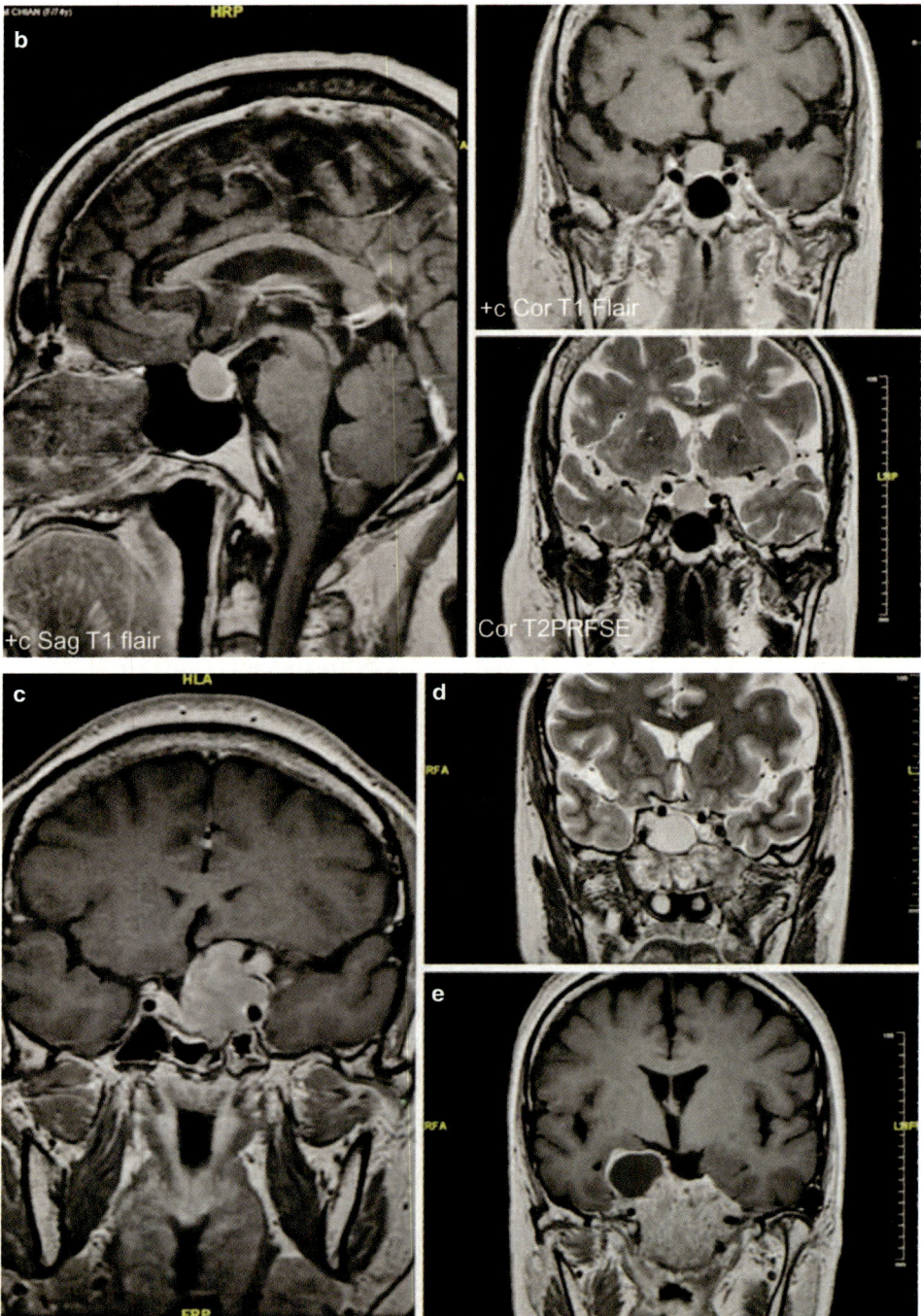

Fig. 20.5: b. MRI images of a 74-year-old lady with pituitary macroadenoma and elevated FSH level. The mass was compressing the left optic nerve but spared the optic chiasm and cavernous carotid arteries, **c.** Suprasellar extension with encasement of left side of cavernous sinus and supraclinoid left carotid artery seen in recurrent pituitary macroadenoma; **d.** Pituitary macroadenoma with cystic component on the superolateral aspect seen with high signal on T2 FRFSE sequence, and **e.** Same tumour seen indenting the left temporal lobe, encasing cavernous sinus, displacing optic chiasm superiorly and with erosion into the sphenoid and clivus

more recently we have moved away from this practice without the use of speculum.[8]

In most instances, instruments and endoscope are channeled via a single nostril to perform surgery but when the view is limited or space is too crowded then the 2-nostril technique is utilized.

Adjunct procedures are sometimes also required, thus patients are usually prepared for it in the event it is required.
1. Graft harvest: Periumbilical fat, fascia lata
2. Hadad flap

Surgical Technique (Step by Step)

Position: Supine, neck in a slightly extended position and head turned slightly away from surgeon (Fig. 20.6).

Anaesthesia: General anaesthesia with orotracheal intubation and throat pack *in situ.*

Prophylatic antibiotic: Given at induction of anaesthesia.

Bladder catheterization; kept till postoperatively to monitor for diabetes insipidus.

Operating room set-up and positions of surgeon and assistant are demonstrated in Fig. 20.7 as practiced in our institution though it may vary elsewhere where neurosurgeon and assistant holding the endoscope stand on the same side.

Primary Pituitary Surgery—Single Nostril, Transseptal Transsphenoidal Surgery

Exposure to Sella (Video 1)

1. Nose is sprayed with cophenylcaine (lignocaine 5% and phenylephrine 0.5% spray) prior to packing performed with cottonoids/neuropatties soaked with adrenaline 1:1000. Packing is done along the floor of the nose and in between septum and middle turbinate.
2. Midface is prepared and draped with modified towels/drapes to allow placement of image-guided surgery tracking system instruments. Additionally the abdomen is also routinely prepared for later fat graft harvest (if required).
3. Preliminary packing is removed and the nose is again inspected with a 0° nasal endoscope and the whole surgery is recorded in a digital media.
4. Both the sphenoethmoidal recesses are packed with cottoinoids/neuropatties soaked in adrenaline 1:1000 (Fig. 20.8a,b).
5. The osteocartilaginous junction is infiltrated with a mixture of mepivacaine and adrenaline 1:100 000 on both sides of the septum (Fig. 20.8c,d)
6. A bipolar diathermy is used to cauterize the site of incision followed by a vertical

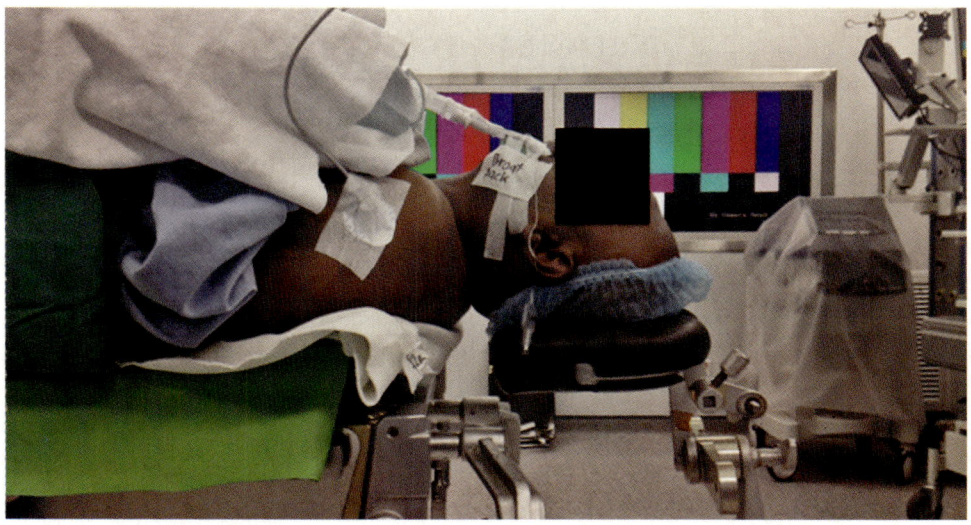

Fig. 20.6: Position of patient during endoscopic transsphenoidal surgery with neck slightly extended

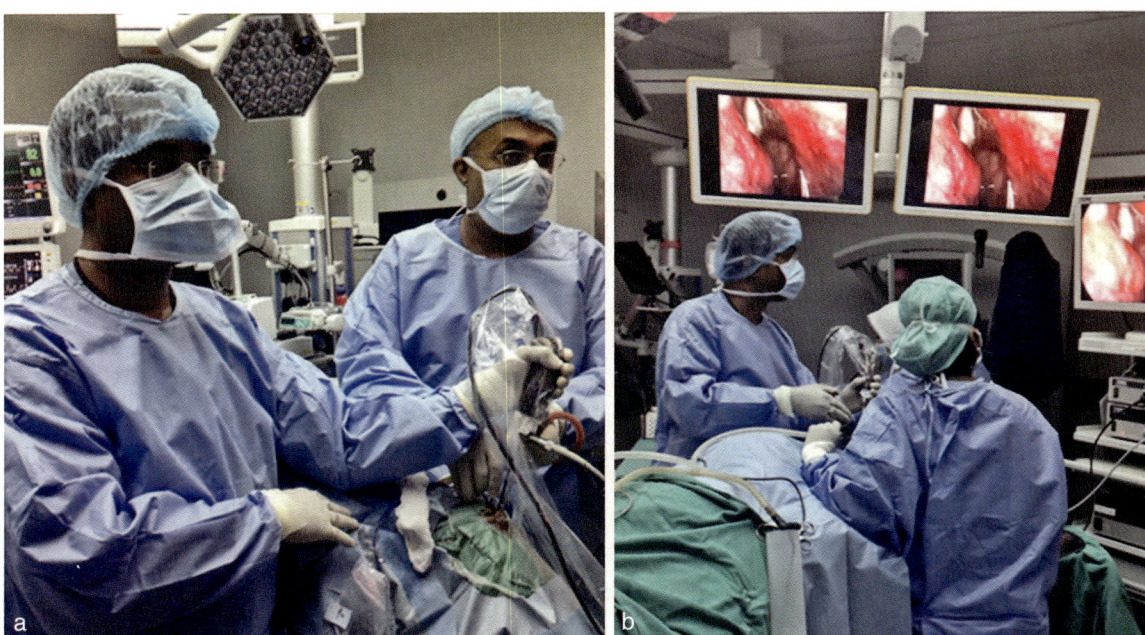

Fig. 20.7: a. Assistant on the left of patient holds the endoscope while neurosurgeon operates instrumentation with both hands; **b.** Operating room set-up showing the positions of surgeon, assistant and monitors

incision at the osteocartilaginous junction (Fig. 20.8e,f).

7. Mucoperiosteal flap is elevated on one side of the septum followed by dislocation of the bony cartilaginous junction, this gives access for flap elevation of the opposite side for (Fig. 20.9a,b).

8. Posterior bony septum is then removed (Fig. 20.9c).

9. Mucoperiosteal elevation is extended till sphenovomerine suture and ostium is located while at the same time exercising care not to damage the posterior septal artery. At this point, the keel of the sphenoid is fully exposed (Fig. 20.9d). See also Fig. 20.10.

10. Kerrison's punch is used to remove the keel of sphenoid (Fig. 20.9e,f) and the anterior wall of sphenoid sinus to give a wide exposure of the sellar and surrounding anatomy.

11. Septations in the sphenoid sinus are carefully removed, paying particular attention of septations running to ICA (Figs 20.11 and 20.12a,b).

12. Exposure is achieved from carotid eminences laterally and from planum sphenoidale superiorly and the clivus inferiorly (Fig. 20.11b,c). Bony dehiscence over CCA is sometimes encountered as seen in Fig. 20.11b.

13. Mucosa over the sellar is cauterized and elevated off the sellar floor (Fig. 20.11d).

14. If the bone overlying the sella is thick, then it is usually drilled away (Fig. 20.11e–f).

Tumour Removal (Video 2)

1. In macroadenomas, the bone overlying the sellar is usually thin enough to be flaked off with either a right-angled probe or freer elevator exposing the dura covering the sella (Fig. 20.12c, d).

2. Right-angled probe is used carefully to lift away dura from the periosteum of the sella turcica before proceeding with a wide bony removal. The lateral limit of bony removal is the cavernous sinus, inferiorly the inferior intercavernous sinus and superiorly the superior intercavernous sinus (Fig. 20.12e,f).

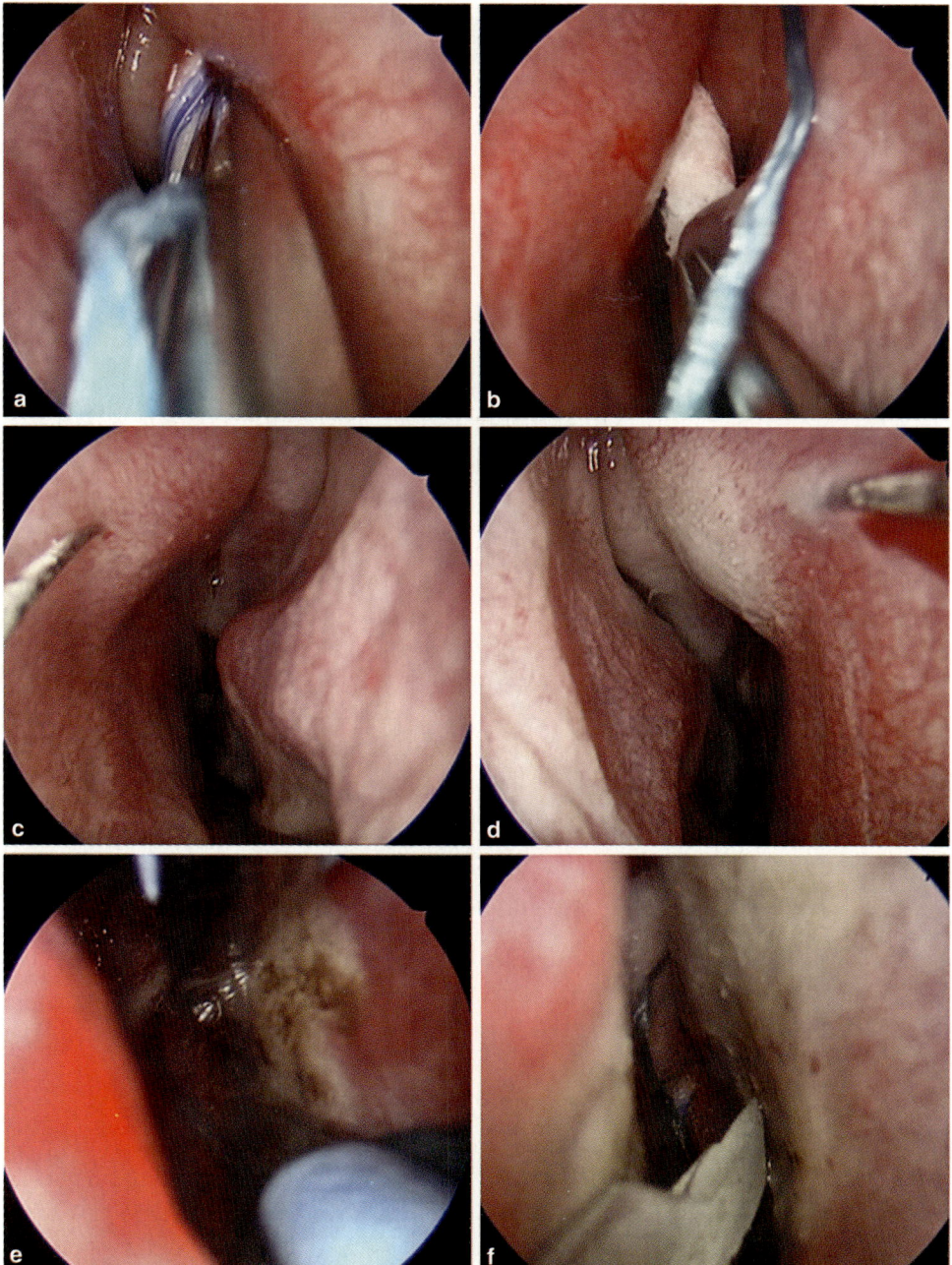

Fig. 20.8: Transseptal transsphenoidal pituitary surgery: Nasal preparation

3. The dura is cauterised at the site of incision. Often cruciate incision is made over the dural covering of the pituitary but occasionally it is also tailored to the content and site of the cystic component. Incision is made lower in a case of superolateral cystic component to prevent early descend of the diaphragm which can obscure the surgical field (Fig. 20.13a–c).

4. A sample of tumour is removed for histopathological examination (Fig. 20.13d).

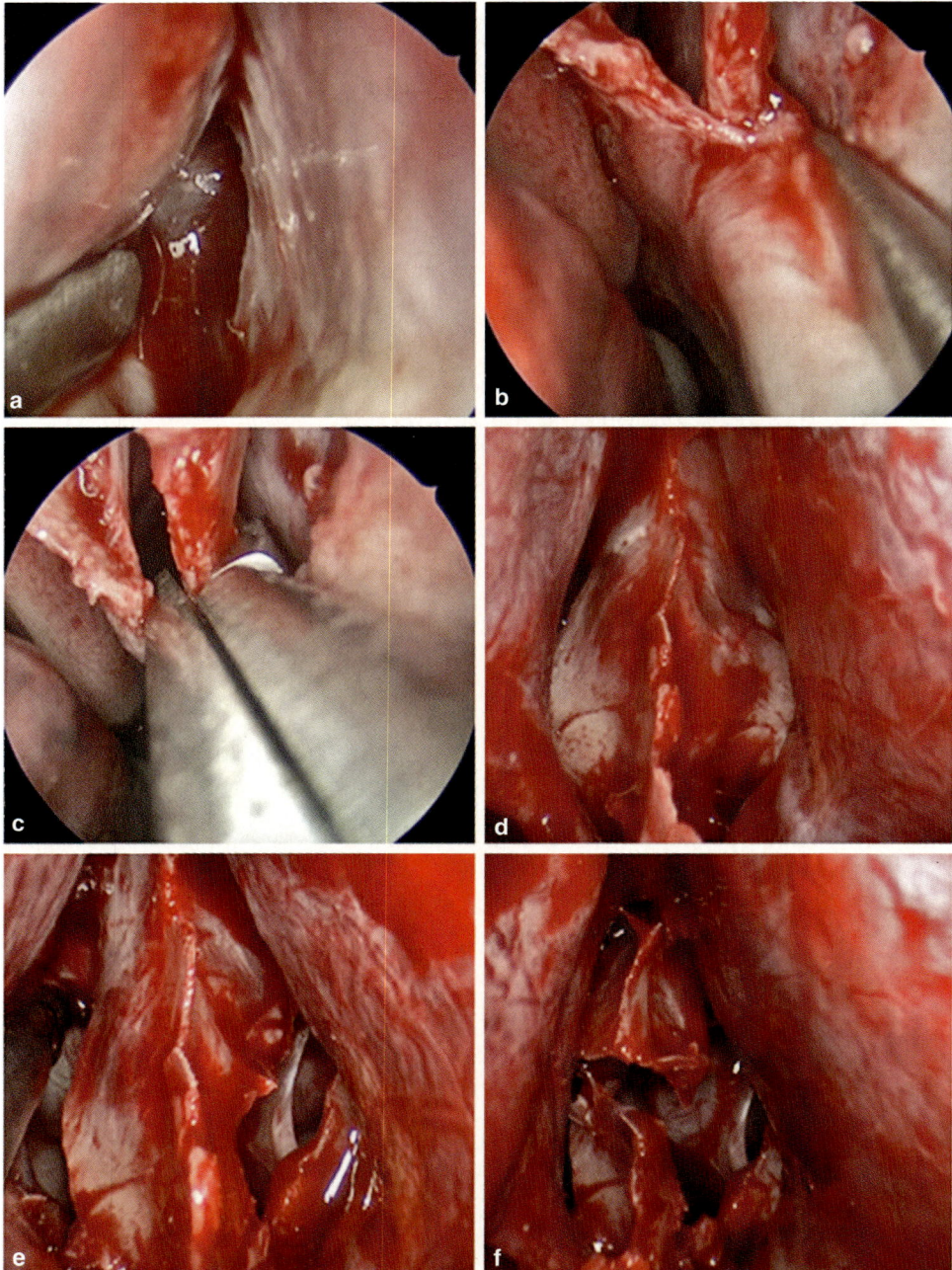

Fig. 20.9: Transseptal transsphenoidal pituitary surgery: Removal of posterior septum and keel of sphenoid

5. The rest of the tumour removal is performed using suction, dissectors and also ring curettes (Fig. 20.13e,f). Tumour removal is performed systemically from inferior to lateral then superiorly, this is also done to prevent early descend of

diaphragm thus obscuring the surgical field.

6. Incision is extended, if residual tumour is suspected (Fig. 20.13g–i). Complete removal of tumour is attempted, paying particualr attention to corners and clefts

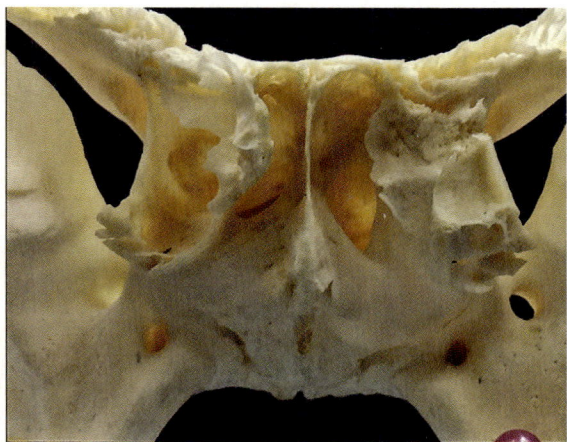

Fig. 20.10: Dry bone specimen demonstrating the keel of sphenoid (sphenoidal rostrum) and the opening into the sphenoid sinus

between the cavernous sinus and diaphragma sellae (Fig. 20.13j,k). In most instances, the dome of diaphragm descends symmetrically once tumour removal is adequate. Inspection is done using the suction to hold up the diaphragma sellae (Fig. 20.13l).

7. If there is no CSF leak, then sellar reconstruction is not required to complete the surgery.
8. The cavity is packed with Gelfoam and Surgicel®.
9. The mucoperiosteal flap of septum is replaced.
10. Merocel packings are placed in both nostrils.

Primary Pituitary Surgery— Double Nostril Technique

A double nostril technique may be utilized in patients with a narrow nostril with limited exposure and the space is crowded for instruments to be moved in and out of the nose in a smooth manner.

In this technique, the surgery proceeds in a similar manner except for removal of the superoposterior mucoperiosteal flap from both sides leaving a large opening in the posterior septum. This can be done easily with microdebrider/shaver (Video 3).

This allows both nostrils to be used for instrumentation.

Revision/Redo Pituitary Surgery

In a surgery for recurrent or residual tumour, it is imperative to check the previous records for preoperative symptoms, pre- and postoperative endocrine status, visual field tests and the operative notes of the previous surgery. This is important to find out what technique has been used in the past, flap reconstruction that has been used, anatomical variants encountered and postoperative complications.[9]

Besides that, imaging (pre- and postoperative T1-weighted post-gadolinium MRI images) will also give additional clues of previous surgery: Tumour size, tumour extension such as suprasellar and cavernous sinus invasion, and the extent of tumour resection.[9]

In a revision surgery, adhesions between septum and turbinates need to be released if present (Fig. 20.14a). If a large posterior septal opening is present, then entry into sphenoid sinus is fast (Fig. 20.14b). However, it must also be determined, if a posterior septal flap was used to reconstruct the sella which is then cauterized and elevated off the bone (Fig. 20.14c,d). Remove debri that may have collected within sphenoid sinus cavity (Fig. 20.14e). Mucosal growth over the anterior face of sphenoid may reduce the view of the surgical field and need to be removed (Fig. 20.14f,g). Equally important is the size of posterior septectomy that may need to be enlarged anteriorly, done easily with a backbiting forceps (Fig. 20.14h).

Bony regeneration over the sellar and adjacent bone has been seen to occur and affect the sellar exposure in revision surgery.[10] In most cases, this requires drilling or piecemeal removal with Kerrison's punch to expose the dural covering of pituitary (Fig. 20.14i–l).

The rest of the surgery proceeds in a similar manner. Intraoperative navigation is often helpful to identify fixed critical structures that serve as a landmark (pituitary fossa, planum sphenoidale, clivus) and also the position of internal carotid arteries (Fig. 20.15).

If available, intraoperative MRI is employed to look for residual tumour.

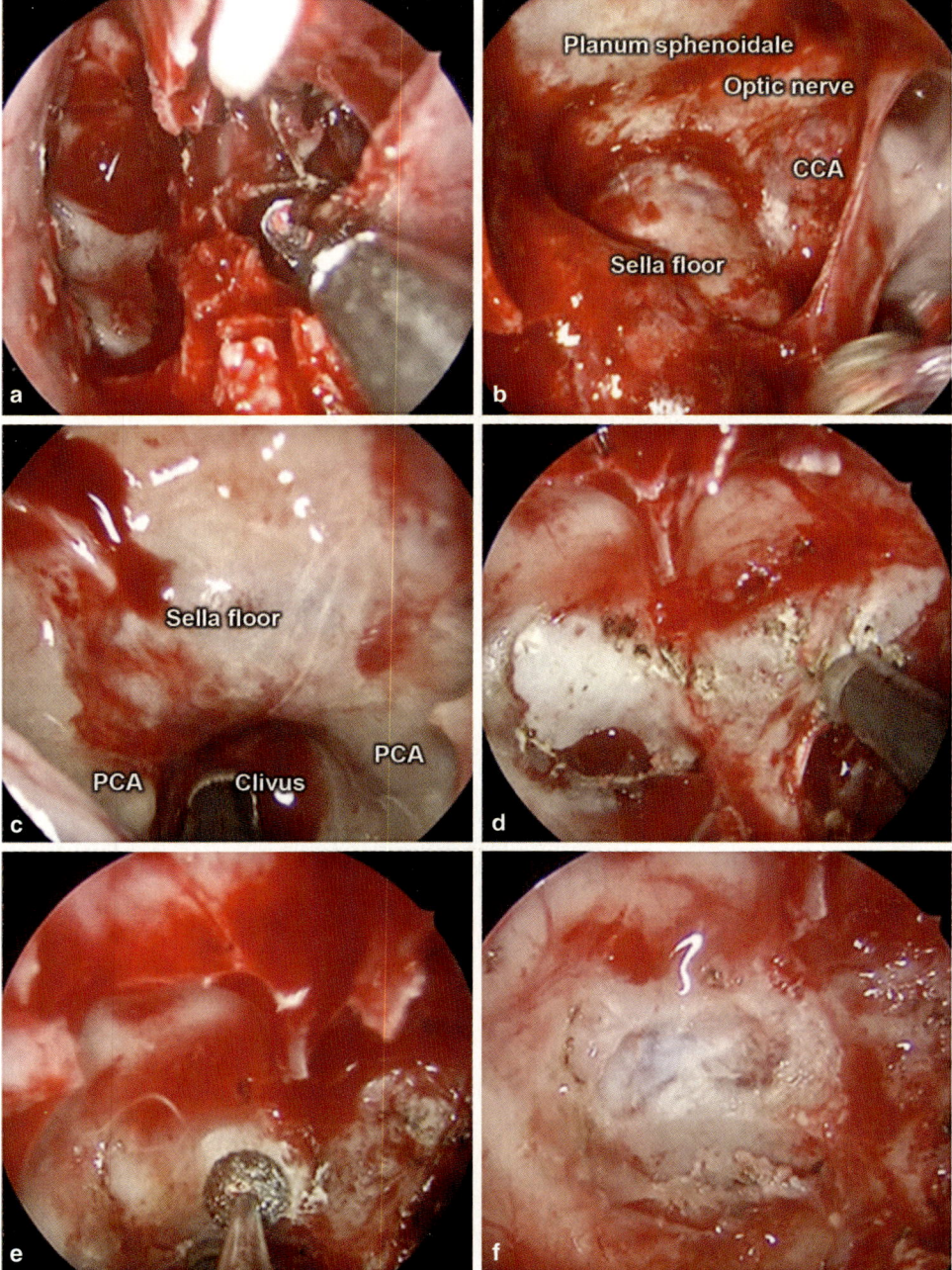

Fig. 20.11: Transseptal transsphenoidal pituitary surgery: Exposure of sella, also showing paraclival carotid artery (PCA) and cavernous carotid artery (CCA)

Postoperative Care

1. Nasal packs are removed within 24–48 hours, longer up to 72–120 hours, if CSF leak repair has been performed.

2. Patient is advised to avoid straining (no sneezing, coughing, straining during defaecation, etc.), if CSF leak has been repaired.

3. Nasal endoscopy and toileting is performed at 1 week postoperatively.

4. Repeat imaging is done to look for residual tumour.

5. Repeat endocrine blood investigations.

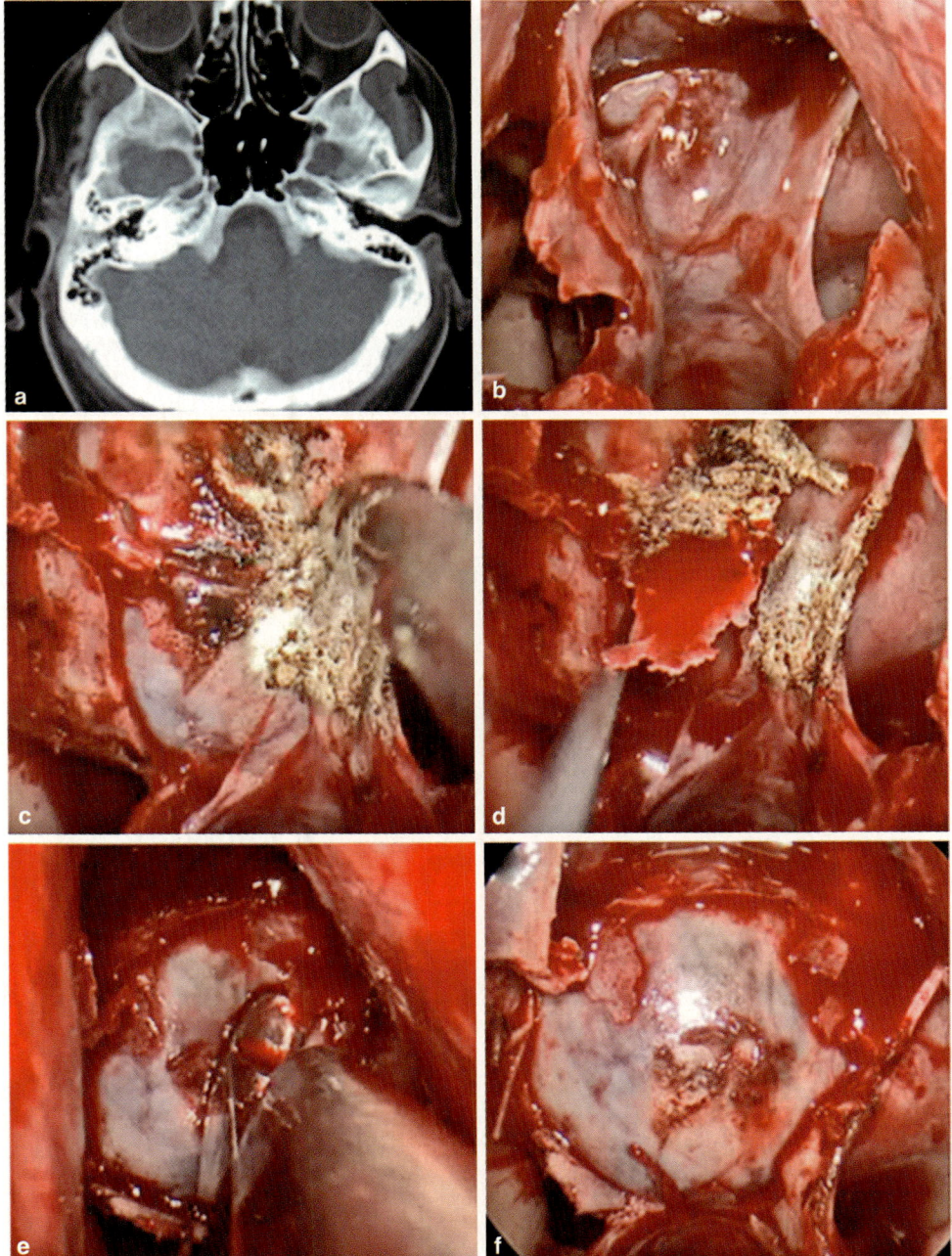

Fig. 20.12: Transseptal transsphenoidal pituitary surgery: Exposure of pituitary

Complications of TSS

1. Bleeding from posterior septal artery, mucosa, exposed bone, dural veins, cavernous sinus, ICA.

2. *CSF leak:* CSF leakage can occur during or after the tumour removal, during the exploration of cavernous sinus and diaphragmatic recesses particularly seen in revision surgery and with suprasellar extension of macroadenoma.[11]

3. Residual or recurrences

4. Hyposmia (seen with excessive coagulation of superior turbinate and superior part of middle turbinate or turbinectomies, if performed).[10]

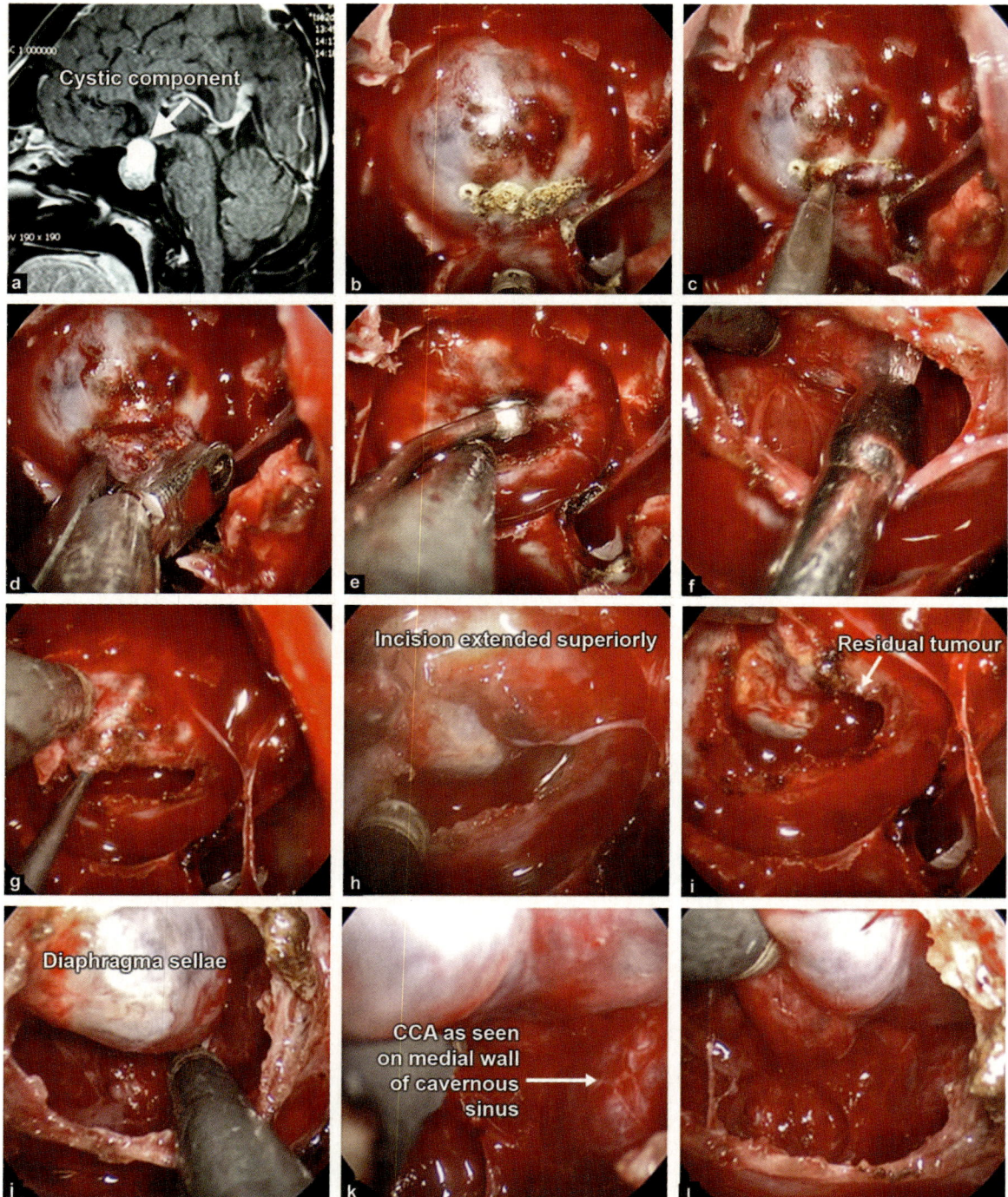

Fig. 20.13: Transseptal transsphenoidal pituitary surgery: Tumour removal

5. *Endocrine complications:*[11]
   a. Temporary diabetes insipidus (DI) can occur due to temporary dysfunction of vasopressin-producing neurons secondary to surgical trauma and thermal injury of cautery or a dysfunction of posterior pituitary gland; however, recovery is reported to occur within 6 months.

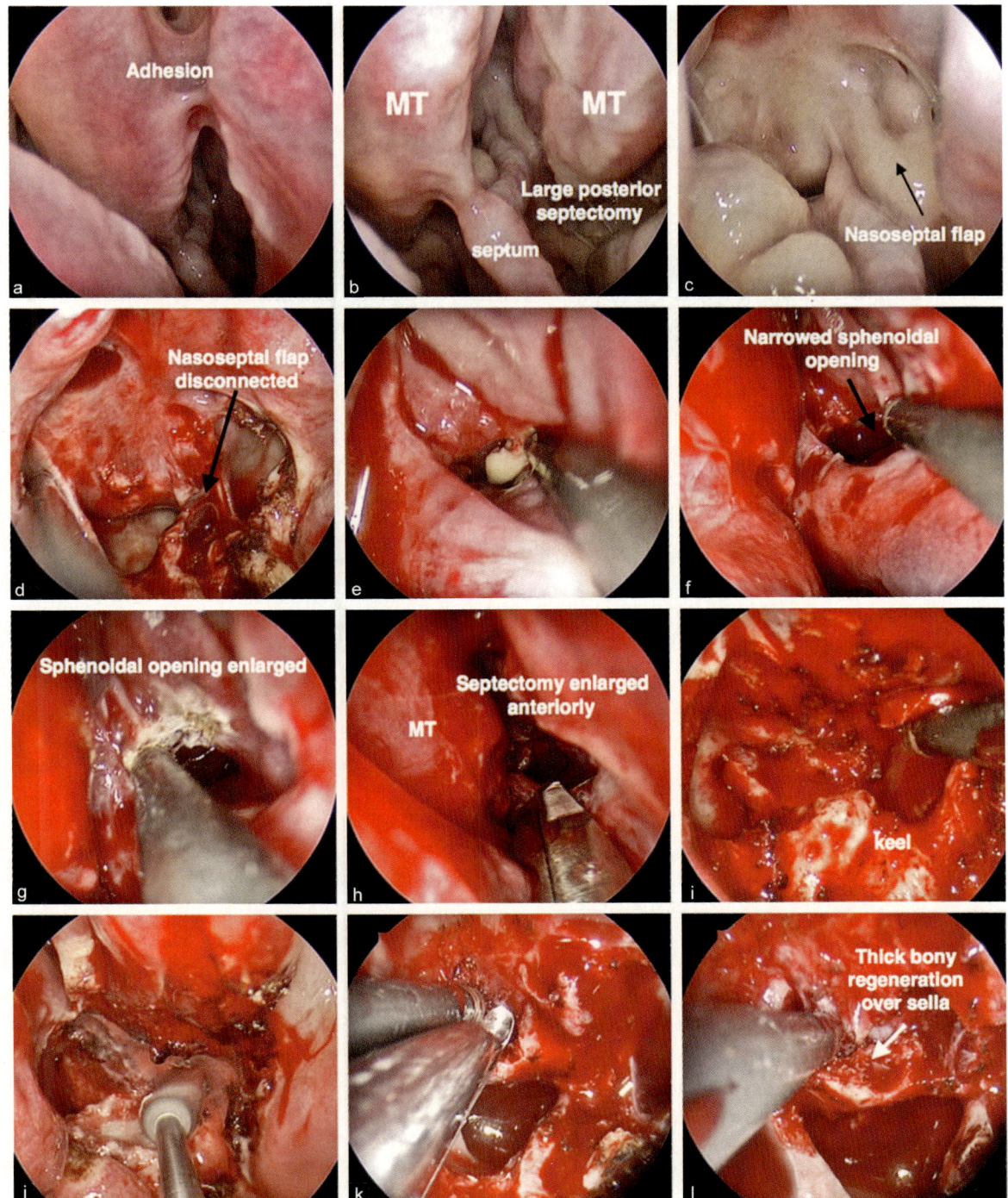

Fig. 20.14: Transseptal transsphenoidal pituitary surgery: Exposure to sella in redo surgery

b. Anterior pituitary deficiency may become apparent postoperatively and is believed to be secondary to excessive use of the tumour aspirator in the sellar cavity, inappropriate manipulation and resection of the normal pituitary gland

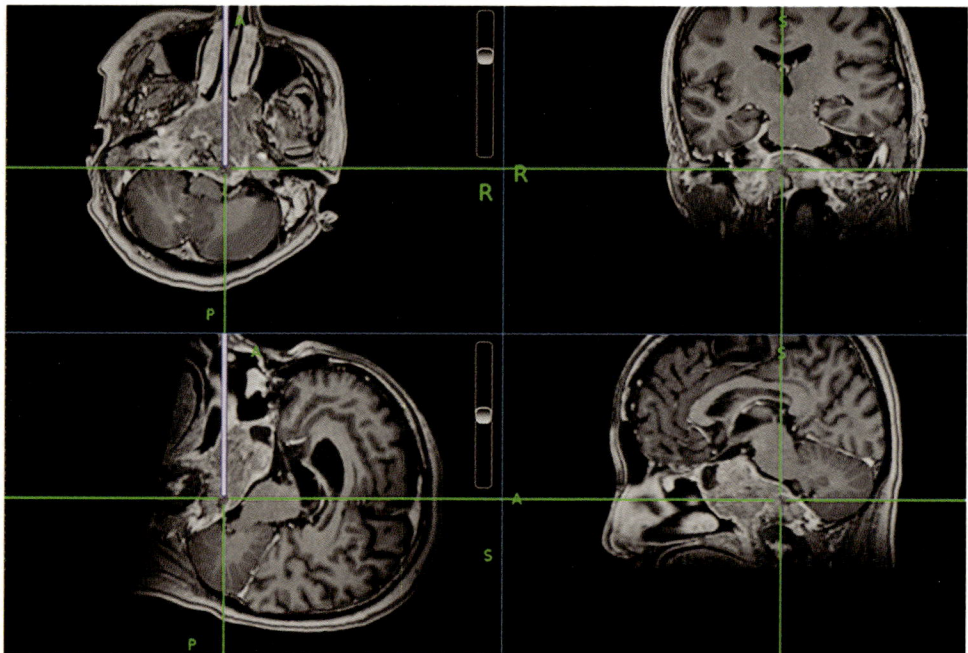

Fig. 20.15: This image is a snapshot while utilizing an intraoperative navigation system used to identify the location of the odontoid peg as tumour was removed from clivus

adjacent to the adenoma and use of bipolar cauterization in sellar cavity after the tumour removal.

Management of Complications

Bleeding

1. Mucosal bleeding can usually be arrested with monopolar or bipolar cauterization.
2. Bleeding from exposed bone may occasionally require bone wax, if cautery is insufficient to control the ooze.
3. Bleeding from dural veins and cavernous sinus can often be controlled with use of Surgicel (fibrillar absorbable haemostat, Johnson & Jonhson) or when inadequate other haemostatic agents can be used, e.g. FloSeal (haemostatic matrix sealant agent, Baxter). In our institution, haemostasis is achieved using Taming Sari, a device designed by the author (ViknesWaran) which allows the delivery of haemostatic agents accurately over the site of haemorr-hage while simultaneously maintaining compression and suction. This is particularly useful in endoscopic surgery through a long narrow tunnel and the device is also able to prevent from haemostatic agent from being washed away by brisk bleeding.[12] (Video 4)
4. ICA injury is a disaster to be avoided; if possible, conventional angiography should be performed immediately followed by endovascular stent-graft placement.

CSF Leak

1. In a small leak, a fat graft can be used to seal the leak site followed by Tisseel glue (fibrin sealant). The sphenoid sinus is packed well with Gelfoam and the Merocel packing is left *in situ* for about 5 days (Fig. 20.16). (Video 5)
2. A larger defect causing CSF leak may require additional graft. In our practice, we use fascia lata and/or Hadad flap. (Video 6)

Pearls and Points for Surgical Procedure

1. For a beginner rhinologist who has been performing basic FESS, pituitary surgery may need adjustments in terms of head positions and orientation of the skull

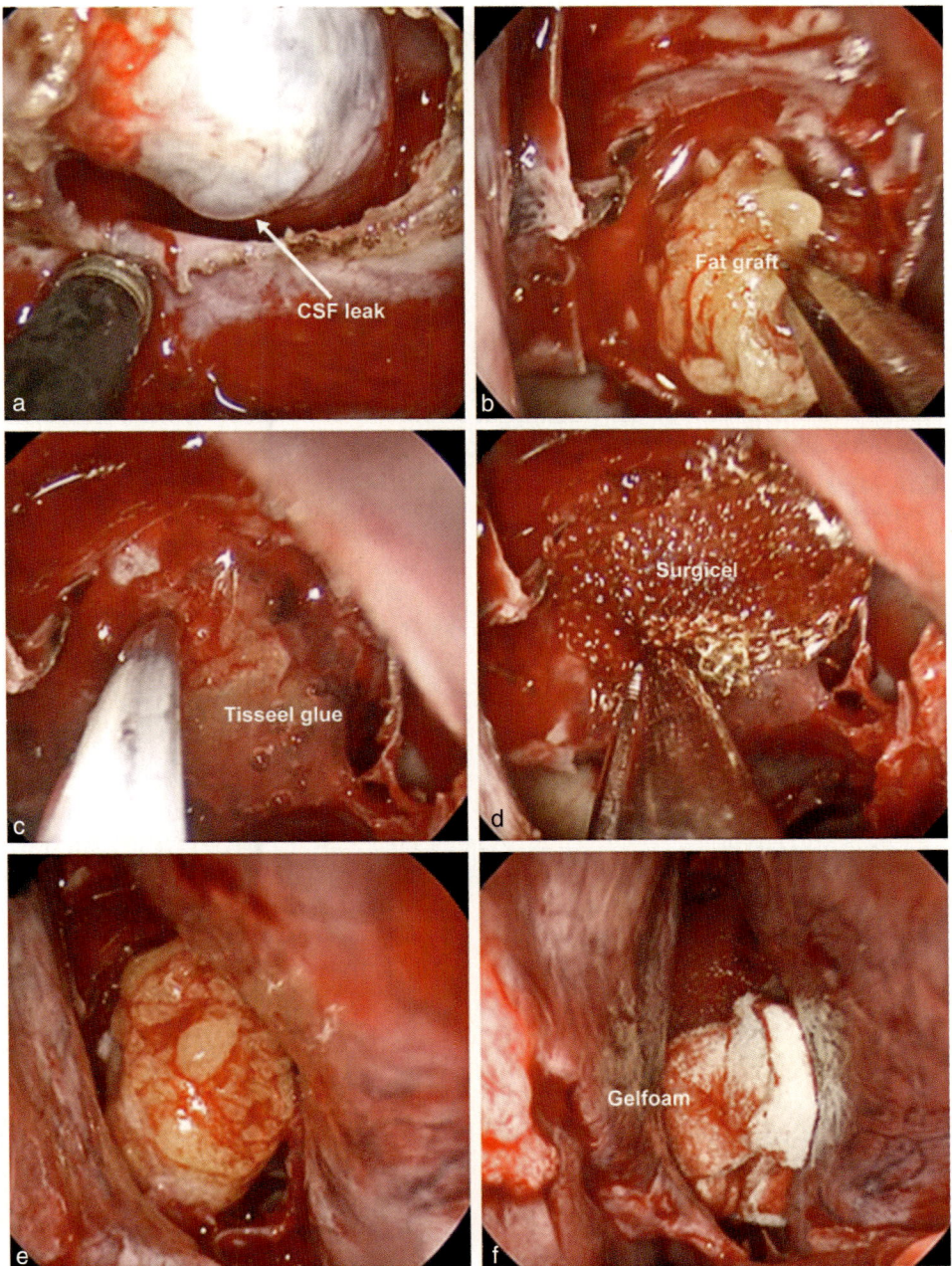

Fig. 20.16: Transseptal transsphenoidal pituitary surgery: CSF leak repair

base besides the 3/4-hand technique in performing surgery.

2. In-depth anatomical knowledge and repeated practice on cadavers are of paramount importance.

3. Study of the patient's radiological images to look for anatomical variants and tumour extent is invaluable during surgery.

4. Use IGS where available.

5. Preserve posterior septal artery in case Hadad flap is required.

6. Septations in sphenoid sinus is carefully removed, in particular those running towards ICA.

7. Careful elevation of dura off periosteum to avoid bleeding and CSF leak.

8. To know the lateral limits and superior limits of surgery.

9. Clefts and corners are thoroughly inspected with use of 0° or when required 30° endoscope to look for residual tumours.

10. Avoid cautery within the sella cavity.

11. Immediate repair of CSF leaks with meticulous graft.

12. Minimize trauma to the nasal cavity.

REFERENCES

1. Buchfelder M, Schlaffer S. Surgical treatment of pituitary tumours. Best Pract Res Clin Endocrinol Metab 2009;23:677–92.

2. Wilson CB. A decade of pituitary microsurgery. The Herbert Olivecronalecture. J Neurosurgery 1984;61(5):814–33.

3. Wilson CB. Extensive personal experience. Surgical management of pituitary tumours. J Clin Endocrinol Metab 1997 82;8:2381–85.

4. de Divitiis E, Laws ER, Giani U, Iuliano SL, de Divitiis O, Apuzzo ML. The current status of endoscopy in transsphenoidal surgery: An international survey.World Neurosurg 2015 Apr; 83(4):447–54.

5. Laws ER Jr, Barkhoudarian B. The transition from microscopic to endoscopic transsphenoidal surgery: The experience at Brigham and Women's Hospital. World Neurosurg 2014; 82, 6S:S152–S154.

6. Gaillard S. The transition from microscopic to endoscopic transsphenoidal surgery in high-caseload neurosurgical centers: The Experience of Foch Hospital. World Neurosurg 2014;82:6S: S116–S120.

7. Patronas NJ, Liu CY. State of art imaging of the pituitary tumours. J Neurooncol 2014;117:395–405.

8. Waran V, Tang IP, Karuppiah R, AbdKadir KA, Chandran H, Muthusamy KA, Prepageran N. A new modified speculum guided single nostril technique for endoscopic transnasal transsphenoidal surgery: An analysis of nasal complications. Br J Neurosurg 2013 Dec; 27(6):742–46.

9. Chang EF, Sughrue ME, Zada G, Wilson CB, Blevins LS Jr, Kunwar S. Long-term outcome following repeat transsphenoidal surgery for recurrent endocrine-inactive pituitary adenomas Pituitary. 2010 Sep;13(3):223–29.

10. Yahia-Cherif M, Delpierre I, Hassid S, De Witte O. Bony regeneration of the sella after transsphenoidal pituitary surgery. World Neurosurgery (2015), doi: 10.1016/ j.wneu.2015.10.073. [Epub ahead of print]

11. Berker M, Hazer DB, Yücel T, et al. Complications of endoscopic surgery of the pituitary adenomas: Analysis of 570 patients and review of the literature. Pituitary 2012;15:288–300.

12. Waran V, Sek K, Bahuri NF, Narayanan P, ChandranHaemostatic Agent Delivery System for endoscopic neurosurgical procedures. Minim Invasive Neurosurg 2011 Oct;54(5-6):279–81.

Videos:

Video 1: Transseptal transsphenoidal pituitary surgery: Exposure to sella.

Video 2: Transseptal transsphenoidal pituitary surgery: Tumour removal.

Video 3: Transseptal transsphenoidal pituitary surgery: Single nostril and double nostril approach.

Video 4: Transseptal transsphenoidal pituitary surgery: Haemostasis using Taming Sari.

Video 5: Transseptal transsphenoidal pituitary surgery: Fat graft repair for minor CSF leaks.

Video 6: Transseptal transsphenoidal pituitary surgery: Sella reconstruction with fascia lata and Hadad flap.

Surgery for Chronic Frontal Sinusitis (Draf Procedure)

DR Nayak

Surgical treatment of frontal sinus is always difficult and challenging and can be devastating unless properly planned and well indicated. Chronic frontal sinusitis is always difficult to treat. Despite various techniques having been adopted in the past two centuries, a clear cut well established technique to manage this condition is yet to be achieved (Ramadan, 2005). Endoscopic frontal sinus surgery, developed in the later part in the evolution of FESS is often unsafe to the patient, and can result with significant rate of failure (Friedman, 2000).

Draf in 1991 develop a new technique to open the frontal sinus intranasally and allowing it to drain and achieved a success rate of 90%. Draf I consisted of an anterior ethmoidectomy with opening of the naso-frontal duct (NFD). Draf II in addition consists of unilateral resection of the floor of the frontal sinus; Draf III is bilateral resection of the frontal sinus floor. The surgery has been further refined by Wormald.

Draf I (Fig. 21.1a and b)

It is done by exenterating the septa of cells in the anterior ethmoid including agger nasi in the frontal recess while preserving the mucosa of the Killian's infundibulum (Fig. 21.2) thus facilitating improvement in drainage. CT scan plays an important role in planning (Fig. 21.1).

Indications for Draf I Procedure

- Orbital and other endocranial complications associated with acute frontal sinusitis not responded to antibiotics.

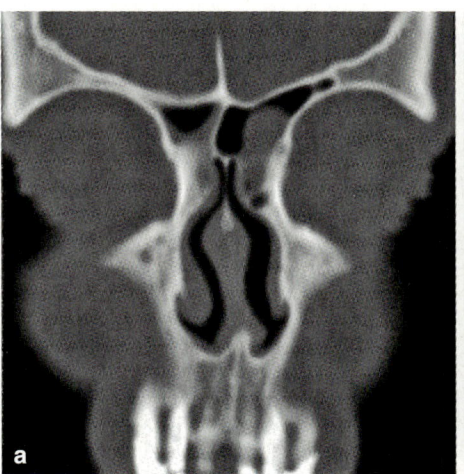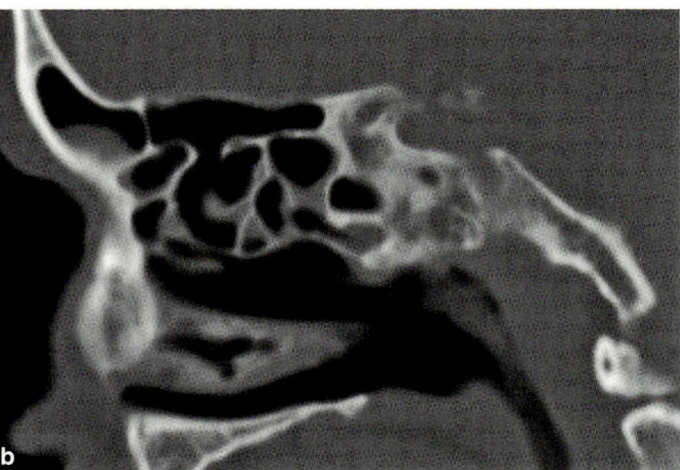

Fig. 21.1: a. Coronal; **b.** Axial CT showing minimal isolated disease in both frontal sinuses. With kind permission from editor OJOLHNS for reproduction

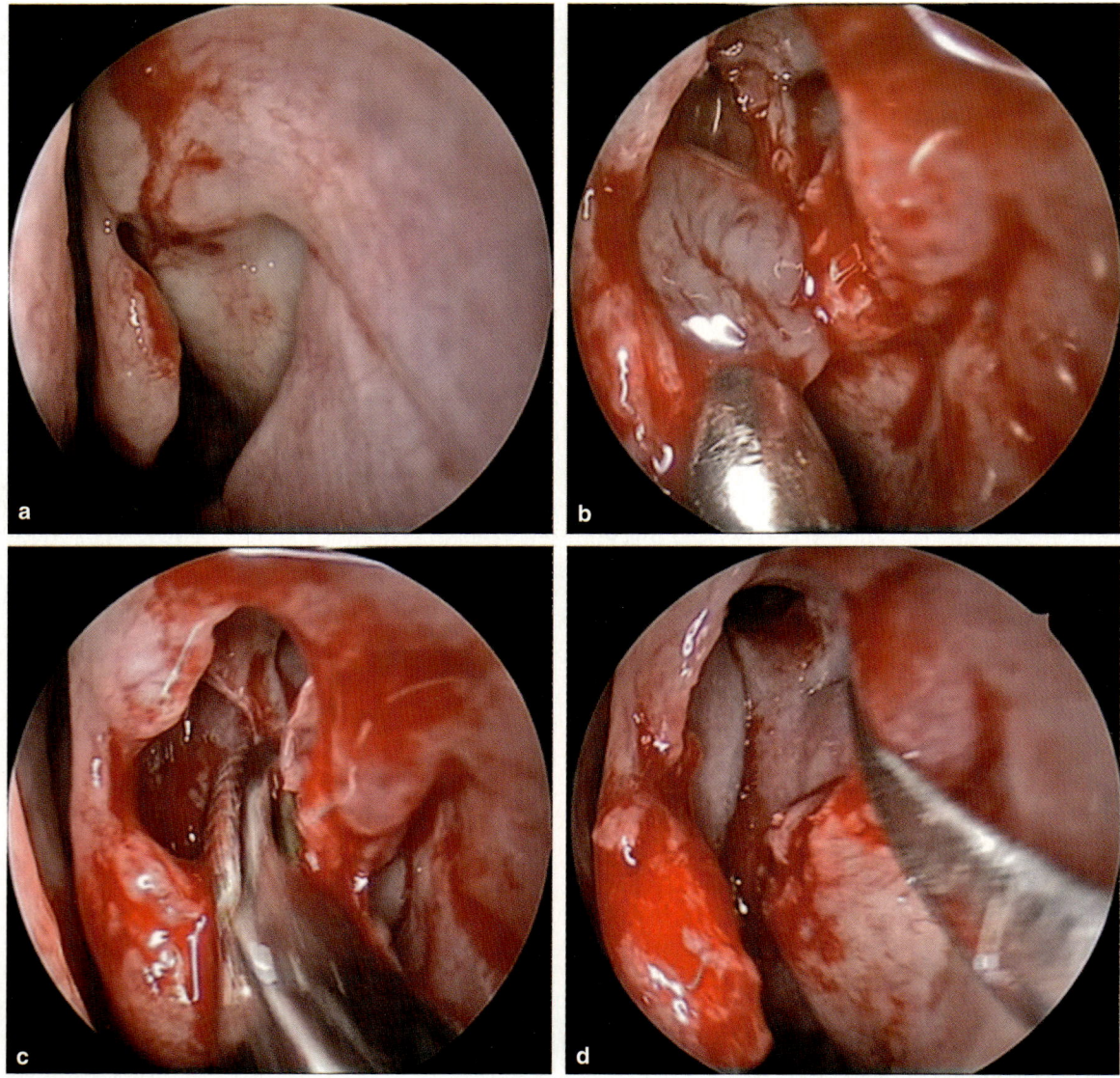

Fig. 21.2: a. Incision for axillary flap and anteriorly based flap, **b.** Drainage of frontal sinus after removal of inferior wall and part of the posterior wall of agger nasi. **c.** Removal of bone along with mucosa attached while preserving mucosa from the back of the posterior wall. **d.** Axillary flap mucosa rotated over raw medial wall, mucosa from the posterior wall of agger nasi rotated ove raw superior wall anteriorly based flap repositioned. Note the intact bulla and mucosa over the posterior wall of the frontal recess and frontal ostium (with kind permission from editor OJOLHNS for reproduction)

- Acute frontal sinusitis having failed to respond to conservative management.
- Chronic sinusitis with frontal sinus involvement with no previous history of frontal sinus surgery.
- Revision endoscopic sinus surgery with incomplete ethmoidectomy.

Draf II Procedure

Draf IIa: In this, surgery is done as in Draf I and further extended by removing the frontal floor between the lamina papyracea and the middle turbinate attachment. All the cells including agger nasi, frontal and suprabullar cell/frontal bulla (Figs 21.3 and 21.4) needs

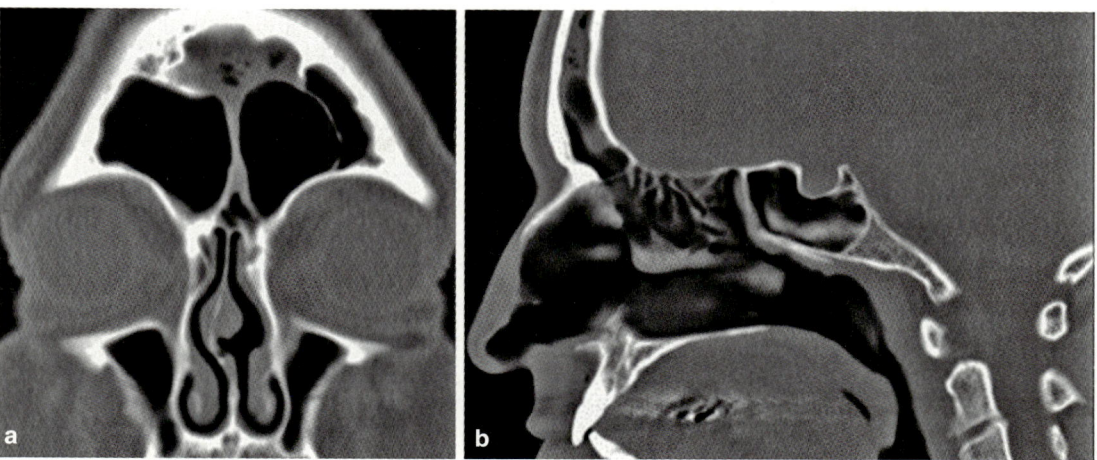

Fig. 21.3: CT scan: **a.** Coronal cut, and **b.** Sagittal cut, showing frontal sinus infection due to obstruction by large frontal bulla cell

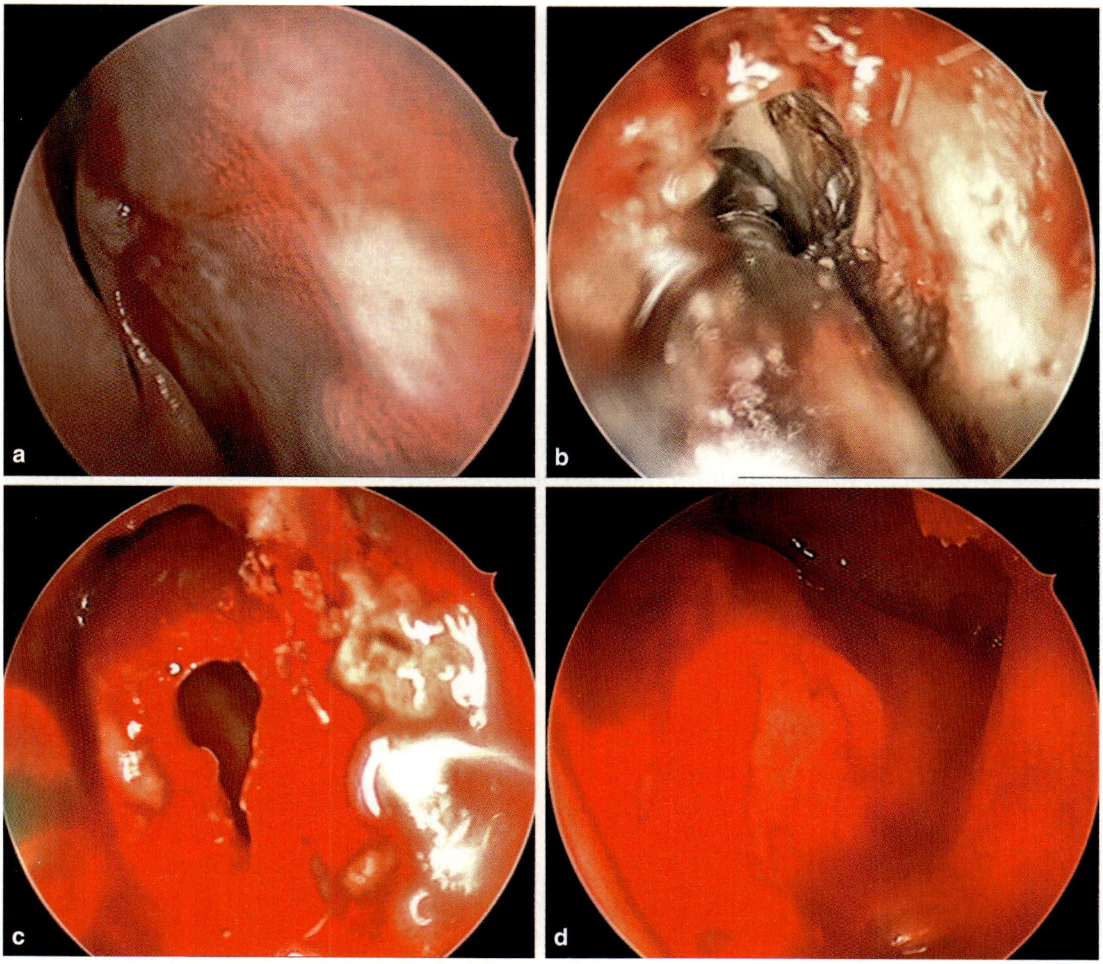

Fig. 21.4: a. Axillary flap incision, **b.** Drilling of frontal beak after identification of frontal recess and ostium, **c.** Exposure of frontal bulla cell and removal, **d.** After removal of frontal bulla cell

to be opened, while outer cell mucosa is preserved to keep the drainage pathway intact. Alternately Stammberger's technique of uncapping the egg can be adopted (Stammberger, 2000). In case of a lateralized middle turbinate as in revision cases, a frontal sinus rescue procedure described by Kuhn in 1996–97 can be done (Kuhn, et al 2000), where, attachment of middle turbinate to lateral wall is separated while preserving the lateral wall mucosa of the middle turbinate. The medial wall mucosa and middle bone is removed along with the mucosa of the corresponding part of the septum. The lateral mucosa from the middle turbinate remnant draped over the raw bony surface of the septum to create a mucosalized frontal ostium.

Draf IIb: Initial procedure is same as Draf IIa, but to increase the size of the ostium drilling can be done further medially till the nasal septum. In this surgery, axillary flap is extended superiorly towards the nasal septum. This flap is elevated superiorly up to 1st olfactory neuron (Fig. 21.4). Then drilling is done over this thick bone over the frontal sinus floor between nasal septum medially to lamina papyracea laterally with the help of angled drill by MedtronicZomed®. Mucosal flap created by axillary flap repositioned.

Indications for Draf II Procedures

Type IIa drainage

- Serious complications of acute sinusitis.
- Medial mucoceles and pyocele involving frontoethmoid.
- Ethmoid tumour surgery (benign tumours) involving frontal recess.
- Extensive chronic frontal sinusitis with no gross mucosal disease.

Type IIb drainage

- If Draf IIa could not achieve an opening of 5–7 mm, a Draf IIb procedure is done.
- Failed Draf I procedure

Draf III (Modified Lothrop)— Out side in approach

This is also known as endonasal median drainage of the frontal sinus. Here the surgery for IIb is further expanded by resecting part of the superior nasal septum and extending further into the opposite frontal sinus floor. In case of distorted landmark, the surgeon can go for outside in approach. Before starting the surgery, one should look into coronal and sagittal imaging to get acquainted with the landmarks. Sagittal imaging is important to analyze the frontal sinus beak (Fig. 21.5). This approach is an evolution of modified

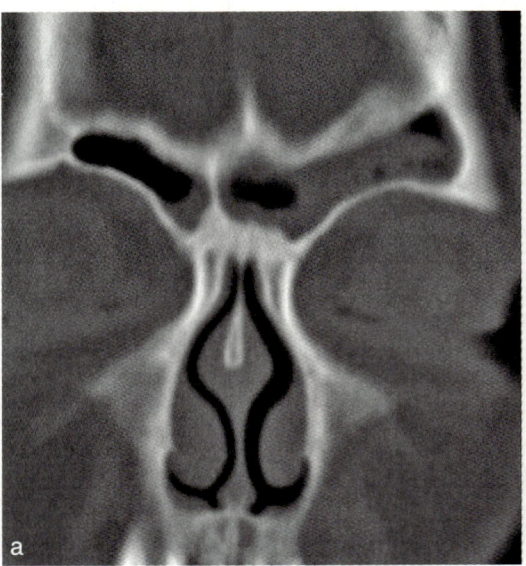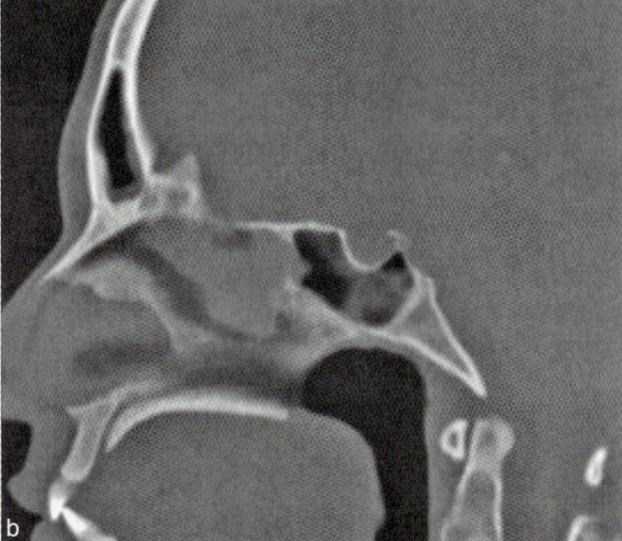

Fig. 21.5: Preoperative CT showing persistence bilateral frontal sinus disease after adequate medical treatment: **a.** Coronal CT, **b.** Sagittal CT

endoscopic Lothrop technique which follows the established landmark and is quite effective in inflammatory disease, mucoceles and CSF leak in relation to frontal sinus (Chin, et al 2012). The incision is given at the midpoint of middle meatus over the maxillary line and extended superiorly. Similar incision started over the septum of about 5 mm anterior to the lateral incision and extended superiorly till it joins the lateral incision along the anterior margin of the nasal process of the frontal bone. Similar procedure is done on the opposite side. Before this procedure, it is important to complete the ethmoidectomy and identify the lamina papyracea, if disease also involves ethmoid. The author does not perform ethmoidectomy as a routine when ethmoid is not diseased. The flap is elevated posteriorly further to reach the 1st olfactory neuron (Fig. 21.6a). While identifying it on either side, one should not get confused with the emissary vein that may be encountered before the neuron. This becomes the posterior boundary of Lothrop cavity. The nasal septal cartilage and bone are removed with roungeur to create a septal window. Drilling starts over the frontal process of maxilla laterally and extending superiorly just anterior to 1st

olfactory neuron and then onto the remnant bony nasal septum attach to the nasofrontal beak.

Drilling is done laterally till the periostium of the frontal process of maxilla is identified to facilitate safe removal of bone, anterior to the frontal recess and axilla that lies medial to this landmark. Drilling is done in an inverted 'U' motion to remove the frontal beak and frontal sinus floor anterior to the 1st olfactory neuron on both side (Fig. 21.6a). Once the frontal sinus floor is opened on one side, further drilling work is then carried out on the opposite side frontal sinus floor, thereby exposing the interfrontal septum (Fig. 21.6b).

The interfrontal septum is reduced superiorly taking care not to injure the skull base (Figs 21.7 and 21.8). Sometimes more than one frontal sinus septum may be noted on CT and should be addressed and interfrontal septal cell accordingly. The frontal cells including that extends into the frontal sinus (Type-3) should be exenterated and removed (Figs 21.7 and 21.9).

Preservation of mucosa of the drainage pathway in continuity with posterior wall is very important for proper drainage. The author prefers to pack both frontal sinus and

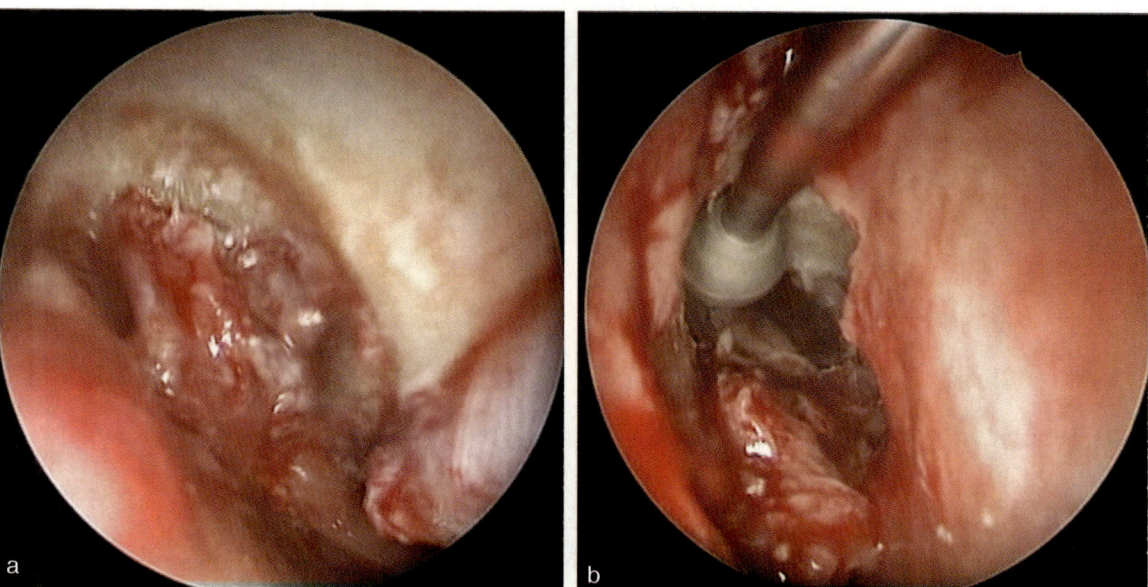

Fig. 21.6: a. Inverted U-shaped drilling anterior to the 1st olfactory neuron, with removal of frontal sinus floor after inferiorly based mucoperiosteal flap elevation. **b.** Opening of left frontal sinus and drilling of the interfrontal septum

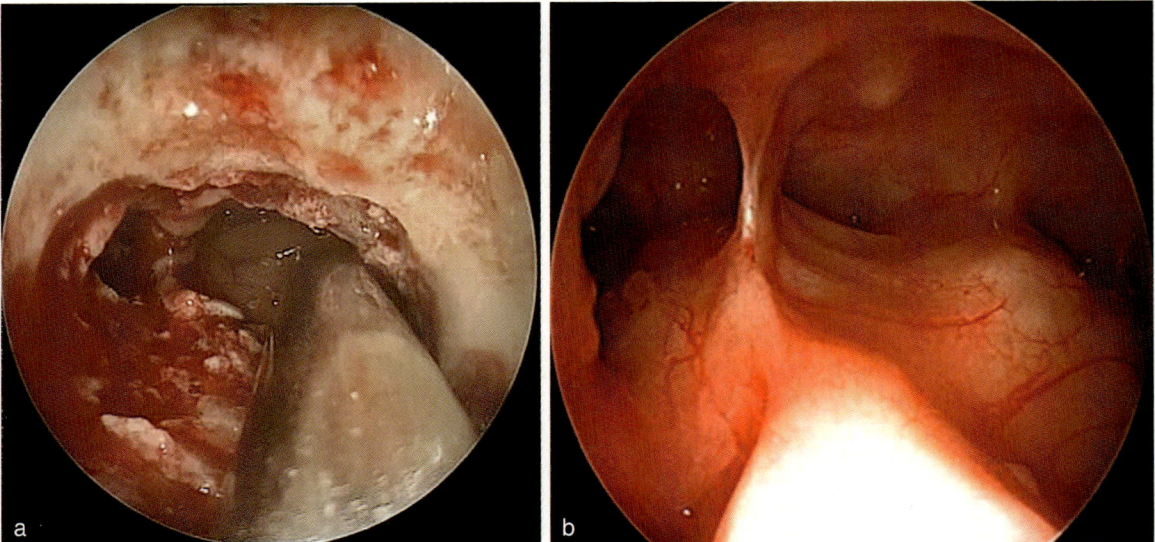

Fig. 21.7: a. Exposed interfrontal septum, that is partially drilled, left frontal sinus and partially opened right frontal sinus, **b.** Postoperative picture of the same patient

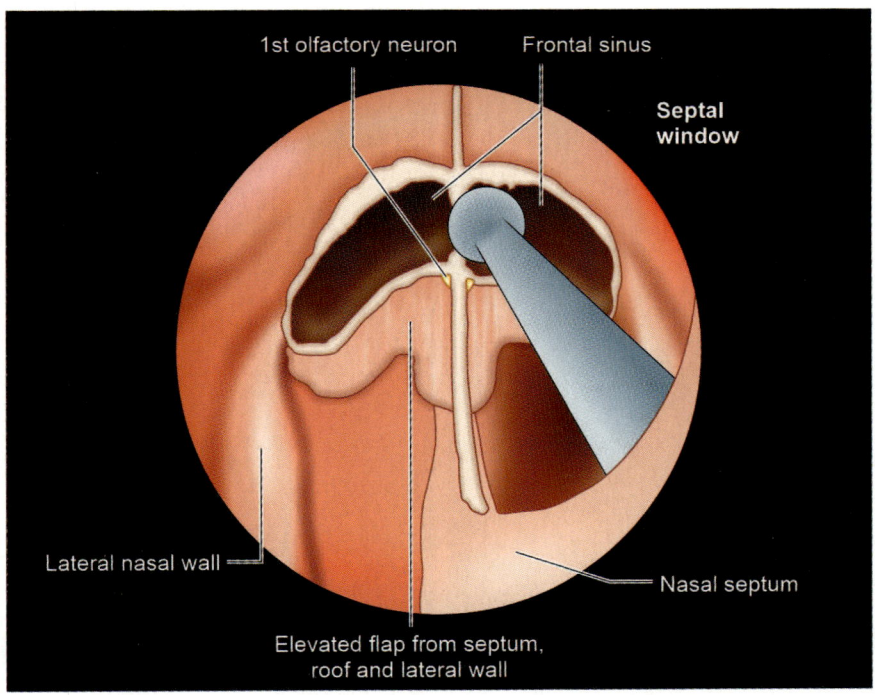

Fig. 21.8: Removal of interfrontal septum

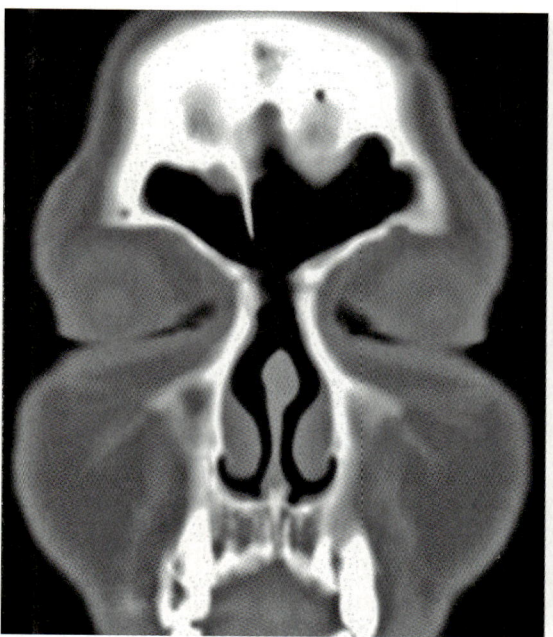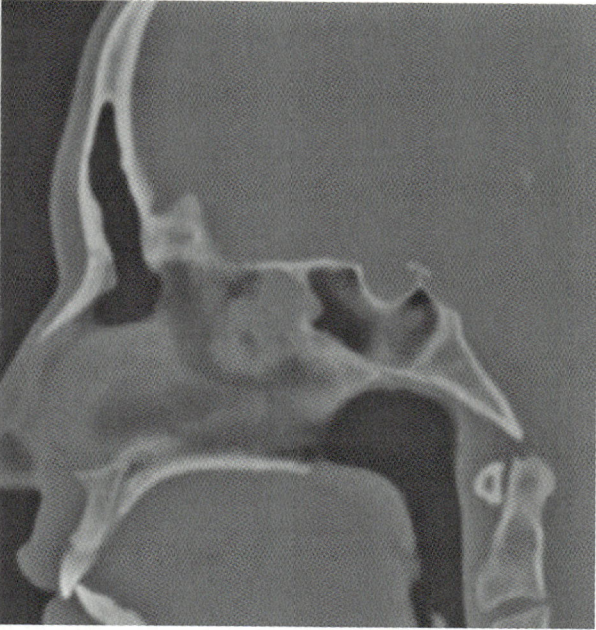

Fig. 21.9: Postoperative CT (note the preoperative CT in Fig. 21.5) after 6 months showing complete clearance of disease with removal of interfrontal septum and frontal beak in the same patient

the drainage cavity with NasoPore®. Alternatively cut glove pieces can be kept in the sinus cavity.

Draf III Procedure—Indications

- Extensive chronic frontal sinusitis with bilateral invovement with failure of Draf II procedure.
- Severe polyposis associated with Samter's triad.
- Primary ciliary dyskinesia, mucoviscidosis or Kartagener's syndrome, etc.
- Benign and malignant tumours of the paranasal sinuses as part of the approach.

Out side in approach to frontal sinus is a quick and easy way to perform a Draf III, and reduces operative time and minimizes complications. By using mucosal flaps and/or free mucosal grafts to cover exposed bone reduces the incidence of stenosis of drainage pathway and synaechia formation (Carney 2017).

Inside Out Draf III Procedure

This approach is ideal for bilateral extensive frontal sinus disease with narrow and crowded nasal cavities and when the frontal out flow tract could be identified on probing (Fig. 21.10a–d). Initial incision over the attachment of middle turbinate is given as in Draf I and the axilla is exposed. Drilling is done over the axilla, exposing the inferior and anterior wall of the agger nasi cell. The posterior and inferior wall of agger nasi cell is removed while preserving the uncinate process and the bulla. The drilling is followed superiorly till the frontal beak, laterally till level of lamina papyracea, medially and superiorly towards the superior attachment of nasal septum. The anterior floor of the frontal sinus is removed under direct vision, while preserving the mucosa of the frontal sinus drainage pathway. The window created by removing the septum superiorly till opposite side middle turbinate with superior attachment could be visualized. The redundant mucosa of the adjacent septum is removed with microdebrider and the adjacent bony septum is drilled out. Frontal sinus cavity inspected, frontal beak is drilled and interfrontal septum removed (Fig. 21.10e). The drilling is carried out to the opposite side frontal sinus. Similar

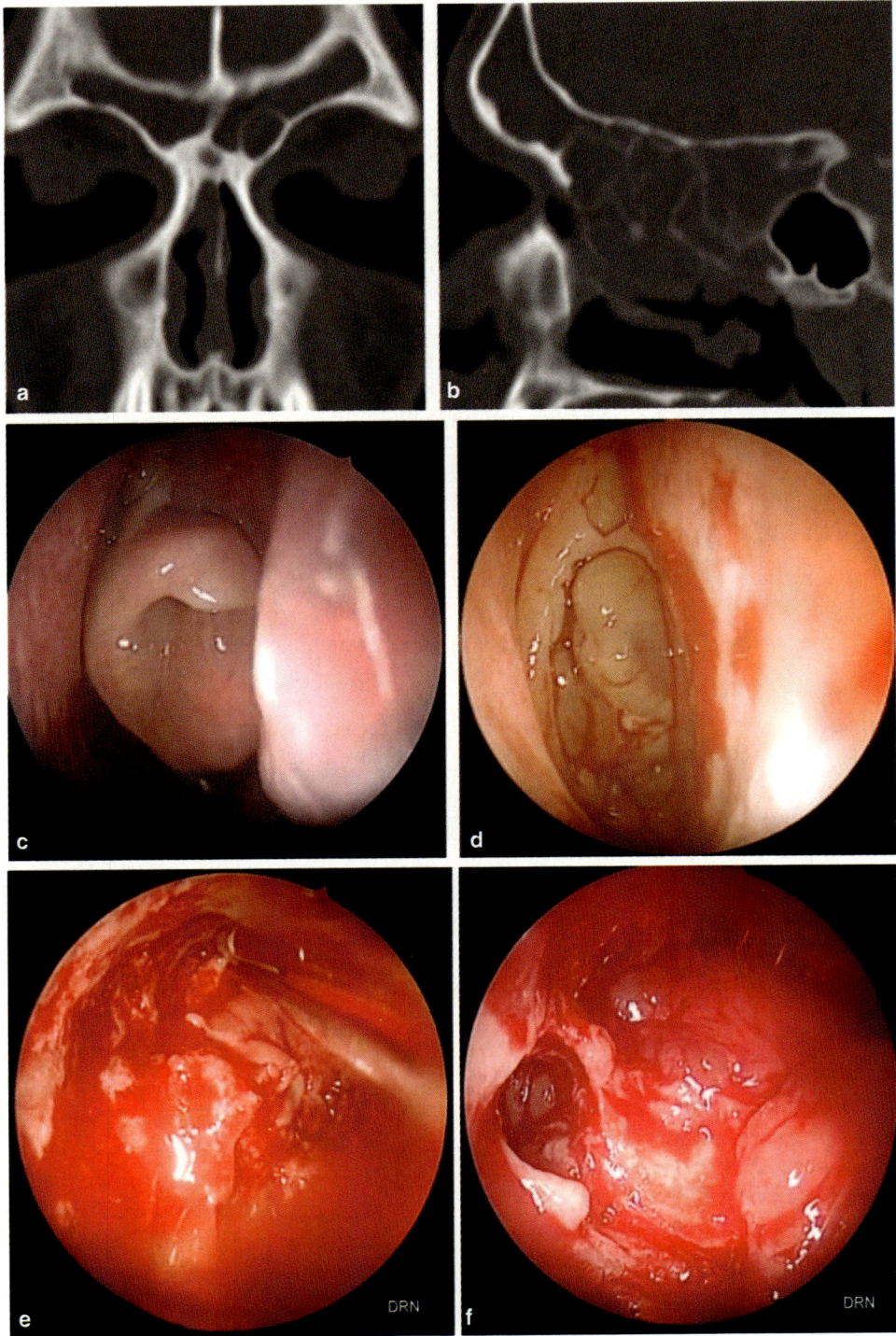

Fig. 21.10: a and b. Ethmoidal polyposis with gross bilateral frontal sinus involvement, **c.** Remnant polypoidal middle turbinate on left side, **d.** Polyps in the middle meatus with missing middle turbinate, showing **e.** Drilling of interfrontal septum after elevation of mucosa, **f.** Completion of Draf III after returning back the mucosal flap over raw bony surface in the interfrontal septum region (Ref: Fig. 9.30 and Video link for surgical steps)

procedure done through other nasal cavity, to identify the frontal recess and frontal outflow tract on the opposite side. Four-hand technique is adopted after creation of window for clearance of disease. Finally drilling is done on the opposite side frontal sinus till lamina papyracea. Both frontal sinuses are converted to a single cavity (Fig. 21.10f, also refer Chapter-9, Fig. 9.30).

Videos: Inside out modified Lothrop (Draf III) procedure. Preoperative image of CT and enoscopy and peroperative pictures are shown in Fig. 21.10.

BIBLIOGRAPHY

1. Carney AS. Am J Rhinol Allergy 2017 Sep 1; 31(5):338–40.
2. Chin, et al. Outside-in approach to modified endosopic Lothrop procedure. Laryngoscope 201;122:1661–69.
3. Draf W. Endonasal Microendoscopic frontal sinus surgery—Fulda concept. Operative Techniques in Otolaryngology—Head and Neck Surgery 1991;2(4):234–40.
4. Freedman M, Landsberg R, Schults RA, et al. Endoscopic technique and preliminary results. Am J Rhinol 2000;14(6):393–403.
5. Kuhn FA, Javer AR, Nagpal K, Citardi MJ. The frontal sinus rescue procedure: Early experience and three-year follow-up. Am J Rhinol 2000;14: 211–16.
6. Nayak DR. A tailor made approach to endoscopic sinus surgery for chronic rhinosinusitis. OJOLHNS 2015;9:2:6–8.
7. Nayak DR, Pai K, Nair S, et al. A short-term subjective and objective analysis of modified endoscopic Lothrop's procedure and its functional outcome: Our experience. Indian J Otolaryngol Head Neck Surg (2016);68 (4):481–86.
8. Ramadan HH. History of frontal sinus surgery in "The Frontal Sinus" edited byKountakis SE, Brent A, Draf W; Published by Springer.
9. Stammberger H. FESS, "uncapping the egg". The endoscopic approach to frontal recess and sinuses. Storz Company Prints 2000.

Endoscopic Medial Maxillectomy and Anterior Skull Base Surgery

DR Nayak, R Balakrishnan, S Nair, NA Reddy

Surgery of maxillary sinus by making an opening in the anterior wall through sublabial incision was credited to Caldwell (1893)[1] and Luc (1897).[2] Denker modified this procedure subsequently by removing the pyriform aperture through an additional transfacial incision communicating it with nasal cavity.[3] These procedures have been extensively performed since then. Canfield in 1906 described a similar procedure through a transnasal pyriform aperture incision.[4] Although open medial maxillectomy was the preferred approach in the past for lesions involving the anterior and lateral wall, the availability of angled and curved instruments including grasping instruments, powered instruments including burrs have made it possible to tackle such cases endoscopically.[5] Transnasal endoscopy has been the preferred approach for benign and early malignant tumours of nose and paranasal sinuses. Endoscopic medial maxillectomy is one of the most essential procedure to deal with such cases especially inverted papilloma. It involves complete resection of the lateral nasal wall with boundaries that are inferior to the nasal floor; superior to the cribriform plate and fovea ethmoidalis; anterior to the anterior maxillary wall, including the nasolacrimal duct; and posterior to within 5 mm of the Eustachian tube (Neil, et al 2007).[6] The resection margin can be extended to incorporate the anterior skull base, pterygopalatine fossa and nasopharynx. The author (DRN) uses 30° endoscope most of the time along with 0° and 70° in certain areas. The endoscopic

medial maxillectomy is indicated in following conditions.[3,5,7–9]

Indications

1. Inverted papilloma
2. Haemangioma
3. Solitary fibrous tumour
4. As an approach for complete removal of juvenile angiofibroma
5. Selected malignant tumour involving maxilloethmoidal complex without transgressing the dura and orbit
6. Invasive fungal sinusitis especially post COVID-19 mucormycosis

Operative Technique

Turri-Zanoni, et al coined the term endoscopic partial maxillectomy and classified the surgery into four types based on the tumour extent.[3]

Type-1 (Fig. 22.1): It is an extended version of middle meatal antrostomy where the natural ostium is enlarged posteriorly till the posterior medial wall of the maxilla by removing medial maxillary and vertical portion of palatine bone, anteriorly inferior half of the uncinate process is removed while preserving the nasolacrimal duct and superiorly up to medial and inferior orbital junction. It gives good access to posterior and superior wall of maxillary sinus. It is best suited for complete removal of antrochoanal polyp. If necessary, an inferior meatal window (antrostomy) can be done in addition to facilitate removal of antrochoanal polyp attached to lateral wall or floor for instrumentation.

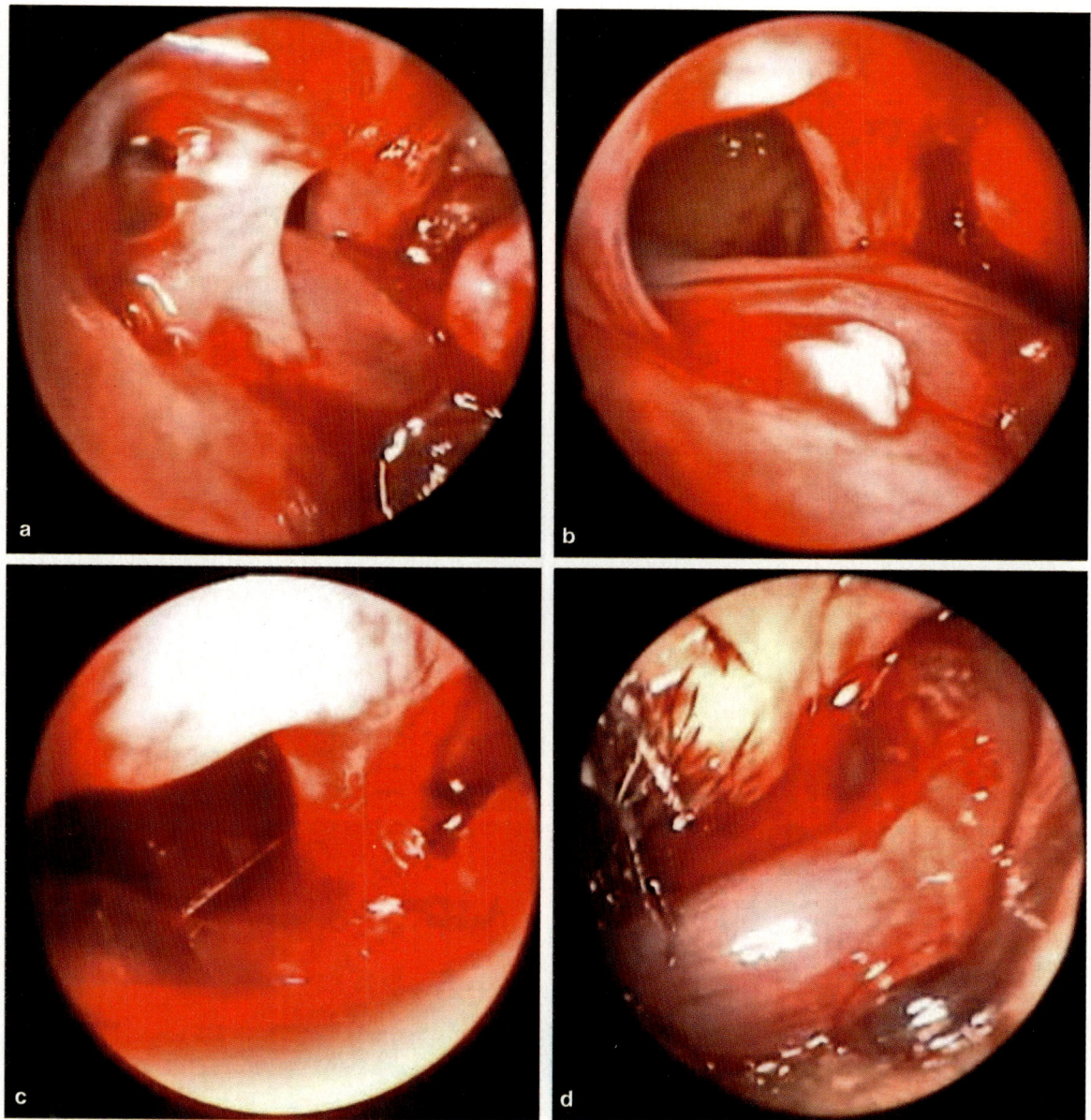

Fig. 22.1: a. Right antrochoanal polyp coming out through the accessory ostium and natural ostium seen anterior to that with a bridge of bone covered with mucosa in between, **b.** The polyp can be seen clearly after removal of the bridge of tissue, **c.** Removal of polyp with gradual traction, **d.** Polyp being pulled out through the anterior nare

Type-2 (Fig. 22.2): In addition to type-1, along with removal of inferior medial wall along with partial or complete inferior turbinectomy, while preserving the nasolacrimal duct. Pterygopalatine fossa can be accessed through this approach by removal of posterior wall of maxilla. It is suitable for angiofibroma with limited extension to pterygopalatine fossa and also pterygoid recess. In selected cases, removal of inferior turbinectomy may not be required. The posterior medial wall of maxilla can be removed by enlarging the maxillary ostium through removal of the palatine bone till sphenopalatine foramen up to the inferior

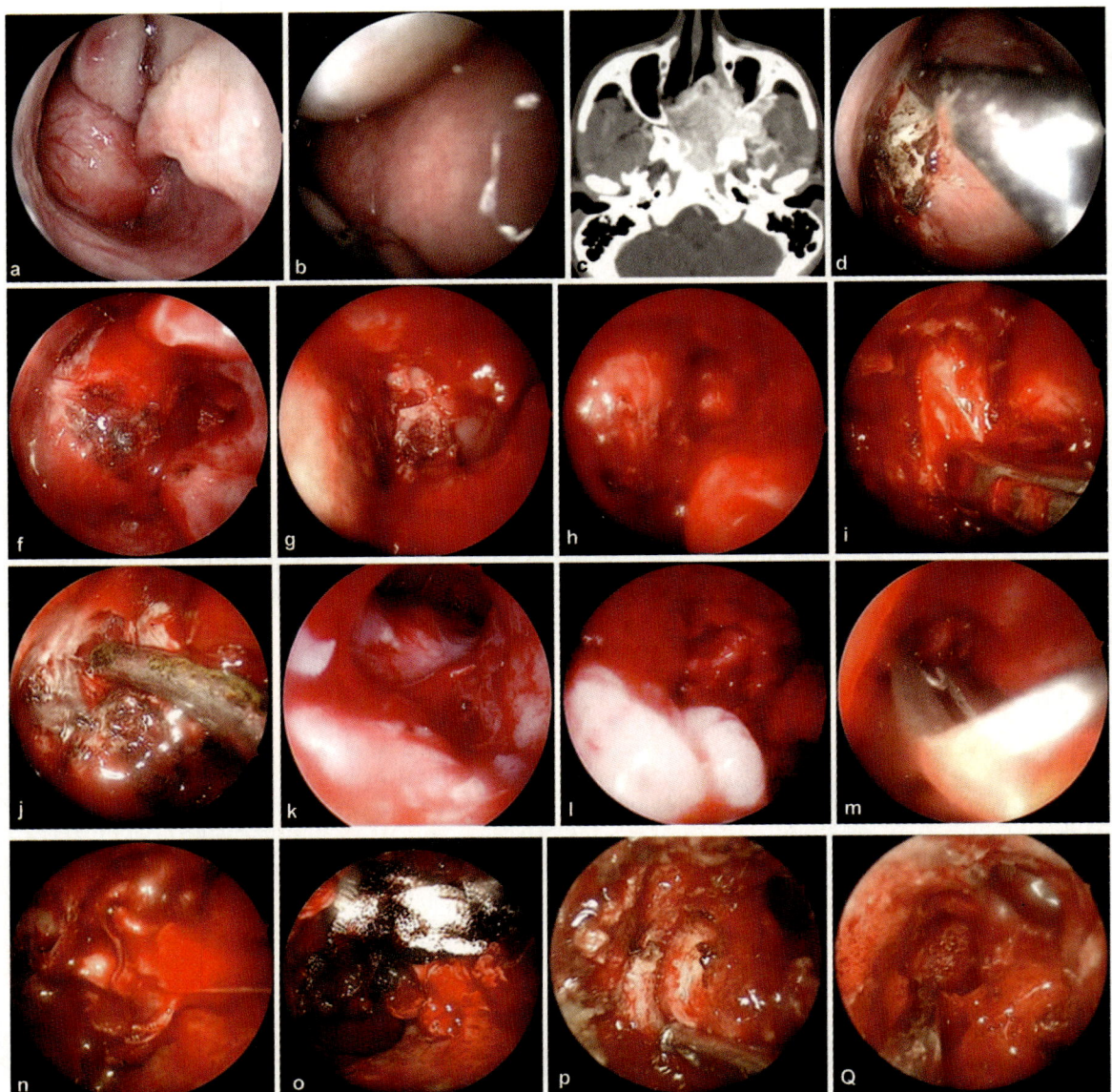

Fig. 22.2: Endoscopic view of **a.** Angiofibroma occupying the posterior part of left nasal cavity, **b.** Seen through the right nasal cavity, **c.** CT scan showing extension of JNA to the left pterygopalatine and infratemporal fossa, **d.** Intraoperative picture showing cauterization of surface and release of secondary adhesions, **f.** Extended middle meatal antrostomy, **g.** Exposure and removal of bone around sphenopalatine foramen and posterior wall of maxilla, **h.** Exposure of tumour after complete removal of bone from posterior wall of maxilla, **i.** Removal of tumour from the infratemporal fossa and pterygopalatine fossa by push pull method by enodoscopic traction and simultaneous digital pressure applied through the check by sublabial approach, **j.** Blunt dissection of tumour from the sphenoid sinus, **k.** After delivery of tumor from the sphenoid sinus, **l.** Separation of tumour from all attachment before removal, **m.** Clipping of branches of sphenopalatine arteries, **n.** Clipped sphenopalatine vessels after tumour removal, **o.** Operated cavity packed with surgicel, **p.** Drilling of pterygoid recess and tumour exposure when involved, **q.** Sphenoid sinus and pterygoid recess after tumour removal

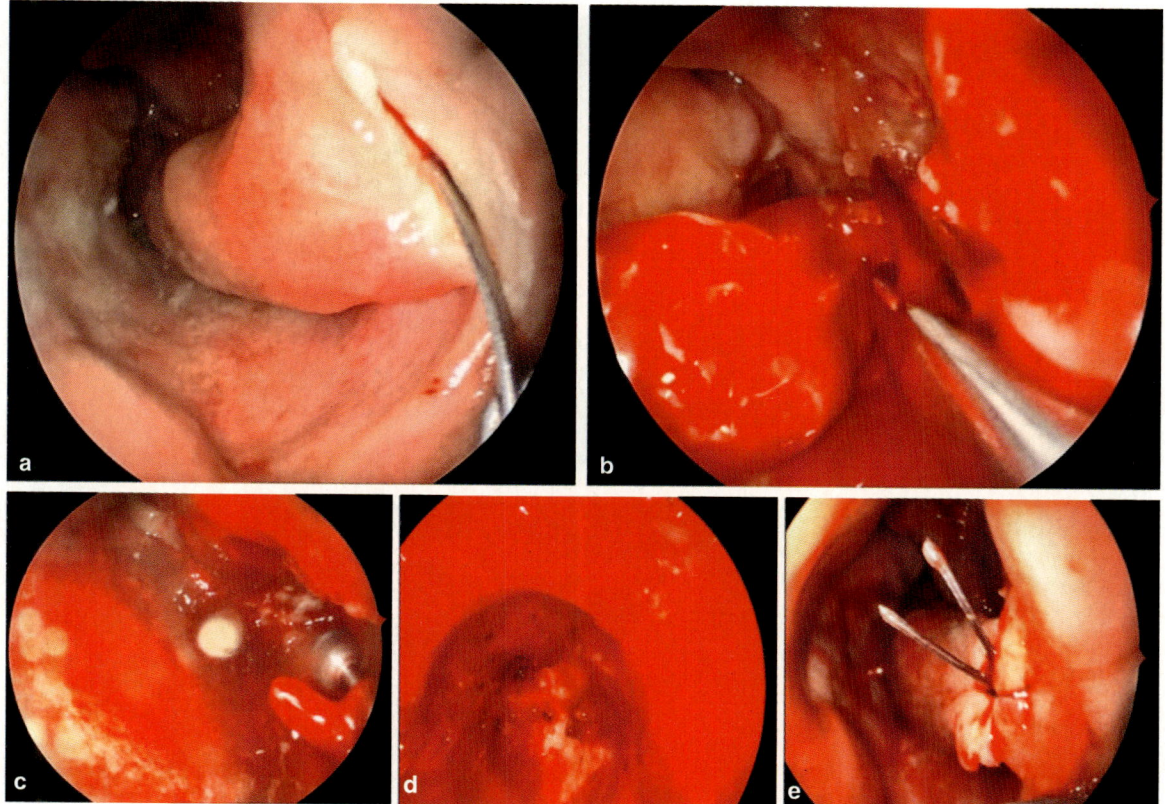

Fig. 22.3: a. Incision over anterior part of inferior turbinate for collumnar cell papilloma, **b.** Inferior turbinat preserved and created as a posteriorly based flap, **c.** Drilling is done to remove medial wall of maxilla, **d.** Complete tumour removal done along with mucoperiosteal layer and entire maxillary sinus cavity wall was drilled with diamond burr to remove residual tissue adherant to the bone, **e.** Inferior turbinate flap sutured back in position

medial of the orbit, posterior wall of the maxillary sinus for tumour exposure.

Type-3a: In this type, the nasolacrimal duct is sacrificed by removing few millimeters of bone anteriorly, that gives improved access to the lateral and inferior wall of maxillary sinus. It is an excellent approach to remove benign tumour like inverted papilloma.

Type-3b (Fig. 22.3): The surgery is similar to type-3a but the drilling is extended anteriorly further over the ascending process of maxilla to remove the pyriform aperture as described by Canfield.[4] This approach gives wide approach to alveolar process and zygomatic recess. Inferior turbinate can be preserved in benign tumour by dividing the inferior turbinate at its anterior attachment and transecting further posteriorly as a posteriorly

based flap. After the complete removal of the tumour, the turbinate is sutured back anteriorly in its position (Fig. 22.3).

Type-4 (Fig. 22.4): In this type, drilling is extended further laterally from the pyriform aperture (modified Denker's approach) to complete removal of anterior wall of maxillary sinus as far as zygomatic arch. Infraorbital nerve can be preserved in this approach while taking care of to preserve the periorbita and anterior superior alveolar nerve.

The endoscopic medial maxillectomy approach can be combined with ethmoidec-tomy, removal of lamina papyracea, frontal sinusostomy including Draf procedure and endoscopic Lothrop procedure, sphenoidotomy, depending on the involvement of the tumour and in case of rhinocerebral mucormycosis

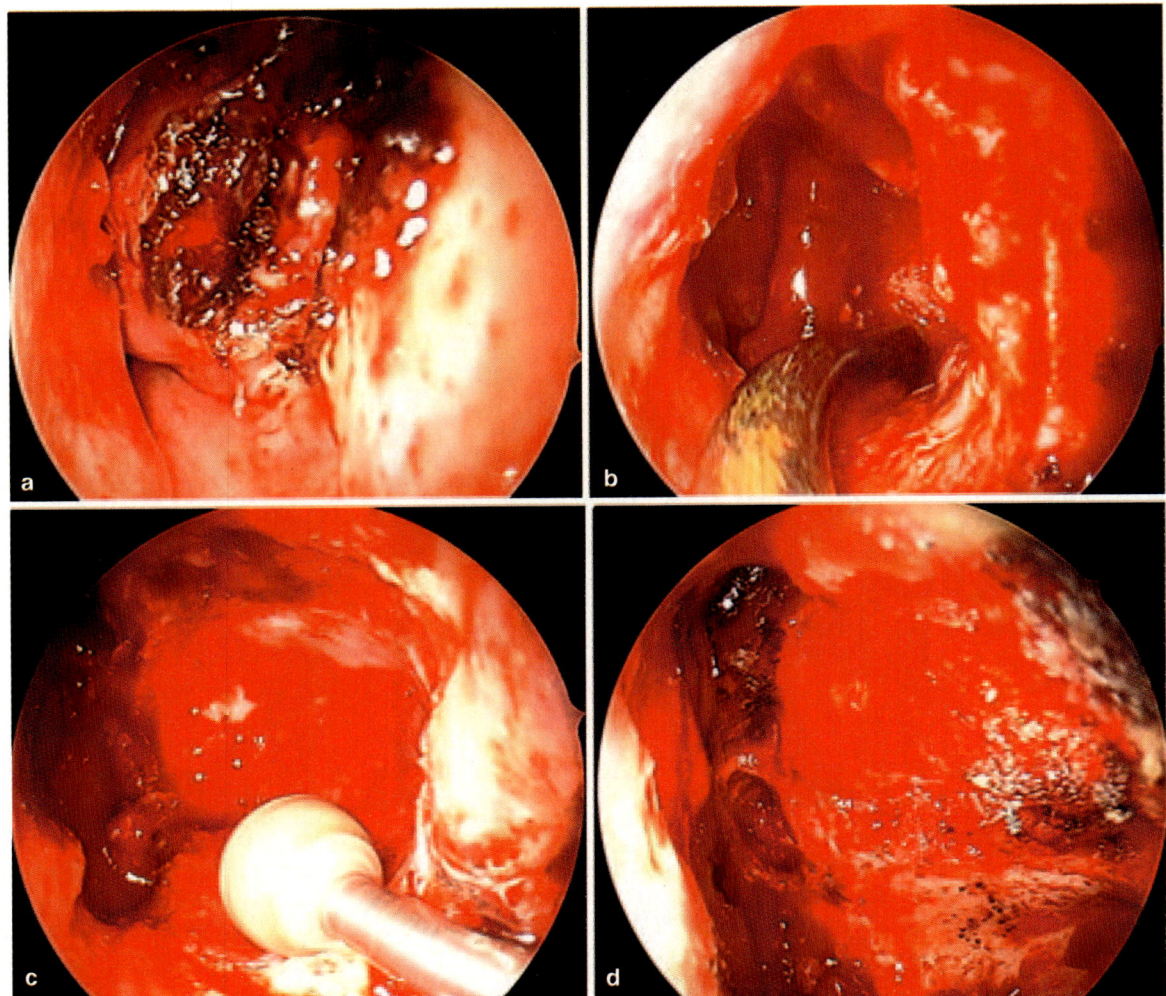

Fig. 22.4: a. Endoscopic view after endoscopic partial removal of the tumour involving maxilloethmoidal complex (inverted papilloma with squamous cell carcinoma, **b.** Medial maxillary wall after removal of inferior turbinate, **c.** Drilling of the floor of the medial wall after removal of the tumour from the maxillary sinus. The anterior wall has been removed partially by drilling the pyriform aperture. **d.** The skull base, roof and posterior wall of maxillary sinus after complete removal of tumour, also note a Draf II frontal sinusotomy done for identification of anterior skull base

(Fig. 22.4). The steps of the surgery include the following (Nayak & Balakrishna 2012, Nayak, et al 2017, Castelnuovo, et al 2006 and 2012[11,12]):

- Disassembling tumour using powered instrumentation and/or cutting instruments which reduces the bulk of the tumour and helps to visualise the margins clearly.
- Removal of the posterior nasal septum and sphenoid rostrum.
- Draf type IIb frontal sinusotomy in the case of unilateral mass with frontal sinus

extension and Draf type III median frontal sinusostomy is performed, if the lesion involves both sides by identifying the cribriform plate (Figs 22.5 and 22.6).

- *Centripetal removal:* Exposure of antero-superior and posterior inferior margin. Endoscopic medial maxillectomy type III.
- Nasoethmoidosphenoidal complex is isolated and pushed towards the central part of the nasal fossa (centripetal technique) and removed.[12]

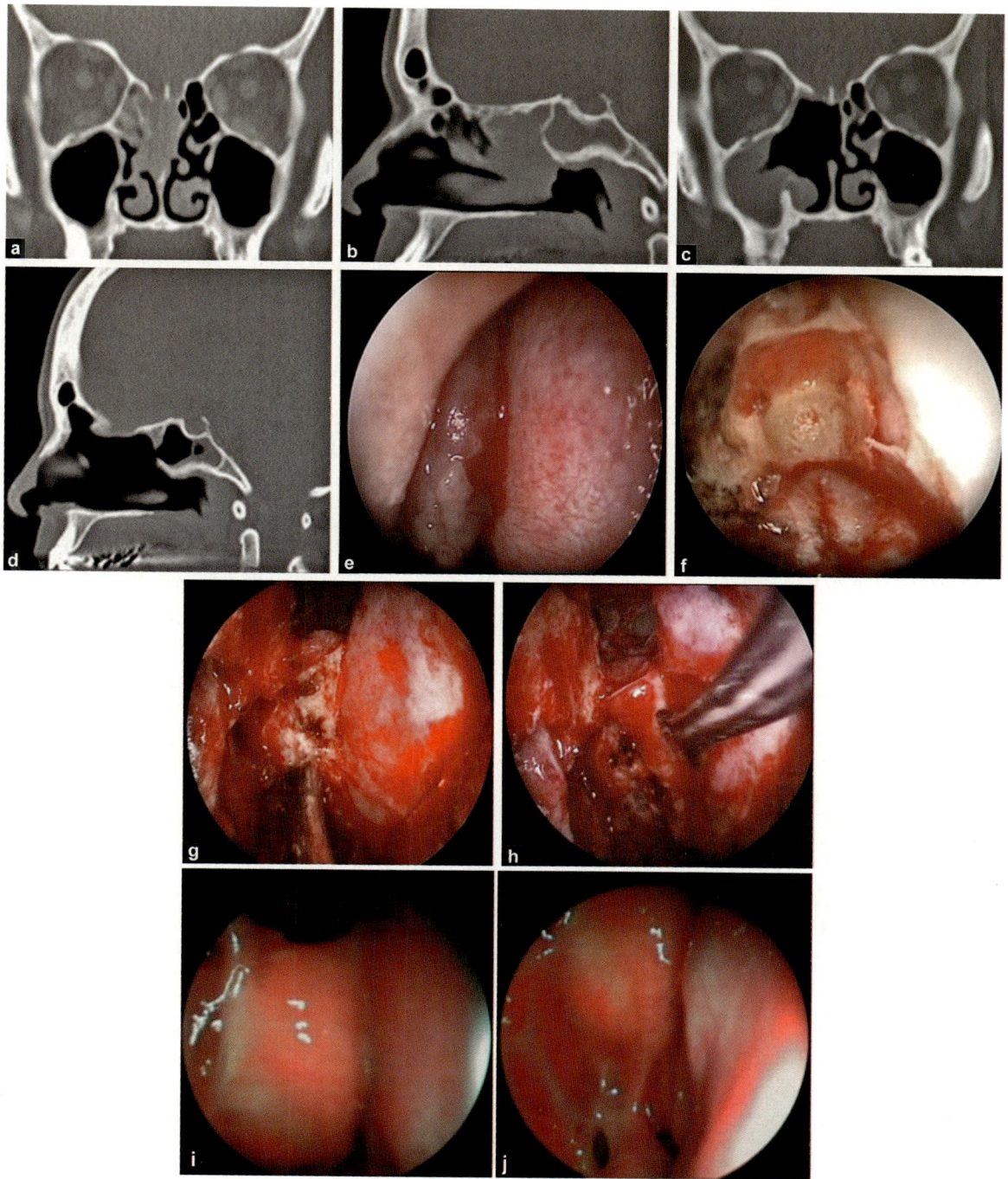

Fig. 22.5: Olfactory neuroblastoma: **a, b.** Preoperative CT, **c,d.** Postoperative CT, **e.** The lesion occupying the superior aspect of nasal cavity, **f.** Exposure of skull floor of frontal sinus anterior to 1st olfactory neuron. Note the tumour along with healthy mucosal margin has been separated, **g.** A Draf II sinusotomy has been performed to identify the skull base and the tumour has been resected completely from dura after removal of adjacent bone, **h.** Reflection of septal flap from opposite side to cover the dura (with kind permission of editor OJOLHNS for reproduction), **i.** Post surgery-post radiation status through septal window, with no disease after 5 yrs with olfaction preservation, **j.** Both sphenoid ostium visible through septal window. Left olfactory cleft can be seen through the septal window

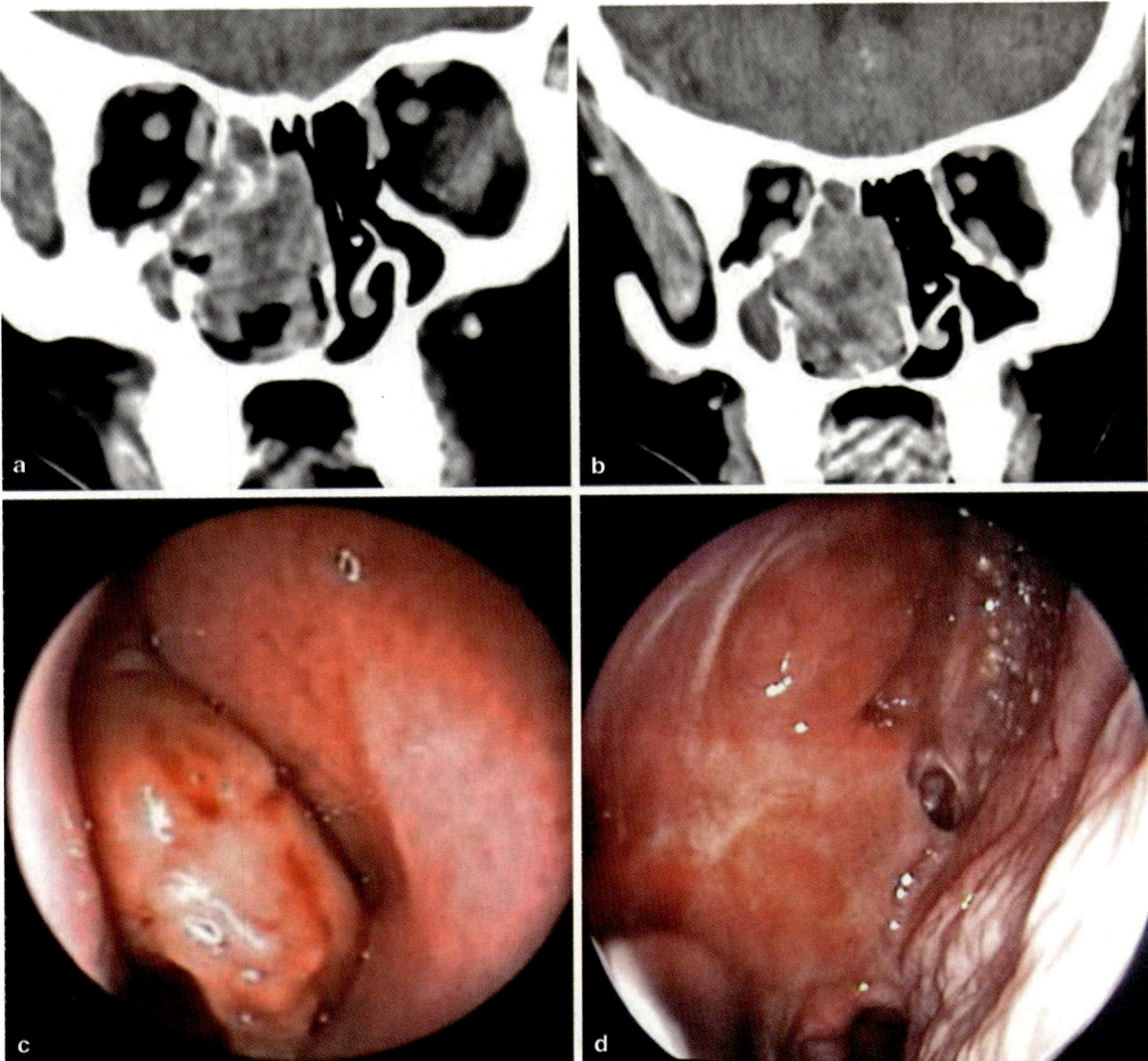

Fig. 22.6: Adenocarcinoma: **a and b.** CT scan paranasal sinus showing the tumour extent, **c.** Intraoperative endoscopic picture before resection, **d.** Postoperative endoscopic picture after one year showing no evidence of disease (reproduced with kind permission of editor OJOLHNS)

- *Skull base removal:* Can be extended to resect anterior cranial base.
- *Reconstruction:* Endoscopic multilayer technique.

The author (DRN) performs endoscopic medial maxillectomy surgery based on the same principle. Since this book is meant for the beginner, basic surgical steps will be discussed. The surgeon should be well-versed with head and neck surgical oncology principles before attempting to tackle

malignant paranasal sinus cancer even though they may be in the early stage.

The endoscopic medial maxillectomy has replaced the open medial maxillectomy, which has traditionally been considered the gold standard treatment for neoplastic disease involving the lateral nasal wall and maxillary sinus (Cunningham & Welch).[5] The surgery is performed under hypotensive general anaesthesia. A complete endoscopic evaluation of the mass is mandatory after a good surface anaesthesia with oxymetazoline hydrochloride and 4% lignocaine before proceeding with the surgery. If the tumour is very bulky and occupying the hole of the nasal cavity, it is essential to reduce the size of the tumour by debunking with a microdebrider/KTP-532 laser. This facilitates better visualization to assess the tumour extent also easy manipulation during resection. Bony cuts ware made with osteotome/drill around healthy area with tumour free margin. A Draf II for unilateral skull base invovment, and Draf III for bilateral to identify the skull base after tumour bulk is reduced.

Removal of nasal septum and sphenoidal rostrum, if tumour is extending posteriorly to nasopharynx. Endoscopic medial maxillectomy type III is performed as describe earlier. Nasoethmoidosphenoidal complex is isolated and pushed towards the central part of the nasal fossa (centripetal technique) and removed. Approach is made around the periphery of the tumour with a disease free margin from the normal tissue. Surgery can be extended to resect anterior cranial base by drilling the crista gali anteriorly and posteriorly separating the cribriform plate and adjacent skull base when transgression of dura is absent (Fig. 22.6). We prefer to resect intracranial extension with tumour transgressing the dura by an open approach (bicoronal craniotomy) along with the neurosurgeon. Reconstruction is done with endoscopic multilayer technique along with nasal septal flap when available (Nayak, et al 2017). Decision making is very important in endoscopic approach. Proper case selection, preoperative planning including reconstruction option and multidisciplinary team (neurosurgeon, radiologist, anaesthesiologist) approach is the key to have a successful surgical outcome (Jain & Medikeri, 2015). Cancer cases must be discussed in a head and neck tumour board involving medical and radiation oncologist for proper treatment planning.

REFERENCES

1. Caldwell GW. Diseases of the accessory sinuses of the nose and an improved method of treatment for suppuration of the maxillary antrum. NY Med J 1893;58:526–28.

2. Canfield RB. The submucous resection of the lateral nasal wall in chronic empyema of the antrum, ethmoid and sphenoid. JAMA 1908; 14:1136–41.

3. Cunningham K, Welch KC. Endoscopic medial maxillectomy. Operative Techniques in Otolaryngology 2010;21:111–16.

4. Luc H. A new method of operation for chronic empyema quick and radical cure of the maxillary sinus (in French). Arch Laryngol Paris 1897; 10:185–207.

5. Nayak D, Nair S, Reddy NA, Balakrishna R, et al. Oncological outcome analysis of transnasal minimally invasive endoscopic resection of sinonasal malignancy not transgressing the dura: a single centre study. OJOLHNS 2017 June; 11(1): 16–24. DOI: 10.21176/ojolhns.2017.11.1.3

6. Nayak D, Nishanth S, Kudva R, Pai K. Solitary fibrous tumors of the nose and paranasal sinuses—our experience. Orissa J Otolaryngology Head Neck Surgery. 2017 Dec; 11(2): 11–14. DOI: 10.21176/ojolhns.2017.11.3

7. Nayak DR, Balakrishnan R. Exclusive endoscopic/endoscopic-assisted minimaly invasive surgery for sinonasal neoplasm—our experience. J Neurol Surg B 2012; 73-A015.

8. Neil T, John DE, Hamid A, et al. Arch Otolaryngol Head Neck Surg/vol 133 (no. 11), nov 2007.

9. Turri-Zanoni M, et al. Transnasal endoscopic partial maxillectomy: Operative nuances and proposal for a comprehensive classification system based on 1378 cases. Head and Neck 2017 April;754–766.

10. Jain S, Medikeri G. Complete endoscopic resection of an ossifying fibroma involving the skull base and orbit with superolateral extension up to the lateral orbital wall. Ceylon Journal of Otolaryngology 2015;4 (1): 36–39.

11. Castelnuovo P, Battaglia P, Locatelli D, et al. Endonasal microendoscopic treatment of the malignant tumours of paranasal sinuses and anterior skull base. Oper Tech Otolaryngol 2006;17(3):152–67.

12. Castelnuovo P, Turri-Zanoni M, Battaglia P. Endoscopic endonasal approaches for malignant tumours involving the skull base. Curr Otorhinolaryngol Rep (2013) 1:197–205.

Endoscopic Endonasal Approach to the Orbit

R Balakrishnan

Introduction

With the advent of Hopkins's rod nasal endoscopes and the evolution of the endoscopic sinus surgery, it is now possible for the endoscopic surgeon to get a good view of the lamina papyracea and the floor of the orbit following complete sphenoethmoidectomy and a wide middle meatal maxillary antrostomy. The medial and inferior aspects of the orbit are easily accessed through these. If an access to the superomedial aspect of orbit is needed, it may even necessitate an endoscopic modified Lothrop's procedure. The lateral and superolateral aspects of the orbit are difficult to approach transnasal endoscopically and an external approach to the orbit may be needed. Various pathological conditions ranging from inflammatory to traumatic and benign neoplastic conditions may be dealt with the endoscopic approach. A transnasal orbital biopsy for histopathological confirmation avoids external approach for the same which has the risk of seeding into the skin. Orbital apex and optic nerve decompression is possible endoscopically via the sphenoethmoids. Orbit could also be used as a passage to access various intracranial lesions at the skull base and various procedures grouped under 'transorbital neuroendoscopic surgery (TONES)' have been described in the literature.[1,2] Good knowledge of the three-dimensional and endoscopic anatomies of the orbit and its relations to the paranasal sinuses and the anterior and middle cranial base is mandatory before venturing to such endoscopic approaches. MR or CT imaging of the orbit helps in proper planning. The possible postoperative visual disturbances, though less common, should be adequately informed to the patient with a proper written or a video consent before embarking on to this approach.

Anatomical Considerations

The paranasal sinuses may be called 'para-orbital' sinuses too. All the paranasal sinuses are related to the orbit (Fig. 23.1). The spheno-ethmoid sinuses are medial to the orbit and are mainly separated by the lamina papyracea and a small posterior portion by the palatine bone and thicker sphenoid bone. The roof of the sphenoethmoid sinuses, i.e. the fovea ethmoidalis and planum sphenoidale slope laterally to form the roof of the orbit. The floor of the frontal sinus is related to the antero-superomedial aspect of the orbit. The maxillary sinus roof containing the infra-orbital canal with its infraorbital nerve and vessels forms the floor of the orbit. The lacrimal fossa with its sac is located just anterior to the anterior attachment of the middle turbinate in the region of the agger nasi and the nasolacrimal duct runs downwards from here.

The lateral wall of the 'Onodi' cell (para-sphenoidal posterior ethmoid cell) and the sphenoid sinus is related to the orbital apex and the optic nerve (Fig. 23.1). The degree of pneumatization of the sphenoid and posterior ethmoid sinuses determines the proximity of the optic nerve and the internal carotid artery

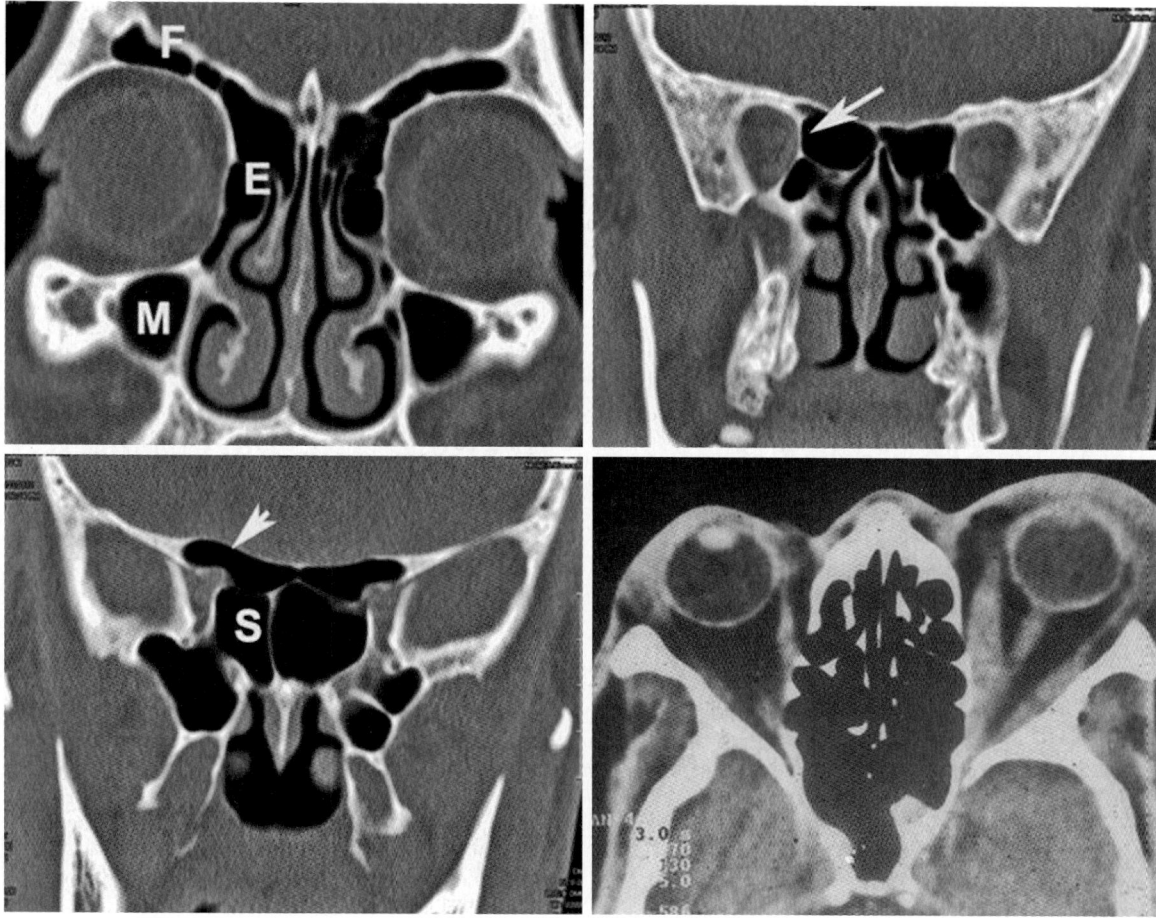

Fig. 23.1: CT images showing the relation of the frontal (F), ethmoidal (E), maxillary (M) and sphenoidal (S) sinuses to the orbit. White arrow: Onodi cell

in their lateral wall. They may just bulge into the sinuses or may be dehiscent or even rarely hang inside the sinus with a mesentery. The knowledge of this variation should be kept in mind and CT imaging is invaluable in diagnosing it preoperatively.

Once identified endoscopically after a sphenoethmoidectomy, the lamina papyracea is raised off the underlying orbital periosteum by a Freer's elevator with its anterior limit being the lacrimal sac and posteriorly till the optic bulge. The removal of medial bony wall of the orbit posteriorly becomes easier with more pneumatization of the sphenoid sinus as the intervening wall becomes thin. In poorly pneumatized sphenoid sinus, this bone may be very thick and may even need use of a drill

or a bone punch. Identification of fovea ethmoidalis and anterior and posterior ethmoidal arteries helps the surgeon, signaling the superior extent of lamina papyracea. Inferiorly, the lamina papyracea may be traced to the roof of the maxillary sinus via a large antrostomy. The lateral extent of this is determined on the exposure needed as per the indication. The bone around the infraorbital nerve is often thick. Extensive removal of the floor of the orbit may risk enopthalmos and consequent diplopia. Figure 23.2 shows the different bones forming the orbital skeleton and the various fissures and foramina.

It should be borne in mind that the floor of the orbit slopes upwards as we move posteriorly. This is because the orbit is wide

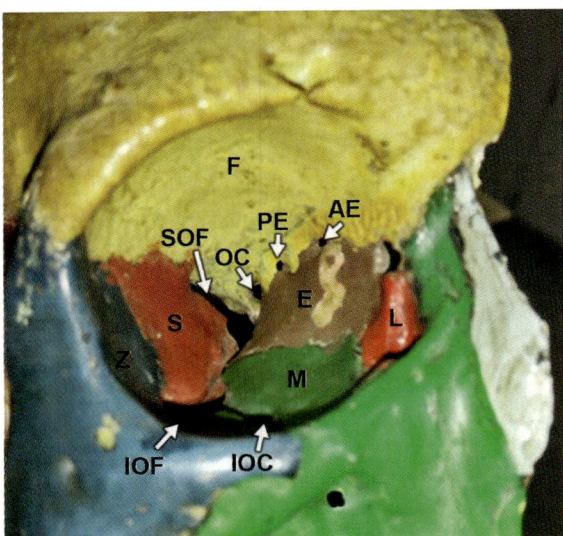

Fig. 23.2: Coloured skull bone depicting the walls of the orbit and certain foramina and fissures. (F: Frontal, E: Ethmoidal, L: Lacrimal, M: Maxillary, Z: Zygomatic, S: Sphenoidal, SOF: Superior orbital fissure, OC: Optic canal, PE: Foramen for posterior ethmoidal artery, AE: Foramen for anterior ethmoidal artery, IOF: Inferior orbital fissure, IOC: Infraorbital canal/sulcus)

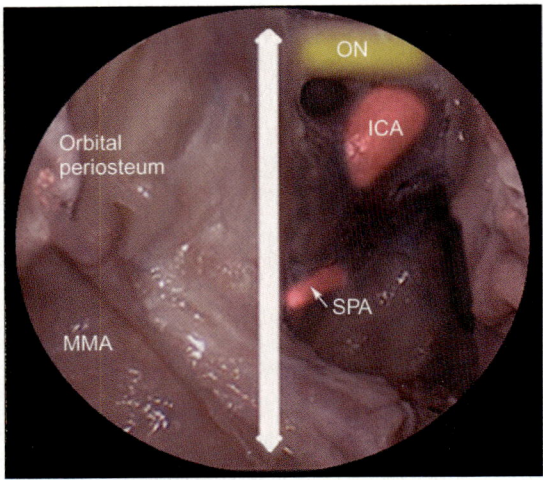

Fig. 23.3: Cadaveric specimen (Rt) showing the medial wall of the orbit after a complete spheno-ethmoidectomy. The vertical white line is the level of imaginary coronal plane corresponding to the posterior wall of maxillary sinus, behind which the sphenoethmoid sinuses are related to the orbital apex. ICA: Internal carotid artery bulge, and SPA: Spheno-palatine artery

anteriorly and tapers towards the orbital apex posteriorly. Endoscopically, as the lamina papyracea is traced downwards, posterior to the posterior wall of the maxillary sinus, the palatine bone is encountered. The spheno-palatine foramen with its artery and its branches could be identified as in Fig. 23.3. An imaginary coronal plane into the orbit as a superior extension of the plane of posterior wall of maxilla demarcates the orbital apex from rest of the orbit. This is important while considering orbital apex/optic nerve decompression. The orbital apex is about 8 cm from the columella.

The inside of the orbit is lined by a relatively tough orbital periosteum. The periosteum may be breeched by the orbital or sinonasal lesion. Identification of the periosteum from the uninvolved site initially is often beneficial. The periosteum may also be breached by sickle knife during lifting of the lamina papyracea. Once breached, the extraconal orbital fat herniates into the operated cavity. Use of suction or microdebrider here may worsen the fat herniation.

The orbital cone is formed by the eyeball with its extraocular muscles. Around the orbital cone is the extraconal fat and inside the cone is intraconal fat with the optic nerve (Figs 23.4 and 23.5). The medial rectus muscle is quite superficial covered by a thin medial extraconal fat and it may be easily injured by sharp instrumentation. Removal of this fat is best avoided and dissection through the fat using ball probe is suitable. To approach superomedial orbit, dissection may be made above the medial rectus but below the superior oblique muscle. It is here the anterior ethmoidal artery is encountered in the orbit. To approach inferomedial orbit, blunt dissection may be made below the medial rectus muscle. To manage intraconal lesions, the corridor between medial and inferior recti muscles is considered safe (Figs 23.4–23.6).

Radiology of the Orbit

Multiplanar HRCT imaging of the orbit and the paranasal sinuses are useful in assessing the vital relations of the sphenoethmoid-sinuses. Of specific interest would be presence of 'Onodi cells', extent of sphenoid pneumatiza-

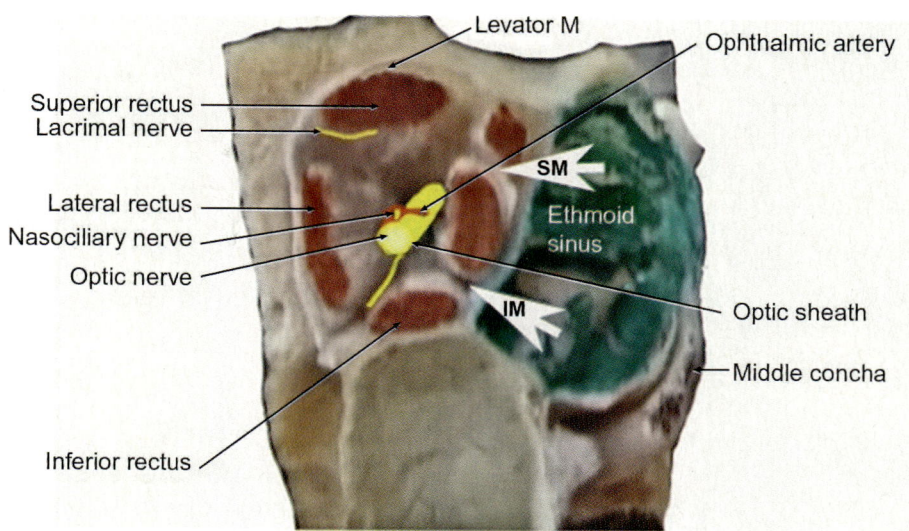

Fig. 23.4: Specimen of the orbit showing the various extraocular muscles and their relation to the ethmoid and maxillary sinus. SM: Superomedial approach between medial rectus and superior oblique muscles and IM: Inferomedial approach between medial rectus and inferior rectus muscles

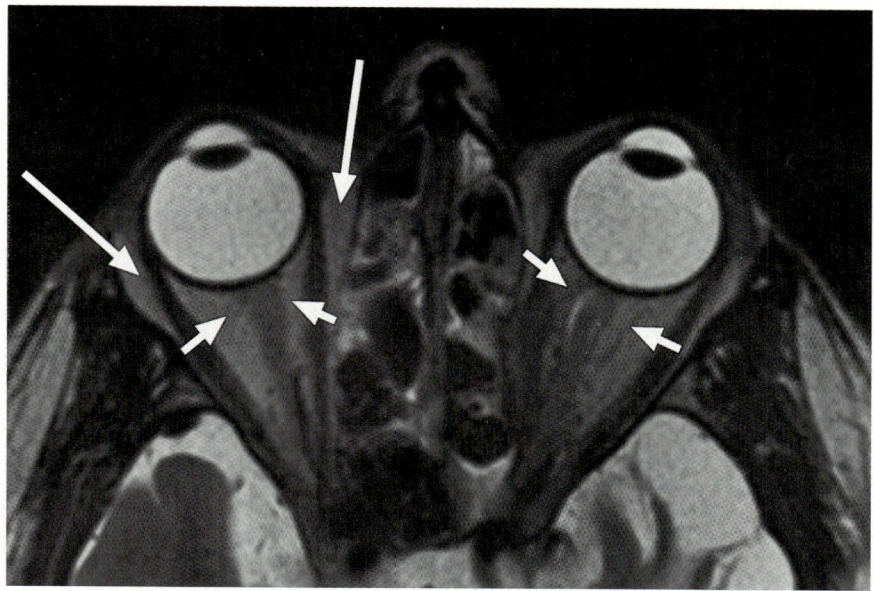

Fig. 23.5: MRI showing the relations of the sphenoethmoid sinuses to the orbital structures. Long arrows: Extraconal fat and short arrows: Intraconal fat

tion, proximity of optic nerve and internal carotid artery and the integrity of lamina papyracea (Fig. 23.1). Contrast scans will be beneficial in neoplastic conditions, vascular lesions, suspected intraorbital abscess or cavernous sinus thrombophlebitis.

MRI is a better tool than CT for assessment of lesions within the orbit as the soft tissue delineation is better. The relationship of the lesion to the extraocular muscles and optic nerve is better delineated in MR imaging with or without contrast (Fig. 23.7).

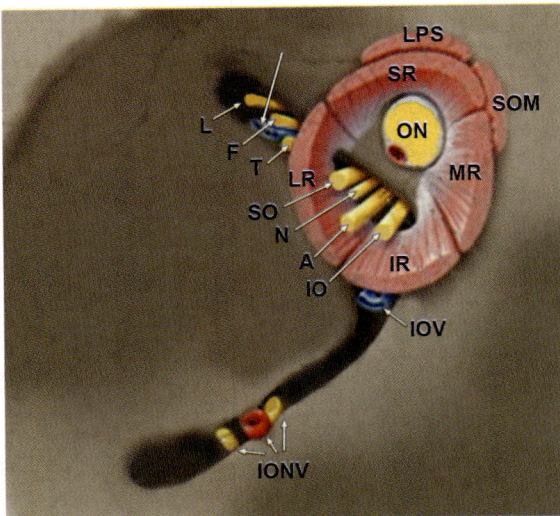

Fig. 23.6: Diagram showing the extraocular muscles arising from the annulus of Zinn and the superior and the orbital fissures with their contents. SR: Superior rectus muscle, MR: Medial rectus muscle, IR: Inferior rectus muscle, LR: Lateral rectus muscle, LPR: Levator palpebrae superioris muscle, SOM: Superior oblique muscle, ON: Optic nerve with the ophthalmic artery, L: Lacrimal nerve, F: Frontal nerve, T: Trochlear nerve, SOV: Superior ophthalmic vein, SO: Superior division of oculomotor nerve, N: Nasociliary nerve, A: abducent nerve, IO: Inferior division of the oculomotor nerve, IOV: Inferior ophthalmic vein, IONV: Infraorbital nerve and vessels

Indications for Endoscopic Approach to the Orbit

Inflammatory
- Orbital subperiosteal abscess
- Orbital abscess
- Orbital cellulitis

Traumatic
- Periorbital or orbital haematoma
- Fracture impaction of optic nerve
- Nasoethmoid complex fractures
- Inferior orbital nerve/inferior rectus entrapment in orbital floor fracture

Endocrine
Severe 'Graves' ophthalmopathy with exposure keratitis and possible visual loss.

Neoplastic

Benign:
- Orbital cyst
- Schwannoma
- Suspected pseudotumour for biopsy/excision of recalcitrant pseudotumour

Malignant:
- Localized malignant lesion in orbit/ethmoid sinus
- Biopsy

Preparation for Surgery

This is same as for any endoscopic sinus surgery. Detailed ophthalmologic workup regarding the visual acuity and field is mandatory prior to surgery. Informed consent should include possible orbital complications like diplopia and impaired vision. Perioperative antibiotic therapy is advised. Adequate medical treatment of underlying nasosinus infection/allergy, if any, helps in reducing intraoperative bleeding.

Surgical Technique (Moe & Berens 2017[3])

Procedure is done under general anaesthesia with controlled hypotension and bradycardia.

Head end raised by 15–30° helps in reducing venous bleed.

Keep the concerned orbit uncovered from the surgical drapes.

Decongestion of the nasal cavity including middle meatus with 1:30000 dilution adrenaline for 5–10 minutes has to be done using cottonoid strips or pieces of Merocel sponge.

'Full-house' functional endoscopic sinus surgery is done on the side indicated, with uncinectomy, middle meatal antrostomy, sphenoethmoidectomy and indicated type of frontal sinusotomy.

Expose lamina papyracea and trace it along the roof of the maxillary sinus through a large antrostomy (Fig. 23.8).

Frontoethmoid suture line is identified by the location of anterior and posterior ethmoidal arteries, which is the superior limit of exposure of the lamina papyracea. The optic bulge, carotid artery bulge and the optic-

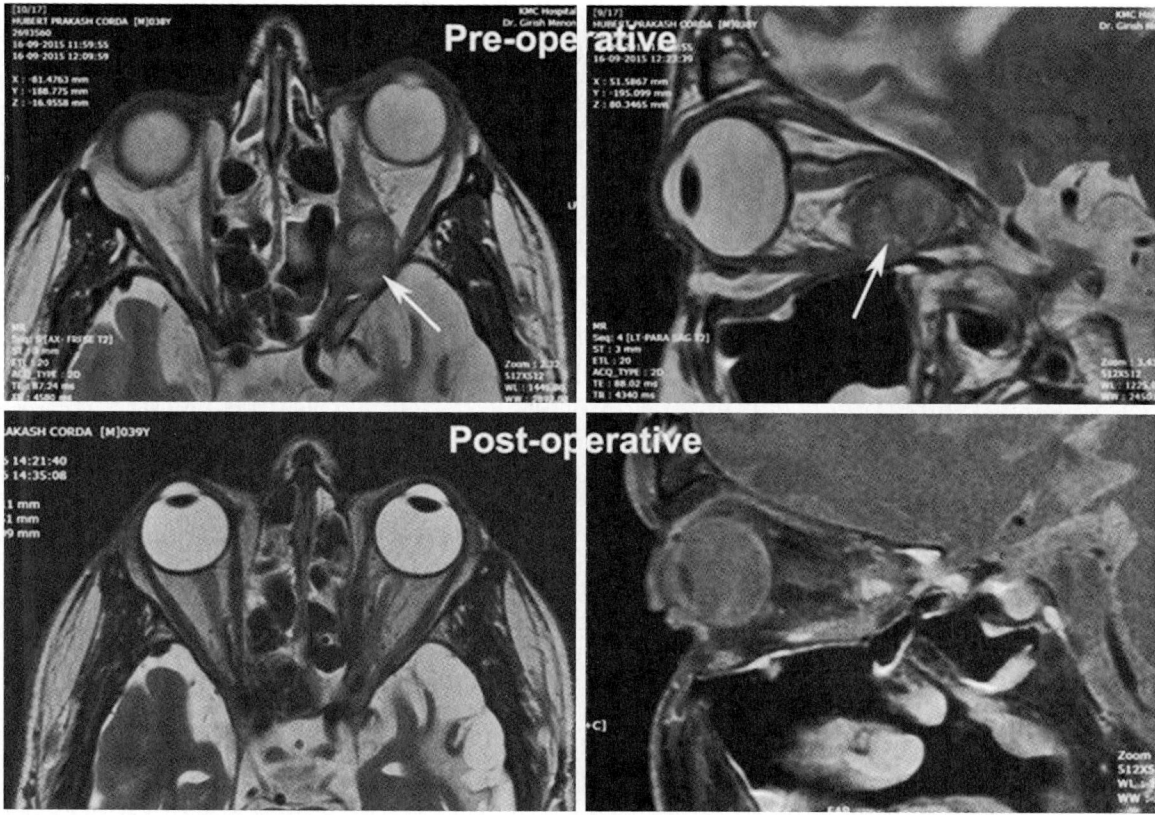

Fig. 23.7: MRI showing pre- and post-operative axial and sagittal images of patient with orbital neoplasm excised endoscopically. White arrows: Intraconal tumour

carotid recess are identified in the lateral wall of the sphenoid sinus/Onodi cells.

Further orbital procedure depends on the indication for surgery.

For subperiosteal abscess, the lamina papyracea needs partial or complete removal to ensure adequate drainage of the abscess loculations into the nasal cavity. This may require exposing the orbital periosteum over the superomedial or inferomedial orbital walls to allow adequate drainage of all abscess septations. The periosteum is left intact without any incisions.

For patients with Graves' ophthalmopathy, the lamina papyracea and medial orbital floor are removed medial to the infraorbital nerve through a wide antrostomy, preserving a bony strut (corresponding to the horizontal ridge of the maxillary antrostomy) with the intension of minimizing the risk of post-operative diplopia. The lamina papyracea is

removed posterior to the level of nasolacrimal convexity and inferior to the border of the fovea ethmoidalis, taking care not to injure the anterior or posterior ethmoidal arteries.

In a standard medial orbital decompression, the posterior lamina papyracea is removed 2 to 5 mm anterior to the optic strut. For maximal decompression, further posterior removal of lamina papyracea may be done with or without optic nerve decompression. The periosteal incisions are given from posterior to anterior using a sickle knife parallel to the superior and inferior borders of the medial rectus muscle, adjacent to the margins of the superior oblique and inferior rectus muscles, respectively. Orbital fat is allowed to herniate through these incisions in a controlled way, preventing a possible post-operative diplopia. Gentle palpation of the orbit externally enables prolapse of orbital fat into the ethmoid sinus cavity and helps

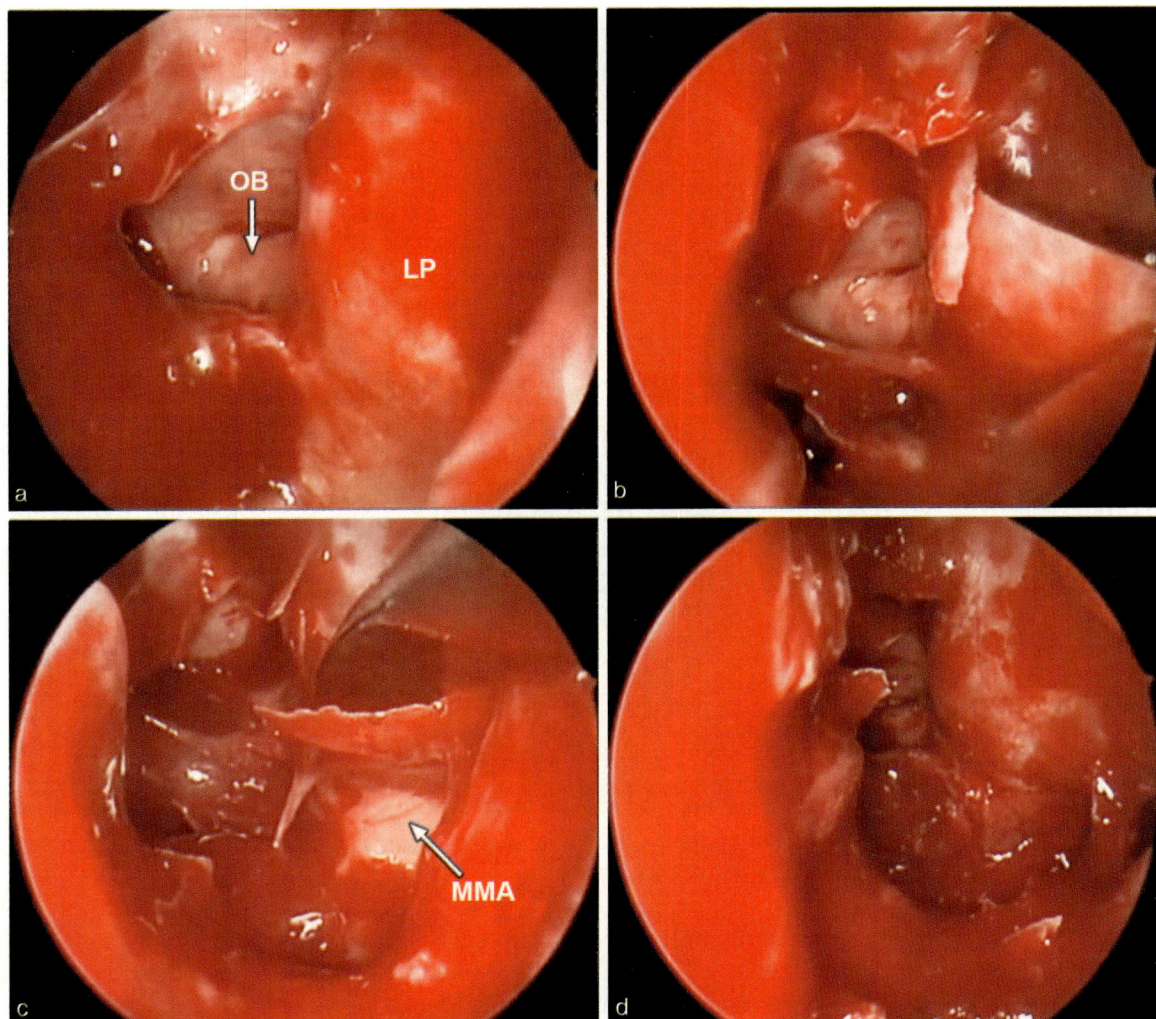

Fig. 23.8: Intraoperative endoscopic pictures showing: **a.** Lamina papyracea exposed after a complete spheno-ethmoidectomy on the left side (LP: Lamina papyracea, OB: Optic bulge), **b.** Lamina papyracea being elevated and removed posteriorly and superiorly, **c.** Lamina papyracea being elevated and removed inferiorly towards roof of the maxillary sinus (MMA: Middle meatal antrostomy), and **d.** After complete removal of lamina papyracea exposing the orbital periosteum

visualize if there are any residual tethering periorbital fascial bands. Multiple passes with the sickle knife or blunt ball-tip probe may be necessary to ensure lysis of all the periorbital fascial bands and ensure maximum decompression. Approximately 3 to 4 mm of decompression is achieved per complete wall decompressed. However, only the medial aspect of the medial orbital floor is decompressed endoscopically. Endoscopic medial and inferior orbital decompression enables approximately 4 to 5 mm of proptosis reduction.

Further reduction in proptosis can be achieved with complete decompression of the orbital floor medial and lateral to the infra-orbital nerve. This can increase the medial/inferior decompression up to 8 mm of reduction. However, this will require a combined endoscopic and external trans-orbital approach using a transconjunctival incision. Care is taken not to occlude the maxillary, frontal, or sphenoid sinus ostia with orbital fat, which can result in secondary ostial obstruction and rhinosinusitis.

For accessing intraconal neoplasm, the intraorbital fat "corridor" between medial and inferior rectus muscles and another corridor between medial rectus and superior oblique may be made use of. Using a trucut forceps, part of the extraconal orbital fat may be removed carefully without avulsion, to gain access to the neoplastic lesion within the intraconal fat. The intraconal fat lobules are carefully dissected/resected to expose the tumour (Figs 23.9 and 23.10). Care should be taken not to injure the nerves and vessels in these fat corridors.

In the upper corridor between the superior oblique and medial rectus muscles, the nasociliary nerve and the distal segment of the ophthalmic artery is seen. Between the above two muscles, the anterior ethmoidal artery enters the ethmoid roof through the foramen at the frontoethmoid suture. Twelve mm posterior to it is the posterior ethmoidal artery. The distal segment of ophthalmic artery identified between the superior oblique and medial rectus muscle, when traced posteriorly, it runs laterally over the optic nerve and in the optic canal it assumes a position infero-lateral to the optic nerve. Anteriorly, the superior ophthalmic vein is seen on the medial aspect of superior rectus muscle. From here as we trace it posteriorly, the vein runs laterally below the superior rectus muscle to assume a position lateral to the muscle (Figs 23.4 and 23.6). Once the intraconal fat lateral to the medial rectus is removed, the tortuous optic nerve is seen. Anteriorly, the optic nerve is surrounded by plexus of ciliary arteries and long ciliary nerves. Posteriorly, the optic nerve is surrounded by the posterior ciliary arteries which are branches of the ophthalmic artery. Of particular importance is the central retinal artery that lies inferior or medial to the optic nerve. The fat corridor between the medial rectus and inferior rectus muscles is relatively safe with fewer vessels and nerves. The inferior ophthalmic venous plexus is seen just superior to the inferior rectus muscle. Haemostasis is achieved using bipolar cautery. Pericapsular dissection around the tumour may need a ball-probe or a curved elevator. An assistant may help in holding the endoscope, permitting the surgeon to use both hands for dissection around the tumour. Crude avulsion of the tumour should not be done to avoid injury to

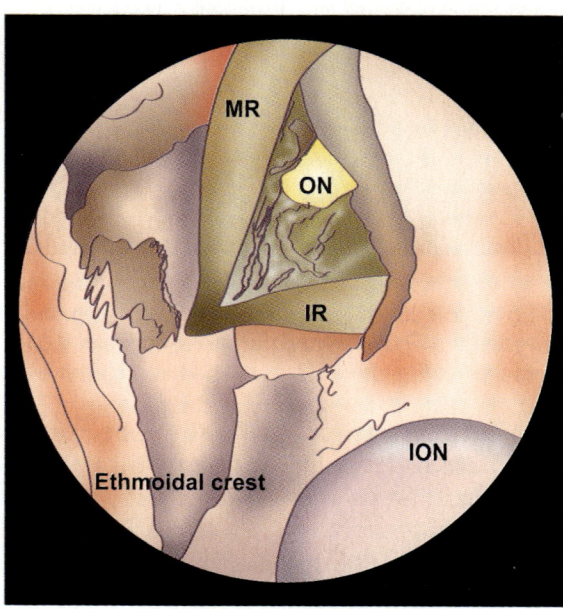

Fig. 23.9: Endoscopic view of the orbit on the left side after removal of the inferomedial extraconal fat and medial intraconal fat between the medial rectus muscle (MR) and the inferior rectus muscle (IR), exposing the optic nerve (ON). ION: Infaorbital nerve

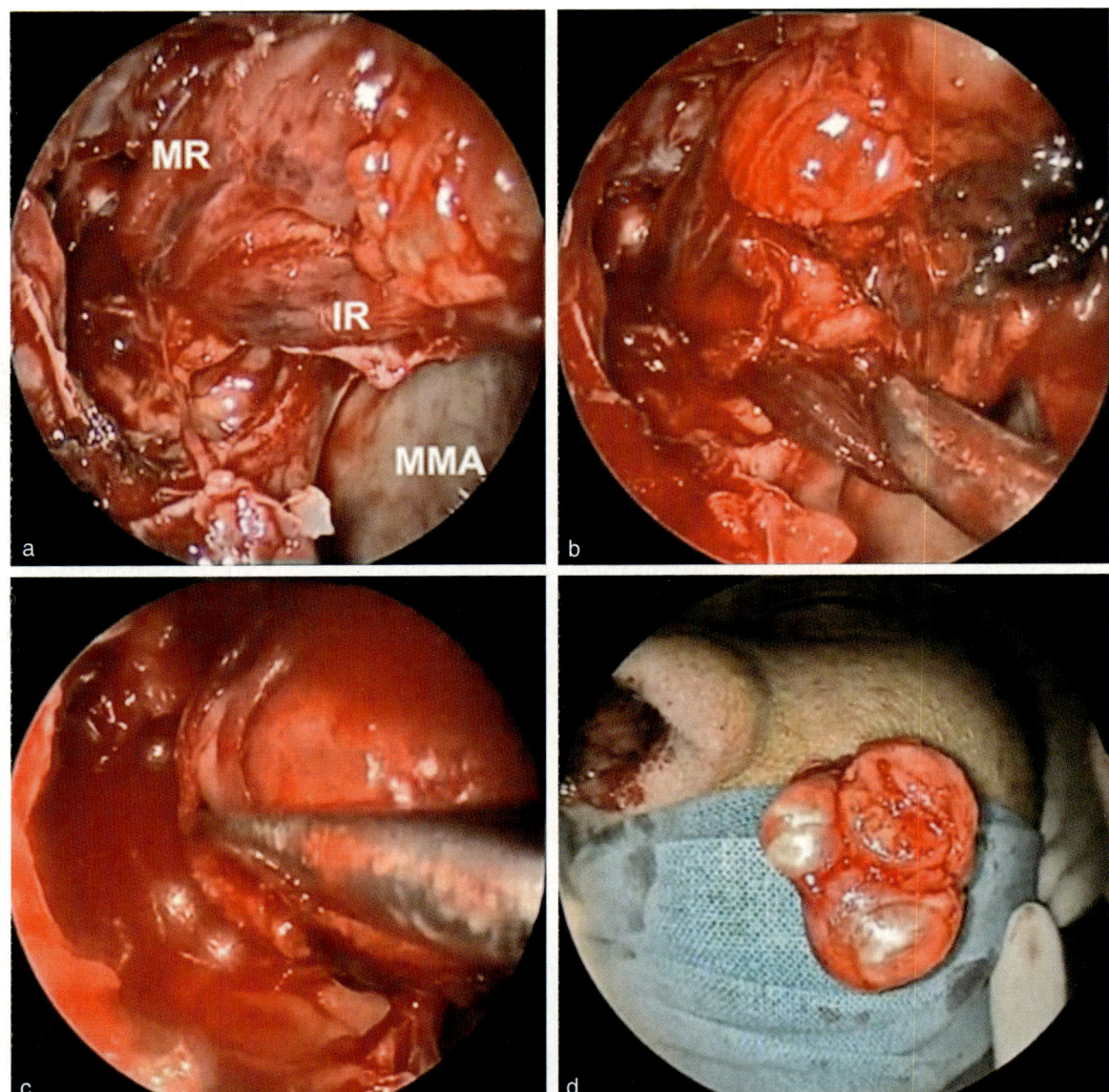

Fig. 23.10: Intraoperative endoscopic pictures showing: **a.** Exposed medial rectus muscle (MR) and inferior rectus muscle (IR) after opening up the orbital periosteum and resecting the inferomedial extraconal fat in the left orbit, **b.** Dissection between the MR and IR and partial resection of the medial intraconal fat, exposing the tumour, **c.** Pericapsular dissection of the tumour, and **d.** The tumour after endonasal endoscopic resection

intraorbital structures. Posteriorly, at the medial aspect of superior orbital fissure, an extraconal vein may be identified that drains into the cavernous sinus. A little anteriorly, a medial connecting vein is usually present that connects the superior and inferior ophthalmic venous systems.

For optic nerve decompression, the thick bone of the optic canal is first drilled using a diamond bur medially, superiorly and inferiorly till a thin bone is left. This thin bone is then removed using a Kerrison punch to achieve a 270° decompression of the optic nerve. Superolateral decompression of the optic canal is technically challenging with increased risk of cerebrospinal fluid (CSF) leak and injury to the optic nerve. Decompression of this wall may be performed using a 2 mm drill and diamond bur under copious irrigation followed by a 2 mm Kerrison punch placed between the anterior cranial fossa dura and the optic canal to dissect the thin bone and unroof the optic canal. The lateral aspect of the optic strut forming the canal floor as well as the base of anterior clinoid is extremely difficult to remove safely via an endonasal approach and can put the ophthalmic artery at risk. The length of the canalicular portion is approximately 8 to 12 mm. The intra-canalicular dura and falciform ligament can be opened endoscopically medial to lateral exposing the intracanalicular segments of the optic nerve. The optic nerve sheath is continuous with the dura mater in this area and thus the nerve is continuous with the subdural space and results in a CSF leak, if left open to the nasal cavity. If the optic nerve sheath is opened, we should be prepared to close the CSF leak. Care must be taken to avoid injury to the ophthalmic and carotid arteries while performing the lateral incision toward the distal dural ring.

Complications

- Diplopia
- Orbital pain
- Diminished vision
- Loss of vision
- CSF rhinorrhoea
- Haemorrhage

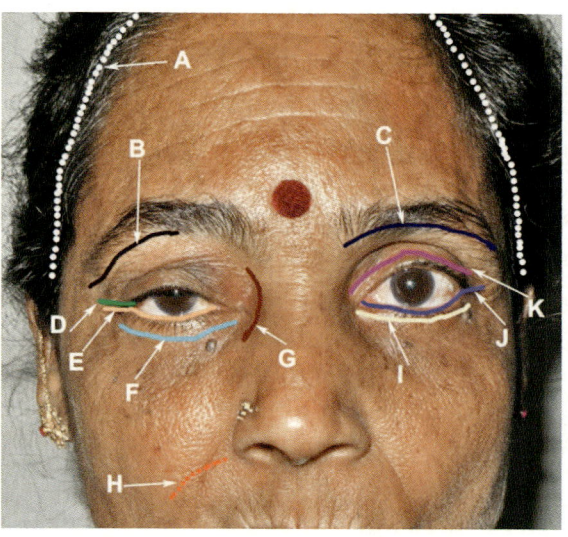

Fig. 23.11: Various incisions used alone or in combination for transorbital endoscopic approach. A: Bicoronal incision meeting in the midline, B: Wright incision, C: Brow incision, D: Lateral canthal incision, E: Transconjunctival inferior fornix with lateral canthal incision, F: Lower rim incision, G: Lynch incision, H: Vestibular incision, I: Inferior eyelid incision, J: Subciliary incision, K: Superior eyelid incision

Transorbital Approaches to the Skull Base

Various transorbital approaches (Table 23.1) have been described to deal with skull base lesions of different locations (Fig. 23.11).[2]

1. Transnasal transorbital endoscopic approach
2. External approaches which may be combined with transnasal endoscopic approach

Table 23.1: Various transorbital approaches		
Transorbital approaches[1]	Approach	Targets
Lateral retrocanthal	Lateral orbit	MCF, ITF, temporal lobe, lateral cavernous sinus, orbital apex, lateral aspect of frontal fossa, lateral sphenoid sinus
Inferior fornix	Inferior orbit	MCF, foramen rotundum, pterygopalatine fossa, sella, parasella, orbital floor/max sinus
Precaruncular	Medial orbit	Bilateral ACF, contralateral MCF, orbital apex, parasella, cavernous sinus, cavernous carotids, optic nerve, and central corridor
Superior lid crease	Superior orbit	Orbital roof fracture, frontal sinus (posterior wall fracture with CSF leak), and anterior fossa pathology

(MCF—Middle cranial fossa, ITF—Infratemporal fossa, ACF—Anterior cranial fossa, CSF—Cerebrospinal fluid)

a. Lynch approach
b. Precaruncular (medial) approach
c. Superior eyelid approach
d. Inferior eyelid approach

3. Purely external transorbital endoscopic approaches
   a. Lateral canthal approach
   b. Superior eyelid approach
   c. Inferior eyelid approach
   d. Swinging eyelid approach
   e. Combined multiportal approach

REFERENCES

1. Dallan I, Castelnuovo P, Franceschini SS, Locatelli D. Endoscopic orbital and transorbital approaches. Endo:Press.

2. Gras-Cabrerizo JR, Martin MM, Lornzo JG, et al. Surgical anatomy of the medial wall of the orbit in human cadavers. J Neurol Surg B Skull Base. 2016; 77:439–44.

3. Moe KS, Berens AM. Transorbital neuroendoscopic approach. In: Bernal-Sprekelsen M, Alobid I (Eds.). Endoscopic approaches to the paranasal sinuses and skull base. Theime Publishers 2017:156–62.

Basics of Rhinoplasty

Aniketh Venkataram, Deeksha Rao

Introduction

Rhinoplasty is considered to be one of the most challenging and unforgiving of all cosmetic procedures. The reason for this is that a difference of even a millimetre is easily noticeable by the human eye, and being the focal point of the face, there is no place to hide your mistakes.

The job of a nose is to be inconspicuous. As an organ, it is not the epitome of beauty. There are poems and songs written about the lips and the eyes, but never about the nose. On the other hand, if the nose is unaesthetic, it distracts from any other beautiful features of the face. Hence, a good rhinoplasty result is one which looks like there never was a surgery in the first place. Whereas a bad result sticks out like a sore thumb.

Add to this, the fact that the nose is functionally important, and a badly done rhinoplasty can compromise a person's ability to breathe, and the challenges of this surgery become readily apparent.

Understanding the Rhinoplasty Patient

Good rhinoplasty patients are those who are clear about what change they are looking for. They understand the limitations of the surgery and have realistic expectations. They are secure in other aspects of life and are looking to overcome this one hurdle which has been holding them back. They can be summarized by SYLVIA (Secure Young Listens Verbal Intelligent Attractive).

Operating on this type of patient can be immensely gratifying as they demonstrate a huge improvement in their self-esteem and confidence after the surgery.

Poor rhinoplasty patients are those who are unsure about what exactly they are looking for. If they do not know themselves, you will never be able to give it to them. They may have other aspects of their lives which are not in balance and may seek surgery as a distraction. Also beware of a patient who is a perfectionist and not willing to accept any flaws. They can be summarized by SIMON (single immature male obsessive narcissist).

Operating on a bad patient can be a miserable experience. Even if you deliver a result that any reasonable, person would judge to be good, as long as they are unhappy it will not matter. It is critical to identify a good patient from a bad one to have a long stable career in rhinoplasty.

Hence, before any surgery, you need to ask two questions:

1. Am I skilled enough to perform this rhinoplasty?
2. Do I want this patient in my practice?

Primary vs Secondary Rhinoplasty

Primary rhinoplasty (Fig. 24.1) is your best chance of getting a good result, and hence should be approached with due responsibility. These patients are usually in a good stable frame of mind. Often times, these patients are operated on by unskilled surgeons who do not

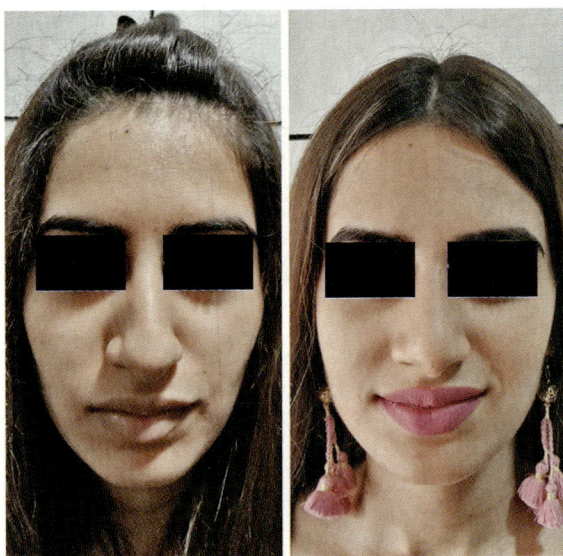

Fig. 24.1: Primary rhinoplasty

give a satisfactory result, and make it much more challenging for the second procedure.[1]

With secondary rhinoplasty (Fig. 24.2), patients can be divided into two groups—those with a poor result, and those unsatisfied with their otherwise acceptable result.

The first group are the ones who need help. However, they need to be evaluated carefully. They are often unsure and hesitant, after having been through a poor first experience.

The second group are those who perhaps should have never been operated in the first place. They have an acceptable result, but their perceived flaws are blown out of proportion in their minds, and they are difficult to please.

PREOPERATIVE EVALUATION

All rhinoplasty patients should be evaluated functionally and aesthetically (Fig. 24.3).

History

The patient is asked about symptoms of unilateral nasal blockade, to rule out deviated nasal septum. Allergic symptoms like excessive sneezing, watering from the eyes and nose, ear and throat itching are asked for. It is important to counsel the patient preoperatively that allergy is a purely medical condition and will not be corrected by a rhinoplasty. History of nasal trauma and previous nasal surgeries should be taken. If this history is positive, then a preoperative CT scan is a must to know if any nasal bone fracture is present and if any septal cartilage is available for reconstruction. If extensive amount of septal cartilage has been removed in their previous surgery, the surgeon has to plan to harvest tragal, conchal cartilage from

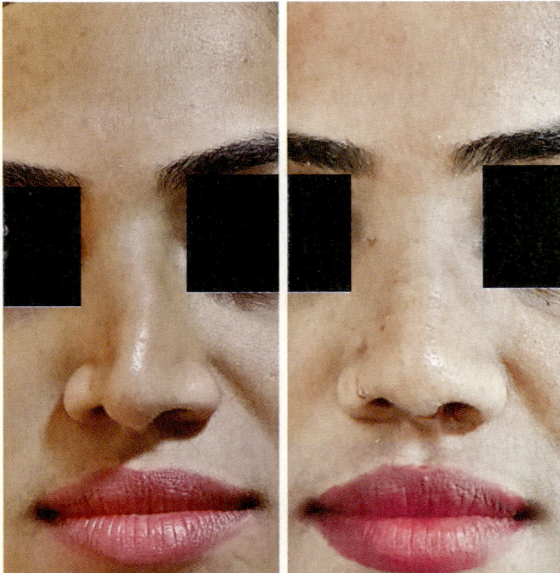

Fig. 24.2: Secondary rhinoplasty

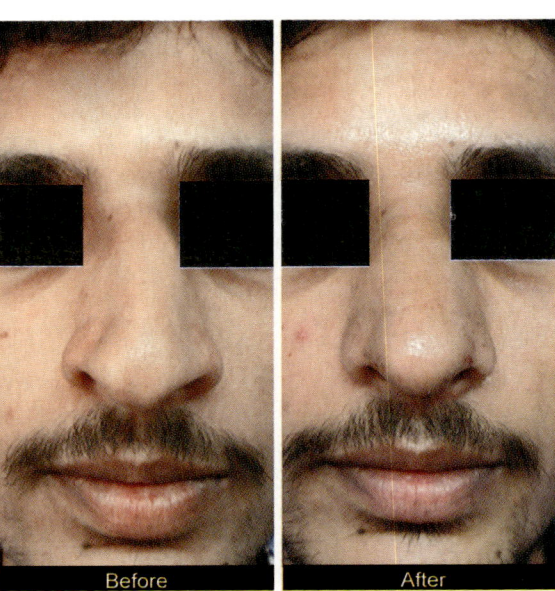

Before   After

Fig. 24.3: Functional rhinoplasty. This patient had severe nasal obstruction and his primary aim of undergoing surgery was to improve his breathing

the ear or rib cartilage for augmentation rhinoplasty cases.[2]

Some patients are not too bothered about the cosmetic appearance of the nose and just want to get a septoplasty to improve their breathing. Such patients must be counselled that a concurrent septorhinoplasty is a better option, as the cartilage harvested during a septoplasty can be used for cosmetic correction. If the patient changes his mind and decides to undergo a cosmetic rhinoplasty in the future, it would become exponentially difficult as the remaining septal cartilage after a septoplasty may not be usable and rib cartilage may be required.[3] Preoperative evaluation of the nasal septum and nasopharynx is paramount before a rhinoplasty surgery. Any physical obstruction diagnosed during this examination, is corrected concurrently.[4]

Functional Examination

We start with a simple rhinoscopy to rule out a deviated nasal septum, presence of spurs, enlarged turbinates. The nasal mucosa is observed, if pale then it indicates allergy. If the nasal mucosa is red with mucoid discharge, a sinus disease should be ruled out and treated accordingly.

Then we progress to a diagnostic nasal endoscopy to rule out any evidence of rhinosinusitis in the form of yellow/greenish discharge. The nasopharynx is examined to rule out any enlarged adenoid tissue.

Aesthetic Evaluation

The importance of proper planning and analysis cannot be overstated. A rhinoplasty surgeon cannot be a slave to one particular method or dogma, and must tailor his approach to each patient to achieve the desired outcome. Moreover, it is important to plan for the long-term, anticipating changes that might occur post surgery.

There is plenty of existing literature on various ideal facial proportions, measurements and angles.[5] However, often there is a lack of clarity on how to convert these measurements and values into an operative plan.

Steps of Analysis

1. *Facial analysis:* This consists of analysis of the patient's face with the established guidelines of aesthetics.
2. *Surgeon's blueprint:* Once the analysis is done, the surgeon analyses all the improvements that can be done for the patient with his order of priority.
3. *Patient discussion:* Rhinoplasty must be a joint endeavour with the patient. The surgeon's blueprint is discussed with the patient, taking the patient's input on their concerns and priorities.
4. *Final blueprint:* The final operative blueprint is decided, based on the surgeon's advice as well as the patient's priorities. In simple words, this is a list of 'what to do'.
5. *Operative plan:* The operative plan is designed to achieve the aims of the blueprint. In other words, this is a sequence of 'how to do'.

Facial Analysis

Facial analysis must be done form the frontal, lateral and basal views. The idea is to identify the external deformities, predict the internal anatomy and determine the appropriate intervention. Here we summarize the essential features to be identified in each view.[6]

Frontal View

The most important things to view are symmetry, balance and tip characteristics
- Horizontal fifths of face—alar base width
- Vertical thirds of face—nasal length
- Skin quality
- Nasal symmetry
  - Dorsal aesthetic lines—deviations—S/C type
- Upper third—bony vault
  - Width—narrow/wide
  - Short or long nasal bones
- Mid vault
  - Narrow/wide
  - Inverted V deformity
- Nasal tip
  - Tip defining points

- Supratip break
- Infratip lobule
- Tip character: Bulbous/pinched/bifid
- Alar rims—notching/retraction
- Alar base width

Lateral View

Should be examined in the Frankfurt horizontal plane. The key is to identify anteroposterior relationships to complete the three-dimensional analysis of the nose:

- Nasofrontal angle
  - High/low radix
- Nasal length
- Dorsum—smooth/depression/hump
- Supratip—smooth/pollybeak
- Tip
  - Projection—over/under
  - Rotation—over/under
- Alar columellar relationship—hanging/retracted

Basal View

The key points to identify are the columella and alar rims:

- Columella
  - Width
  - Flaring
  - Columella lobule ratio
- Nostril—symmetry/flaring
- Alar base width
- Ala cheek junction

Other Features

It is important to also evaluate other features of the face which might need concurrent treatment. The most important of these is the chin (Fig. 24.4). A weak chin can make a nose look much larger than it really is. A chin augmentation may be needed for such patients to achieve facial balance. Lip or forehead augmentation may also be needed in some cases.

Surgeon's Blueprint

Once the analysis is done, the surgeon creates a list of improvements that he feels can be

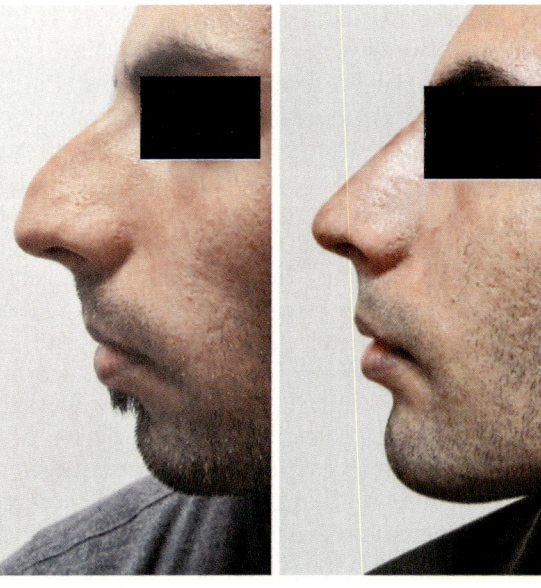

Fig. 24.4: The importance of facial balance. This patient originally came for a rhinoplasty, but was counselled for a simultaneous chin augmentation and upper lip augmentation to achieve facial harmony

made, keeping in mind the aesthetics for the patient's particular race. He also ranks his priorities for these improvements.

Patient Discussion

Very often, an improvement that the surgeon deems necessary might not be a priority for the patient, and something the surgeon deems minor, might be the patient's biggest concern. Ultimately, it is the patient's satisfaction that is paramount. Hence, the surgeon's blueprint must be discussed with the patient and adjusted according to the patient's wishes and priorities. At the same time, it is important not to acquiesce to the patient's every request, as something the patient desires might be detrimental in the short and long run. It is also important to keep in mind the secondary effects of every surgical manoeuvre.

Final Blueprint

Keeping all these factors in mind, the final blueprint is agreed upon which should ideally be an ideal balance of the patient's desires and surgeon's advice.

A TYPICAL RHINOPLASTY PROCEDURE

Preoperative Preparation

Intravenous antibiotics are given. A southpole or RAE tube is preferred to avoid lateral traction which can affect judgement. Throat pack is ensured. Eye ointment is placed and eyes are not taped, so that facial aesthetics can be assessed during surgery.

Infiltration

Lidocaine with 1 in 100000 adrenaline solution is preferred. This is injected in the following sequence:

- Infraorbital vessels
- Angular vessels
- Picture frame block around the nose
- Columella and incision
- Tip
- Dorsum
- Lateral walls
- Septum

A good amount (30cc) is used to aid in hydrodissection as well as for haemostasis. The nose is then packed with ribbon gauze soaked in the same solution

Incision

The transcolumellar incision is placed at the narrowest part of the columella. It is typically in the form of an inverted V (Fig. 24.5). This is then extended vertically 1 mm behind the margin to reach the soft triangle. The soft triangle is carefully preserved and the incision continued along the lower margin of the lateral crus. It is important not to make a rim incision and to follow the crus instead.[7]

Exposure

The incision is deepened. There are two ways of doing this:

- Some surgeons prefer to dissect over the lateral crura and then swing medially and finish with the columellar incision
- Others prefer a columella first technique, and lift the columella off the medial crura before moving to the lateral crura

Either method is acceptable. But the dissection should be deep on the cartilages, preserving tissue on the skin. At the same time, Indian cartilages are a little brittle compared to western counterparts and it is important not to damage the cartilages during dissection. One of the trickiest areas is the soft triangle, and it is important to take your time here to avoid damaging this landmark, which can cause postoperative notching (a telltale sign of a prior surgery).

Once the lower laterals are dissected, the dissection is carried superiorly onto the upper laterals and the nasal bones. Again the aim is to stay as deep as possible. Perichondrium should be raised. If infiltrated properly there should be little bleeding during this dissection, which is easily controlled with electrocautery

Septal Exposure (Fig. 24.6)

The anterior septal angle is identified, and an incision made gently to reach the surface of the cartilage. With a blunt dissector, the perichondrium is gently dissected off. This plane can easily be misidentified. The correct plane is achieved when a transluscent blue of the cartilage is seen and a clear plane easily obtained. The plane is developed posteriorly on the whole septum. This is then extended superior and tunnels created below the upper lateral cartilages. Take your time during this step, as mucosal perforations are easily made inadvertently.

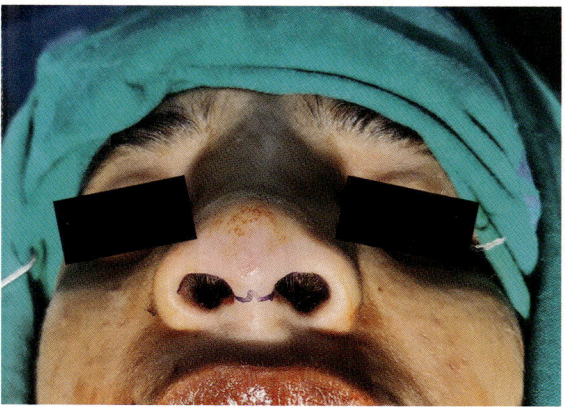

Fig. 24.5: Inverted V incision

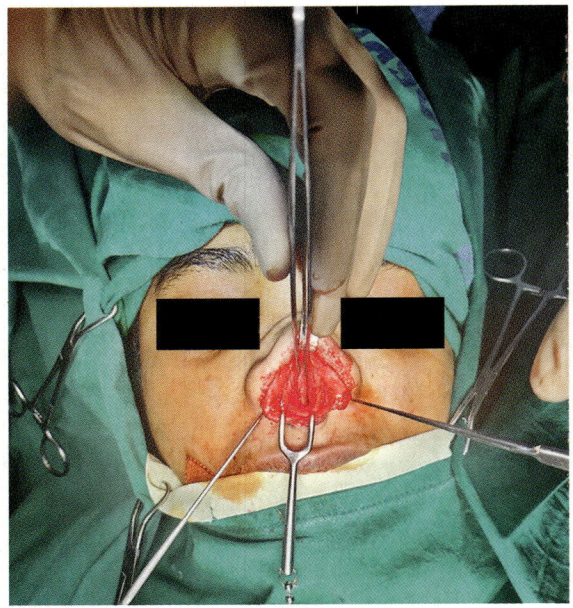

Fig. 24.6: Septal exposure

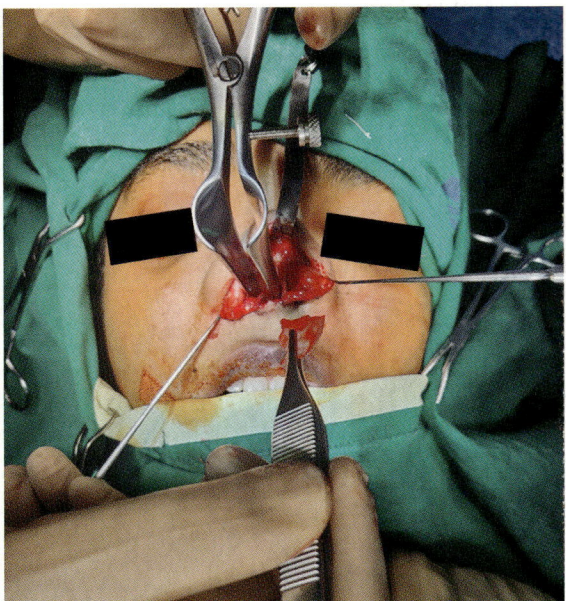

Fig. 24.7: Septal harvest

Dorsal Reduction

The dorsum is reduced first before septal harvest. This is done to ensure adequate remnant septum. The dorsum is reduced in component fashion in an incremental manner. For component reduction, the septum is freed from the upper lateral cartilages using straight scissors. This cut is made flush with the septum, preserving as much ULC length as possible.[8]

First the bony dorsum is rasped. Then the septum is reduced with scissors. Finally, the upper lateral cartilages are reduced with scissors. Component reduction is preferable to using an osteotome for beginners as it allows greater control and judgement although it may take a little more time.

Septum

Next the septum is harvested (Fig. 24.7), if needed. Markings are made leaving behind a 10 mm L strut. The horizontal and vertical incisions are made with a knife. The cartilaginous septum is then gently dissected off the bony septum. A suction dissector is ideal for this manoeuvre. If any bony spurs are present, they are trimmed during this step.

A harvested septum is adequate for spreader grafts, columellar strut and mild dorsal augmentation.[9]

Osteotomies

The aims of osteotomy are to close the open roof after dorsal reduction and narrow the bony base. They can be medial, lateral and transverse. Lateral is subdivided into low to low and low to high. These descriptions are made with low referring to close to the maxilla, and high as meaning coming up onto the nasal bony dorsum. Low to high is easier and avoids a transverse osteotomy but can leave a step deformity which is palpable. Low to low with a transverse osteotomy is ideal for most cases. A medial osteotomy is usually not needed, if bony reduction has been done. In the absence of the same, they might be needed. Osteotomies can be external or internal. We prefer external as it allows proper visualization of the osteotomy line and a proper transverse osteotomy. With internal, most osteotomies end up becoming low to high.[10]

Prior to osteotomy, the markings are made. Low to low is marked at the junction of the nasal process of the maxilla with the body of the maxilla. Transverse is marked at the level

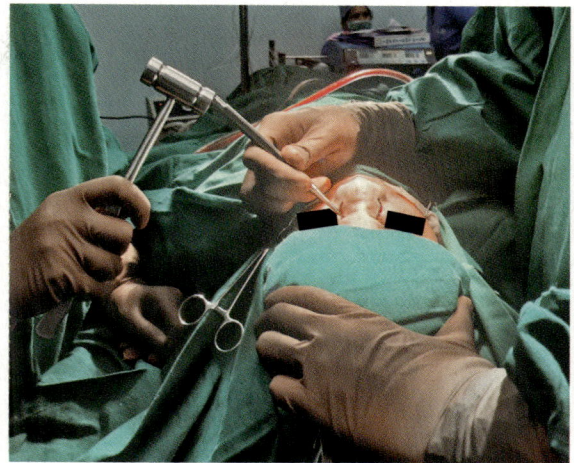

Fig. 24.8: Lateral osteotomy

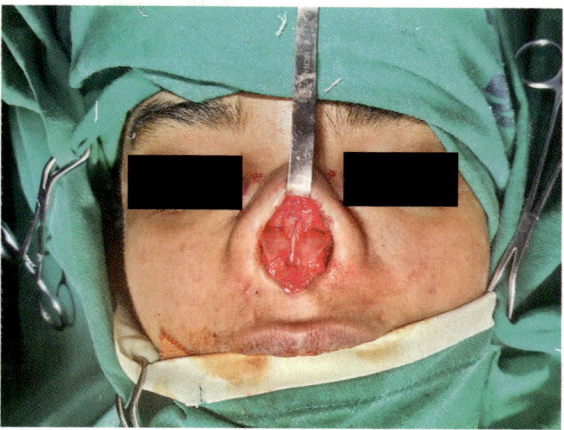

Fig. 24.9: After dorsal closure

of the medial canthus. Infiltration is done, usually a couple of steps before to allow vasoconstriction.

A stab incision is made in the middle of the osteotomy line. A 2 mm or 3 mm osteotome is inserted and used to strip the periosteum from the bone (Fig. 24.8). The bone is broken gently along the line, leaving 1 mm intervals. Then with firm digital pressure, the osteotomy is completed and the bone moved in. This is then adjusted as needed.

Spreader Grafts and Dorsal Closure

Spreader grafts are linear grafts of cartilage around 25 mm long, 1–2 mm wide placed between the septum and ULC prior to closure. They help to keep open the internal nasal valve, and keep the dorsum straight. They are fixed in place with needles and sutured with 5-0 PDS to close the dorsum (Fig. 24.9). Their only downside is they not allow the dorsum to be narrowed completely. The threshold for using spreader grafts should be low. You rarely regret doing them, but the regret of not having done them can cause issues.[11]

Spreaders can also be used asymmetrically, with one side larger than the other to correct deformities. They can be raised slightly above the septum to raise the dorsum. They can be extended and fixed to a columellar strut to improve tip aesthetics and support. They are a very versatile technique indeed.

Dorsal Augmentation

Dorsal augmentation is one of the toughest steps in rhinoplasty and should not be attempted by novices. It is done after dorsal closure. For dorsal augmentation, material has to be obtained and fashioned into a construct. The challenging aspect of this step is that there are multiple options, each with its pros and cons:[12]

- *Septum:* The septum is the preferred donor site, but it is usually inadequate as it is also needed for spreader grafts, strut, etc.
- *Conchal cartilage:* The advantages of conchal cartilage are a hidden donor site and relatively easier harvest. The drawback is its curved shape. It usually has to be sutured as a bilayer to flatten it and be usable. It also might not be enough for large augmentations.[7,13]
- *Rib cartilage:* It has plenty of donor material. Its disadvantages are a scar on the chest wall, and a harder harvest. It is used in two ways:
  - *Solid cartilage grafts*—these are easier to fashion but they have a tendency for warping in the long term.[14]
  - *Diced cartilage in fascia*—these have less warping but need more technical expertise to fashion.[15]
- Implants—silicone/medpor—of not needing harvest and ease of procedure. However, most rhinoplasty surgeons do not prefer this, for their potential for long-term

extrusions which can be a stain on your reputation.

Cephalic Trim (Fig. 24.10)

The cephalic part of the lateral crura can be removed in order to help rotate the lower lateral cartilages (Fig. 24.11), if they are too cephalically oriented and help narrow the tip.[16]

Marking is done, leaving 6 mm of lateral crus. This is especially important in Indian patients where the cartilage strength is less than ideal. Infiltration is done to separate the underlying mucosa form the cartilage. An incision is made and the excess cartilage removed. This cartilage is ideal for tip onlay grafts. It does not work as well for structural grafts such as the columellar strut. If this cartilage is not needed for the tip, then it can just be slid below the preserved LLC so as to not interrupt the scroll ligament.

Tip

Tip work consists of columellar strut, tip sutures and tip grafts.[17]

Columellar Strut (Fig. 24.11)

A columellar strut is important to maintain tip projection and rotation. If the tip is over projected, medial crural overlap is done prior to strut insertion.

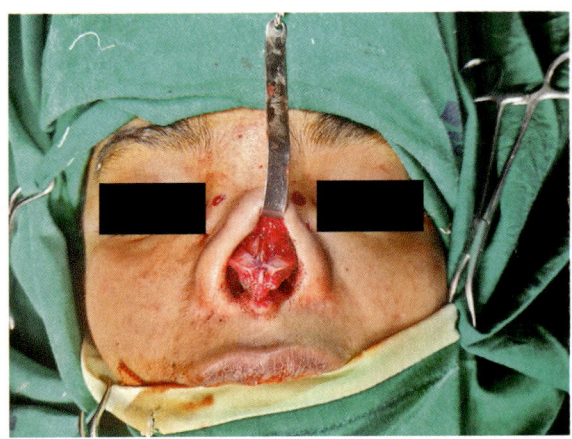

Fig. 24.11: Tip sutures and columellar strut

The strut is fashioned from septal cartilage to approximately 20 mm × 3 mm × 4 mm. A pocket is dissected between the medial crurae, the strut is inserted, but not directly on the ANS to avoid clicking. It is then sutured in place with the medial crurae with 5-0 PDS.

Tip Sutures (Fig. 24.11)

The tip is sutured to narrow the tip and correct any asymmetries.[18]

Intradomal suture: This is done at the intermedial crus, or sometimes a little laterally to increase projection. It is done as a horizontal mattress and tightened to narrow the dome.

Interdomal suture: This is done to bring the domes together. It is done at the cephalic end of the medial crus just below the dome.

Domal equalization: This is done to correct any domal asymmetry. It is done as an inside out suture on the cephalic end of one dome and an outside in suture on the cephalic end of the other dome.

Tip Grafts

Tip grafts are used to increase tip definition and projection. They are particularly useful in thick skin. They are fashioned from the cephalic trim cartilage and sutured at the caudal portion of the dome. It is important not to place them too superiorly or it will move the tip defining points too high.[19]

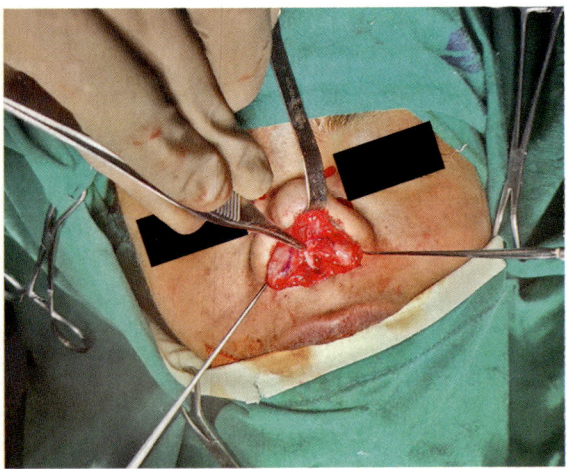

Fig. 24.10: Cephalic trim

Base

Nasal base reduction can be done by alar reduction or nostril sill reduction or both.[20]

Alar reduction: This is done in patients with a high degree of alar flaring. A crescentic piece of tissue is marked at the alar junction, excised and sutured.

Nostril sill reduction: This is done to reduce the overall nasal base width. A 3 mm crescent is marked in both nostrils, skin excised and sutured (Fig. 24.12).

Closure

Once ready to close, the nose is examined in detail from all angles. Complete haemostasis is checked. The columellar incision is closed with 6-0 prolene. The intranasal incision is closed with 5-0 vicryl rapide.

Doyle splints or quilting sutured can be used. Intranasal packs are what we prefer. Taping is done on the nose. Then either a POP or premade splint is placed over the nose.

Postoperative Course

The patient is usually kept overnight or can also be discharged after a few hours of observation.

Early: The nasal packs are removed the next day after surgery and lavage done. The patient is instructed to keep the passages clear with saline drops and keep the incisions clean with antibiotic ointment. The POP splint and sutures are removed on the seventh day.

Late: The patient is advised to be patience as the result takes time to be fully apparent. This is particularly important in thick skin types.

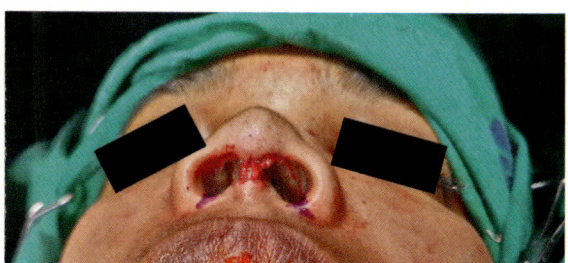

Fig. 24.12: Marking for nostril sill reduction

Complications

Complications of rhinoplasty include:

- *Haemorrhage:* This can be avoided with meticulous haemostasis and proper packing. If occurred, it should be evacuated or it will compromise the result.
- *Infection:* This is thankfully rare with the use of postoperative antibiotics.
- *Septal problems:* Haematomas, abscesses, perforations
- Nasal obstruction
- Unsatisfactory result

It is important to understand that the steps elucidated above constitute the framework for a typical rhinoplasty procedure. Each step is customizable as per the needs of the patient. No two patients are the same and no two procedures are the same.

This chapter serves as a good introduction to the world of rhinoplasty. There are innumerable variations and modifications possible which cannot be covered. To be successful in rhinoplasty, it is important to understand your patient and grow as a surgeon in an incremental manner.

REFERENCES

1. Broer PN, Buonocore S, Morillas A, Liu J, Tanna N, et al. Nasal aesthetics: A cross-cultural analysis. Plast Reconstr Surg 2012;130:843e–850e.
2. Burres S. Tip points: Defining the tip. Aesthetic Plast Surg 1999;23:113–18.
3. Conrad K. Cartilage delivery and open rhinoplasty as two preferred approaches to the nasal tip. J Otolaryngol Suppl 1986;15:1–24.
4. Daniel RK. Diced cartilage grafts in rhinoplasty surgery: Current techniques and applications. Plast Reconstr Surg 2008;122:1883–91.
5. Gunter JP, Cochran CS, Marin VP. Dorsal augmentation with autogenous rib cartilage. Semin Plast Surg 2008;22:74–89.
6. Hamra ST. Crushed cartilage grafts over alar dome reduction in open rhinoplasty. Plast Reconstr Surg 1993;92:352–56.
7. Lee M, Callahan S, Cochran CS. Auricular cartilage: Harvest technique and versatility in rhinoplasty. Am J Otolaryngol 2011;32:547–52.

8. Lee MR, Unger JG, Rohrich RJ. Management of the nasal dorsum in rhinoplasty: A systematic review of the literature regarding technique, outcomes, and complications. Plast Reconstr Surg 2011;128:538e–550e.

9. McCollough EG, Devinder M. Systematic approach to correction of the nasal tip in rhinoplasty. Arch Otolaryngol 1981;107:12–16.

10. Powell N, Humphreys B. Proportions of the aesthetic face. Thieme Stratton, New York, 1984.

11. Rohrich RJ, Adams WP Jr. Te boxy nasal tip: classifcation and management based on alar cartilage suturing techniques. PlastReconstr Surg 107:1849–63; discussion 1864–68, 2001.

12. Rohrich RJ, Hollier LH. Use of spreader grafts in the external approach to rhinoplasty. Clin Plast Surg 1996;23:255–62.

13. Rohrich RJ, Janis JE. Osteotomies in rhinoplasty: An updated technique. Aesthetic Surg J 2003; 23:56–58.

14. Sajjadian A, Rubinstein R, Naghshineh N. Current status of grafts and implants in rhinoplasty: Part I. Autologous grafts. Plast Reconstr Surg 2010;125:40e–49e.

15. Tardy ME Jr, Dayan S, Hecht D. Preoperative rhinoplasty: Evaluation and analysis. Otolaryngol Clin North Am 2002;35:1–27.

16. Toriumi DM. Autogenous grafts are worth the extra time. Arch Otolaryngol Head Neck Surg 2000;126:562–64.

17. Toriumi DM. New concepts in nasal tip contouring. Arch Facial Plast Surg 2006;156–85.

18. Toriumi DM. Rhinoplasty. In: Park SS (eds) Facial plastic surgery: The essential guide. Thieme Medical Publishers: New York, 2005; 223–53.

19. Williams EF 3rd, Lam SM. A systematic, graduated approach to rhinoplasty. Facial Plast Surg 2002;18:215–22.

20. Woodard CR, Park SS. Nasal and facial analysis. Clin Plast Surg 2010;37:181–89.

Nasopharyngeal Angiofibroma—Transnasal Endoscopic Excision

DR Nayak, R Balakrishnan, D Nayak M

Definition

Nasopharyngeal angiofibroma is defined as histologically benign tumour seen in the posterior part of the nasal cavity and naso-pharynx which is extremely vascular and locally aggressive tumour that is seen exclusively in adolescent males.

Introduction

It presents with paroxysms of profuse painless and unprovoked epistaxis and nasal obstruction. This tumour, due to its topographical location close to the pterygopalatine fossa, infratemporal fossa, orbit and anterior and middle cranial fossa, can present with various clinical manifestations. This makes its surgical management more difficult and challenging. Control of intraoperative bleeding is mandatory to achieve successful surgical result.

Progress in the field of diagnostic technology like contrast enhancement CT imaging, contrast MRI, interventional radiology like digital subtraction angiography (DSA) with highly selective embolization techniques and nasal endoscopy have helped the surgeon plan an appropriate approach aimed at complete excision of the tumour. Advances in the anaesthetic gadgets and availability of better surgical tools like endoscopes, laser and bipolar cautery have helped better tumour resection even in advanced cases.

Historical Perspective

Although generally regarded as a rare tumour it has been recognized for a long time and has been quoted by Tapia Acuna (1956) as such a lesion being removed by Hippocrates in the 5th century BC. The name "angiofibroma" was given by Friedberg in 1940. Chelius (1847) described the fibrous nature of an intranasal lesion that occurs around the time of puberty (Schiff 1959). Legouest (1865) first reported its predilection in males and was supported by Finerman in 1951. Bensch & Ewing (1941) thought it originates from embryonic fibrocartilage in the base of skull. Chauveau (1906) first introduced the term of juvenile nasopharyngeal fibroma as it occurred mainly in children. Friedburg 1940 suggested the name of angiofibroma. It has since been termed juvenile nasopharyngeal angiofibroma (JNA) or juvenile nasopharyngeal fibroma. Martin, et al (1948) suggested the hormonal theory. They thought that this tumour results from deficiency of androgen activity or over-production of oestrogen. They expressed the view that these growths are principally angiomatous rather than fibromatous and explained their subsequent development on the basis of hormonal stimulation. They found that treatment with testosterone proportionate resulted in regression of the tumour in some cases. In favour of this hormonal theory, Karatay, et al. (1963) have shown that 17-ketosteroids and 17 OH (17-21 dihydroxy-20-ketosteroids) were diminished in the daily output in the urine of these patients, and folliculin was increased two or three times.

Sternberg (1954) felt that the vascular network was an integral part of the tumour and thought that the tumour was a distinctive type of haemangioma which in part behaved like cutaneous haemangiomata of childhood. These later tend to undergo spontaneous regression with age. Harma in 1958, placed nasopharyngeal fibromata amongst the hyperplastic tissue reactions of fibroangiomatous structure similar to granuloma pyogenicum, or granuloma gravidum. He assumed that it is caused chiefly by a hormonal factor active for a short duration during puberty. Osborn (1959) considered these tumours to belong to the group of malformations. He stressed the similarity of the vascular findings in these tumours to the nasal erectile tissue and considered them to be malformations of the blood vessels like hamartomata. Schiff (1959) put forward the hypothesis that these growths were due to an alteration in pituitary activity, i.e. in the androgen-estrogen axis, and he proposed that the tumour is basically vascular and the fibrous tissue component is a desmoplastic or connective tissue response to the ectopic, sex-sensitive vascular tissue. Capps, et al. (1961) suggested that the tumour in females is of different nature. Apostol (1965) stated that the tumour reported in females is almost always due to faulty diagnosis and in cases the diagnosis is confirmed by repeated biopsy; a sex chromosome study should be indicated.

Walike and MacKay (1970) found that diethylstilbestrol alters the endothelial lining of the vascular spaces under electron microscopic study and stated that it may stimulate the process of fibrosis and regression of an angiofibroma. Apostol (1965) stated that this tumour reported in females is almost always due to faulty diagnosis and in cases the diagnosis is confirmed by repeated biopsy; a sex chromosome study should be indicated. Handousa et al (1954), Mishra & Bhatia (1967), Gupta and Gupta (1971), Girish (1973) and Patil (1982) found that angiofibroma can extend extra-nasopharyngeally to areas like cheek, infratemporal fossa, orbit, maxillary sinus, nose and to the intracranial structures through natural foramina or through bony erosions on rare occasion.

Anatomical Considerations

Knowledge of anatomy of the nasopharynx and posterior part of nasal cavity and its vital relations like cranial base, pterygopalatine and infratemporal fossa and orbit is mandatory to understand the possible extra-nasopharyngeal extensions of the tumour and in its surgical management.

Nasopharynx is situated behind the nose and above the lower border of the soft palate and Passavant's ridge. It is lined by pseudo-stratified columnar ciliated epithelium (respiratory epithelium). The walls are rigid and non-collapsible.

Anteriorly: It opens into the right and left nasal fossae through the posterior choana divided by the posterior end of the septum.

Superiorly: It is bounded by the base of skull (anteroinferior surface of the body of sphenoid bone and basilar part of the occipital bone).

Inferiorly: It is limited by the soft palate, while in the posterior aspect it communicates with the oropharynx at the nasopharyngeal isthmus which is bounded by:

- The lower border of soft palate
- The posterior wall of pharynx (Passavant's muscle).

Lateral wall: It has some of the important areas of nasopharynx. It contains the pharyngeal opening of the auditory (eustachian) tube as tubal elevation (torus tubarius) that bounds the tubal opening. The salpingopharyngeal fold of the mucous membrane runs downwards from the posterior margin of tubal elevation. Another fold passes from the anterior edge of the tubal opening onto upper surface of soft palate caused by levator palatini muscle. Behind the tubal elevation lies the pharyngeal recess called "fossa of Rosenmüller".

Posteriorly: Prevertebral muscles covering the clivus and the 1st and 2nd cervical vertebrae.

Incidence: Exact cause of nasopharyngeal angiofibroma is not known. The heavy male predominance has drawn intrigue into the hypothesis of an imbalance in the pituitary androgen-estrogen axis. It constitutes about

0.05 to 0.5% of all head and neck tumours occurring in 1 of 150,000 individuals (Coutinho-Camillo, et al 2008).

Age and sex: Though it is common in adolescent males it may be occasionally seen in adult males. The term angiofibroma was first introduced by Friedberg in the year 1940. JNA are seldom seen in children below the age of 8. According to Fiji and Davis (1950), the onset of this disease is definitely limited to the period of adolescence which varies from 9 to 19 years (Lund, et al. 2010). This tumour exclusively occurs in adolescent males. There have been some cases of females reported; however, these are very, very few. Martin (1978) reported a case of angiofibroma in a female. Fiji and Briant (1970) reported the sex incidence a male to female ratio of 14:1. Paul (1993) reported from University of California a series of 58 patients of whom 4 were females. Apostole (1965) said that when such a case is reported in females it should be viewed with suspicion. Morrison in 1955 stated that this tumour is rare in girls because the skull development ceases at an early age in girls than that in boys and that the periosteal changes are less likely to occur.

Etiopathogenesis

- **Girgis & Fahmy (1973)** observed cell nests of undifferentiated epithelioid cells or "Zell ballen" at the growing edge of angiofibromas. This appearance was more or less similar to that of paraganglioma. They considered JNA to be a paraganglionoma. Origin from nonchromaffin paraganglionic cells of the terminal branches of the maxillary artery has also been suggested.

- **Maurice and Milad (1981)** interpreted angiofibroma to be hamartoma arising from misplaced genital erectile tissue. Testosterone acting on a hamartomatous nidus of inferior turbinate tissue mislocated in the nasopharynx similar to the midline erectile tissue like penis. There is evidence of increased androgen receptors of tumours and successful tumour regression after antiandrogen therapy.

- **Shikani AH and Richtsmeier (1992)** transplanted the tumour into the subdermal space of athymic mice and also cultured it *in vitro*, to study the effect of hormonal manipulation. The tumour did survive in male and female athymic mice but has failed to grow. Androgen treatment of the mice of either sex did not alter its survival or growth behaviour. The *in vitro* tissue culture grew fibroblastoid cells that were not stimulated by androgen supplementation. This study suggested that factors other than androgens are at least complementary, if not essential, in promoting the growth of juvenile nasopharyngeal angiofibroma in tumour models, and that androgens were not, in and of themselves, sufficient growth stimuli.

- **Gardiello (1993)**, suggested that angiofibromas as extracolonic manifestation of familial adenomatous polyposis (FAP) and tumour growth from normal nasopharyngeal fibrovascular stroma.

- **Nagai, et al (1996)** investigated 20 patients of JNA and found basic fibroblast growth factor (bFgc) over-expressed in 2 out of 17 cases platelet derived growth factor A (PDGF-A) in one out of 12 cases, PDGF-B was over-expressed in 4 out of 8 cases, insulin like growth factor (IGF-2) in 9 out of 17 cases, transforming growth factor β-1 in one out of 18 cases, vascular epithelial growth factor (VEGF) in 4 out of 20 cases.

- **Hwang (1998),** found immunohistological detection of androgen receptor expression in 18 out of 24 JNAs.

- **Dillard, et al (2000)** found by immunohistochemical investigations, activated TGF-β1 in stromal and endothelial cells in 19 JNAs and suggested a possible role of TGF-β1 in the pathogenesis of JNA.

- **Gautham and Ogale,** et al (2002) found loss of Glutathione-S-Transferase Mu1 gene (GSTM1) known to be associated with increased risk of developing malignancy of upper resiratopry tract has been detected in 3 of 8 JNAs.

Some Recent Theories of Etiopathogenesis of JNA

- **Abraham, et al (2001) and Rippel, et al (2003)** analyzed adenomatous polyposis coli (APC)-β catenin pathway and found high frequency of β-catenin gene mutations in Exon3 resulting in cellular and nuclear accumulation of stabilized β catenin in JNA.
- **Bernard Schick (2002)** published first evidence of genetic imbalances in angiofibroma. Chromosomal gains and losses showed high level of agreement for genetic causation. Schick, et al (2005) indicated chromosomal losses on chromosome 17 imply p53 gene and Her-2/neu gene losses in JNAs.
- **Brieger (2004)** describing the various inconsistent studies on molecular basis of JNA suggested future studies targeting Wnt-pathway with its key player β-catenin to explore the actual molecular basis of JNA genesis. They found high vessel densities along with strong proliferating and VEGF-expressing vessel endothelium cells associated with VEGF-expressing and proliferating stromal cells.
- **Valazano, et al (2005)** documented for the first time the association between a somatic and a germline APC mutation in an FAP related JNA.
- **Schuon, et al (2007)** on immunohisto-chemical evaluation found the subcellular distribution of several angiogenic factors and showed that increased levels of basic fibroblast growth factor (bFGF), transforming growth factor-b1 (TGFb1), and VEGF receptor-2 (VEGFR-2) are associated with high vessel densities in JNA.
- **Henrich, et al (2007)** using comparative genomic hybridization analysis for JNA found autosomal genomic alterations in 6 out of 22 cases of JNA.
- **Coutinho-Camillo, et al (2008)** analyzed the imprinting status and expression levels of the IGFII and H19 genes in angiofibroma.
- **Farag, et al (2009)** found specific thermo-stable androgen receptors in the tissues of nasopharyngeal angiofibroma which had high affinity toward DHT more than testosterone.
- **Gramann, et al (2009)** studied the expression of the fibrillar collagen and found a prominent collagen-type VI expression in JNAs. The collagen-type VI may exert an important growth stimulus in this tumour. However, they confirm in another study in 2009, that collagen type II expression is practically absent in JNAs. This refutes the theory that JNAs originate in cartilage tissue.
- **Zhang, et al (2011)** on immunohisto-chemical analysis found biological distinctions between juvenile nasopharyngeal angiofibroma and vascular malformation.
- **Liu, et al (2015)** found high levels of hormone receptors and vascular endothelial growth factor (VEGF) compared with normal nasal mucosa. The interaction between hormone receptors and VEGF may be involved in the initiation and growth of JNA.

Pathology

Though it was earlier thought to be arising from the roof of the nasopharynx, it is now confirmed to have its origin from a point above the superior margin of the spheno-palatine foramen and the base of medial pterygoid plate. Thus it tends to spread laterally into the pterygopalatine fossa.

The proposed origin of the JNA is located along the posterior-lateral wall in the roof of the nasopharynx, usually in the region of the superior margin of the sphenopalatine foramen and the posterior aspect of the middle turbinate. Fetal histology confirms large areas of endothelial tissue in this region. Rather than invading surrounding tissue, this tumour displaces and distorts, relying on pressure necrosis to destroy and push through its bony confines. Intracranial extension is noted in 10–20% of cases. Several studies have been done to find out the reason for the aggressiveness, but flow cytometric evaluation suggests tumour ploidy cannot be used to predict the clinical course of angiofibromas (Barnes, et al. 1992).

Gross:

- Lobulated, firm, non-encapsulated mass
- Usually pink-gray or purple-red
- Sessile or pedunculated
- Secondary attachments usually, complicating resection in continuity.

Histopathology

Consists of bland spindle cell with band of collagen with proliferative irregular thin-walled endothelial lined blood vessels without muscular layer (Fig. 25.1a). The tumour stroma contains tumour cells with stellate and spindly fibroblasts (Fig. 25.1b). At times focus of haemorrhagic area can be noted due to embolization (Fig. 25.1c).

The characteristic histological feature includes:

- It has no capsule.
- Tumour composed of thin-walled vessels of varying caliber in a mature connective tissue stroma.
- The vessels are primitive embryonic in type and typically have a single endothelial cell lining without a muscularis or elastic layer, which probably explains the tumour's propensity for haemorrhage.
- Discontinuous vascular basal laminae, focal lack of pericytes, and pronounced irregularity of the smooth muscle layers. In thick smooth muscle layers and pads, the orientation of muscle cells is frequently disturbed, and the individual cells differ in size and shape. Occasionally, the muscle layers disperse peripherally into individual cells, creating the impression of vessel-independent smooth muscle cells within the stroma (Beham, et al. 2000).

Tumour Extensions and Pathways

The tumour originates from the superior margin of the sphenopalatine foramen where the sphenoid process of the palatine bone meets the pterygoid base and the horizontal ala of vomer (Safadi, et al 2018). The anatomical position of the nasopharynx and its different structural relations facilitate the spread and extensions of this tumour locally through natural foramina and fissures (Conley 1968). Because of the expansive character of the tumour, it frequently erodes the floor of the sphenoid sinus and other rigid boundaries of the nasopharynx. It exerts considerable unimpeded pressure by its slow growth and causes bony resorption and can even involve the orbit, spread into pterygopalatine fossa and infratemporal fossa and then into the cheek (Taneja and Kolhi 1967). Intracranial extension of this tumour has been reported initially by Thomson, et al (1948), and by Chhangain (1968). The tumour can spread to various anatomical sites in and around the sphenopalatine foramen from where the tumour originates. Since the tumour does not have a definitive capsule, it invades locally and behaves like a locally malignant tumour. The tumour extends usually along the path of least resistance and the thin plates of bone can easily be eroded to facilitate the tumour expansion further. Safadi, et al. (2018) described three distinct pattern of bony involvement. They are:

1. Bone remodelling due to expansion, thinning, and displacement (anterior

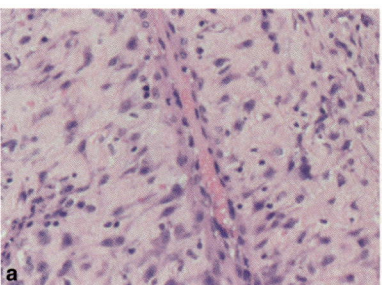 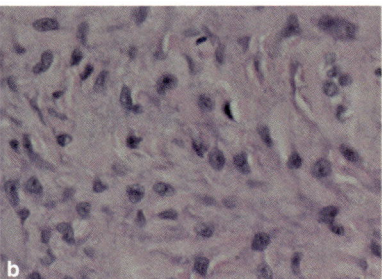 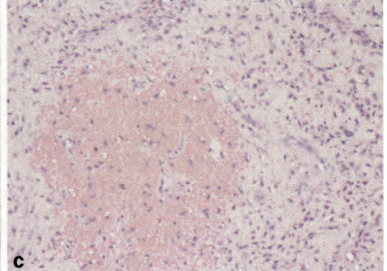

Fig. 25.1: a. Bland spindle cells with bands of collagen and proliferating vessels (H&E, x100), **b.** Tumour cells with stellate and spindly fibroblasts (H&E, x400), **c.** A focus of haemorrhagic necrosis/ infarct-? therapeutic embolization induced (H&E, x100)

displacement of the posterior maxillary wall, enlarged vidian canal, and inferior orbital fissure).

2. Cancellous bone invasion (pterygoid base)
3. Bone resorption and destruction of greater wing of sphenoid bone destruction by large tumour invading the middle cranial fossa.

TUMOUR SPREAD

Medial Spread

This is the earliest and the commonest extension where the tumour after originating from the sphenopalatine foramen enters the nasal cavity, nasopharynx and the ethmoid sinuses. This is associated with secondary attachments to the roof of the choana, posterior part of middle turbinate, nasal septum and the nasopharynx as the tumour enlarges further.

Anterior Spread

It occurs late and the tumour extends anterior to the pterygoid plate to involve pterygopalatine fossa from where it can erode the posterior wall of the maxilla and thus can enter the maxillary sinus. Pterygopalatine fossa involvement is seen in 70% of cases (Antoneli, et al. 1987). Further lateral extension allows the tumour to involve the infratemporal fossa via the pterygomaxillary fissure by eroding the pterygoid plates and later it can extend into the cheek. Posteriorly the tumour erodes the pterygoid plate and enters the pterygoid fossa and can erode medial pterygoid plate and can extend to parapharyngeal space (Szymanska 2015).

Posterior Spread

In the sphenopalatine foramen, the tumour destroys the median pterygoid plate which forms the posterior margin of the foramen and then the lateral pterygoid plates and enters via the vidian canal. Sphenoid sinus involvement occurs following involvement of vidian canal (Zanation, et al. 2012). Rarely the tumour can extend posterolaterally to the pharyngeal recess (Safadi, et al 2018).

Superior Spread

Superiorly JNA spreads through the infra-orbital fissure (IOF) to involve the orbit and through the superior orbital fissure (SOF) and foramen rotundum until it reaches the cavernous sinus.

Intracranial Spread

Intracranial extension may be classified as medial or lateral to the cavernous sinus and internal carotid artery (ICA), depending on the route of extension (Szymanska 2015). It occurs commonly through the sphenoid sinus from where it can extend laterally to involve the cavernous sinus and superiorly to the sella and the middle cranial fossa. The tumour can extend anterolaterally from the sphenoid to the posterior ethmoids, orbital apex and the anterior cranial fossa. From the orbital apex the tumour can directly extend to the middle cranial fossa. The tumour from the pterygopalatine/infratemporal fossa can erode the greater wing of sphenoid and extend through foramina rotundum, ovale and lacerum into the middle cranial fossa. From the middle cranial fossa, the tumour can extend into the parasellar region but often remains extradural and lateral to sphenoid sinus.

Thus there are two common ways of intracranial extension. The first is through the skull base at the attachment of pterygoid process, lateral to the internal carotid artery. The second is through the sphenoid sinus and into the region of the cavernous sinus (Batsakis 1979). Golabek (2019) found the superior orbital fissure to be the most common route for intracranial extension in patients with extensive involvement of the infratemporal fossa. Mattei, et al (2011) highlighted various routes of extension to the intracranial space as follows:

• Directly through invasion of the cavernous sinus after sphenoid and sella turcica invasion,

• Through the foramen rotundum,

• Through the middle fossa after invasion of the infratemporal fossa,

• Through the superior orbital fissure, or

- Through the pterygoid canal after invading the pterygopalatine fossa and the pterygomaxillary fissure.

The directions of extension are lateral, forward, upward and downward.

A. *Lateral extension may occur in following routes.*
   1. Nasopharynx—through sphenopalatine foramen—pterygopalatine fossa—maxillary antrum.
   2. Pterygopalatine fossa—through infraorbital fissure—orbit.
   3. Pterygopalatine fossa—through pterygomaxillary fissure—cheek, temporal region.
   4. Pterygopalatine fossa—fascia basalis at sinus of Morgagni. Infratemporal fossa.

B. *Forward extension takes following ways:*
   1. Nasopharynx—through choana—nasal cavity—maxillary sinus—orbit
   2. Nasal cavity—ethmoid sinus—breaking lamina papyracea—orbit.

C. *Upward extension occurs in the following ways:*
   1. Nasopharynx—sphenoid sinus—pituitary fossa.
   2. Nasopharynx—eroding greater wing of sphenoid into middle cranial fossa.
   3. Nasopharynx—through cribriform plate— anterior cranial fossa.
   4. Nasopharynx—foramen lacerum—middle cranial fossa.

D. *Downward expansion:* May occupy oropharynx

Clinical Features

The chief symptoms of this tumour are nasal obstruction, epistaxis, and change of voice called 'dead speech', fetid nasal discharge and other symptoms like proptosis, deafness and pain in the ear (Taneja and Kollhy 1967, Safadi, et al 2018). The symptoms can be classified according to the site of involvement and extensions.

Nasal and nasopharyngeal: Nasal obstruction is the predominant symptom found in 80–90% of cases (Bruce, et al. 1974, Hardillo, et al 2004) followed by epistaxis in 70–80% of cases (Briant 1970, Witt, et al. 1983)

- Constant and progressive nasal obstruction which is initially unilateral and later can be bilateral
- Profuse painless paroxysms of unprovoked epistaxis—initially unilateral
- Fetid anterior nasal discharge
- Anosmia/hyposmia
- Rhinolalia clausa
- Mouth breathing, snoring and sleep apnoea
- Nasal deformity in extensive cases

Extranasopharyngeal Symptoms

Facial
- Frog face deformity
- Cheek swelling is due to its involvement of pterygomaxillary fissure and extension to infratemporal fossa and cheek.
- Proptosis suggests involment of the orbit through inferior orbital fissure or direct erosion of the lamina papyracea through the ethmoids.
- Facial pain can be due to secondary sinusitis.

Otological: Due to Eustachian tube dysfunction
- Blocked feeling in the ear
- Deafness
- Discharge
- Tinnitus

Oral and oropharyngeal:
- Palatal swelling involving the soft palate
- Postnasal discharge
- Postnasal profuse bleeding
- Difficulty in swallowing
- Dry mouth due to mouth breathing

Ophthalmological: Rare but can be due to orbital apex and cavernous sinus involvement:
- Eye pain
- Epiphora
- Diplopia due to proptosis
- Blindness rarely.

Neurological
- Multiple cranial nerve paralysis, if the tumour involves the cavernous sinus
- Trigeminal neuralgia
- Diplopia due to involvement of abducent and trochlear nerves.

- Extensions into the orbital apex and optic chiasma can cause blurring of vision and blindness.
- Intracranial extensions can cause increase intracranial pressure and lead to headache, blurring of vision and projectile vomiting.

General

Sexual underdevelopment: Martin, et al. (1948) observed that JNA patient have initial sexual underdevelopment and tumour regresses with the development of secondary sexual character.

Clinical Signs

Anterior rhinoscopy: May show the characteristic pinkish globular mass in the posterior part of the nasal cavity between the middle turbinate and the septum. The septum is often pushed to the opposite side.

Posterior rhinoscopy can reveal the nasopharyngeal mass which appears pink to purple in colour, globular with dilated vessels on its surface.

Oral cavity may show prominence of the soft palate when the tumour occupies the nasopharynx. Digital palpation and probe tests are contraindicated. The swelling over the cheek can be palpated and suggests infra-temporal fossa extension.

Proptosis suggests orbital extension and type of proptosis depends on the route of spread. Visual acuity and field can be affect due to optic nerve/chiasma involvement when tumour extends to cavernous sinus.

Otological examination may show retracted or bulging drum with or without fluid level and features of conductive hearing loss. This is due to the compression of the eustachian tube orifice causing its dysfunction/ obstruction.

Neurological findings depend on the cranial nerves involved. II, III, IV and V cranial nerves involvement should be looked for. Headache, blurring of vision and projectile vomiting suggest raised intracranial pressure (Papilledema may be seen in such cases.)

Incidence of clinical presentation:

Nasal obstruction 80–90% (Biller, et al 1974, Hardillo et al, 2004)

Epistaxis/blood stained discharge 75–80% (Thomas et al, 1983, Bryant et al, 1970)

Nasal/facial deformity 34%

Rhinolalia clausa 24% (Biller et al 1974) 48.2% Hardillo, et al. 2004)

Headache 34.48% (Hardillo, et al, 2004)

Ophthalmological 7% (Wittt el, 1983) 13%—visual; changes

Otological 3.2% (Witt, et al. 1983)

Neurological 3.4% (Bryant, et al. 1970), 10% (Witt, et al, 1983)

General under-development: 22.5%. (Witt, et al. 1983, Bruce, et al 1974)

Investigations

- Diagnostic nasal endoscopy is very important in initial diagnosis because of classical presentation and will show a hyper-vascularized globular lobulated mass with a smooth surface covered with dilated blood vessels, typically bulging behind the posterior part of the middle turbinate, obstructing the choana or completely filling the nasal cavity (Fig. 25.2). It also helps in postoperative follow-up.
- Contrast CT scan imaging of the paranasal sinuses (axial, coronal and reconstructed sagittal sections)
- Gadolinium contrast magnetic resonance imaging (MRI) is the ideal method for a multiplanar evaluation of the lesion with relation to important soft tissue structures like orbit, dura, internal carotid artery, cavernous sinus (Nicoli 2003) and is complimentary to CT scan in evaluation and management (Fig. 25.3).
- Digital subtraction angiography (DSA) has been considered to be an ideal technique to identify the feeding blood vessels and also for the early detection of residual lesions (Scholtz, et al 2001). It also helps in selective embolization between 24 and 48 hrs before surgery, if planned for (Fig. 25.4).

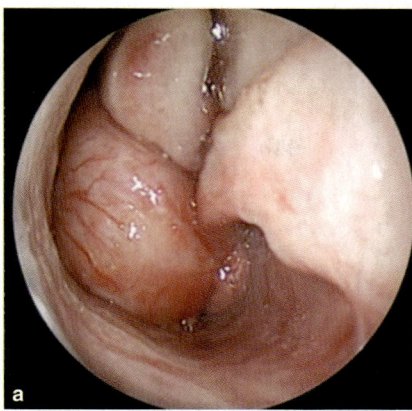 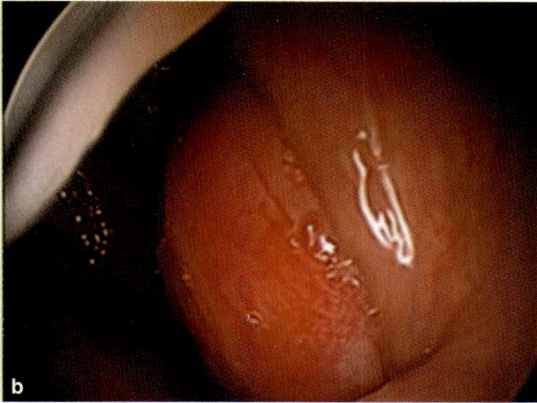

Fig. 25.2: Nasal endoscopic picture showing: **a.** Nasopharyngeal angiofibroma occupying the posterior part of the nasal cavity, compressing the middle turbinate, inferior turbinate and left tubal orifice, **b.** Posterior part of the septum being pushed on the right side by the same tumour, while right tubal orifice is visible

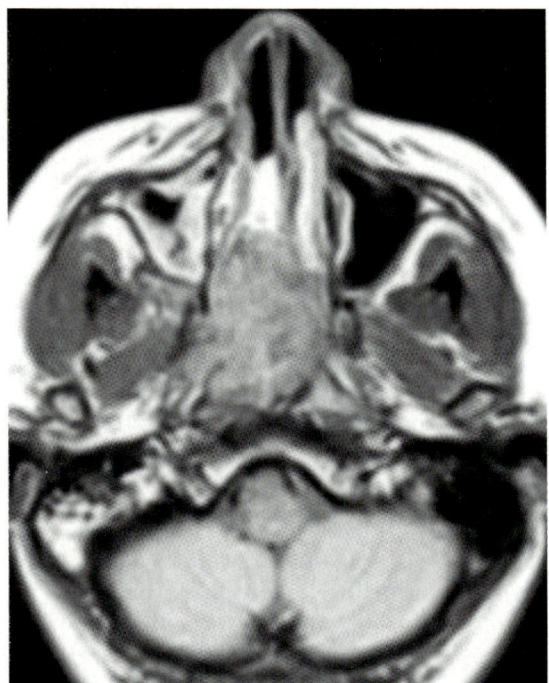

Fig. 25.3: MRI scan showing nasopharyngeal tumour involving left pterygoplatine fossa, pterygoid recess and entire nasopharynx with extension to left nasal cavity

TUMOUR STAGING

Tumour Stage and Extent

- *Sessions staging 1981*
  - Stage IA—Tumour limited to posterior nares and/or nasopharyngeal vault

  - Stage IB—Tumour involving posterior nares and/or nasopharyngeal vault with involvement of at least 1 paranasal sinus
  - Stage IIA—Minimal lateral extension into pterygomaxillary fossa
  - Stage IIB—Full occupation of pterygo-maxillary fossa with or without superior erosion of orbital bones
  - Stage IIIA—Erosion of skull base (i.e. middle cranial fossa/pterygoid base); minimal intracranial extension
  - Stage IIIB—Extensive intracranial extension with or without extension into cavernous sinus
- *Fisch staging 1983*
  - Stage I—Tumours limited to nasal cavity, nasopharynx with no bony destruction
  - Stage II—Tumours invading pterygo-maxillary fossa, paranasal sinuses with bony destruction
  - Stage III—Tumours invading infratemporal fossa, orbit and/or parasellar region remaining lateral to cavernous sinus
  - Stage IV—Tumours invading cavernous sinus, optic chiasmal region, and/or pituitary fossa
- *Andrew's modification of Fisch staging (1989)*
  - I—Limited to the nasopharynx and nasal cavity, bone destruction negligible or limited to the sphenopalatine foramen

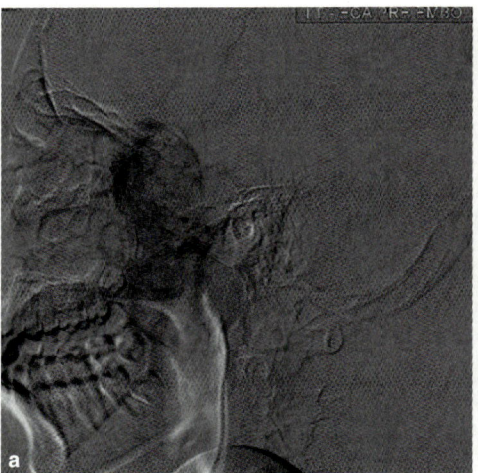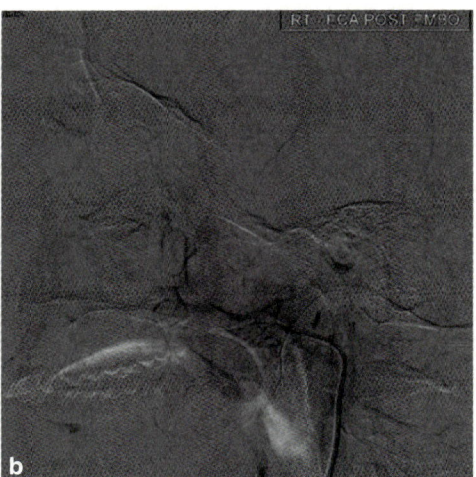

Fig. 25.4: Digital subtraction angiography image: **a.** Tumour blush in the nasopharynx, **b.** Absence of tumour blush after embolization of left internal maxillary artery.

– II—Invades the pterygopalatine fossa or the maxillary, ethmoid, or sphenoid sinus with bone destruction
– IIIa—Invades the infratemporal fossa or the orbital region without intracranial involvement
– IIIb—Invades the infratemporal fossa or orbit with intracranial extradural (parasellar) involvement
– IVa—Intracranial intradural tumour without infiltration of the cavernous sinus, pituitary fossa, or optic chiasm
– IVb—Intracranial intradural tumour with infiltration of the cavernous sinus, pituitary fossa, or optic chiasm

• *Radowsky staging system (1996)*
– IA: Limited to nose or NP
– IB: Extends into one or more sinuses
– IIA: Minimal extension into medial PMF
– IIB: Full occupation of PMF with local mass effect
– IIC: Extension into ITF, cheek, or posterior to pterygoid plates, erosion of skull base
– IIIA: Minimal skull base involvement
– IIIB: Extensive intracranial extension, with or without invasion into cavernous sinus

Common Surgical Approaches

• *Transpalatal:* This approach was developed by Wilson (1951). It is suitable for tumour limited to nasopharynx. A 'U'-shaped incision is made about 2.5 cm anterior to the junction of soft and hard palates and the incision may be wound round the maxillary tuberosity to reach small extensions in the pterygopalatine fossa. Part of the hard palate bone can be removed for better exposure of the tumour, the junction of soft and hard palate extend further anteriorly. This gives good exposure of the nasopharynx but has risk of developing oronasal fistula which should be kept in mind.

• *Lateral rhinotomy* approach with medial maxillectomy gives good exposure and is suitable for extensions to maxillary sinus.

• *Denker's modification of Caldwell-Luc operation* is suitable for extensions into the maxillary antrum.

• *Sardana's approach (1964):* Modified the transpalatal approach with sublabial extension and separating the pterygoid plates from maxilla to facilitate removal of infratemporal extension along with nasopharyngeal part.

• *Midfacial degloving approach (Maninglia 1986):* This gives good cosmetic results as it avoids facial incisions.

- *Le Fort-I osteotomy approach (Sasaki, et al 1990):* It is similar to mid-facial degloving approach and avoids facial incision. This gives good exposure for extranasopharyngeal extensions (Singh, et al. 2011)
- *Transmandibular approach to skull base (Biller, et al 1981):* Transmandibular lip-splitting approach gives excellent exposure of the infratemporal fossa, pterygoid muscles and is suitable for very large tumours with multiple extensions including pterygopalatine fossa, infratemporal fossa and cheek. It has a disadvantage of external scar.
- Infratemporal fossa approaches for extensive tumours with intracranial extension to middle fossa (Fisch type C) are rarely being done nowadays and has been replaced with extended endoscopic approach.
- Facial translocation approach (Janeka, 1997)
- Craniotomy, if extensive intracranial extension is present.
- Endoscopic endonasal approach for small and medium-sized tumours with limited extensions to pterygopalatine fossa, early infratemporal fossa and sphenoid sinus could be treated successfully with judicious use of +/− modified Denker's approach. In recent days, tumour extending intracranially are successfully dealt with endoscopic approach.

Other Modalities of Treatment

Radiotherapy, chemotherapy and hormonal therapy have been tried but none are curative. Radiotherpy/Gamma knife can be indicated in unresectable tumours with extensive intracranial extensions or unfit for surgery due to clinical comorbidities (Roche, et al 2007, Fonseca, et al. 2008). One has to note that radiation therapy can induce malignancy and cataracts, as reported by Cummings, et al.

- Chemotherapy

Prognosis

- Depends on the stage
- Early diagnosis favour complete resection
- Prognosis good, if completely excised.

Endoscopic Management of JNA

The evolution of endoscopic endonasal surgery, better understanding of the skull base anatomy and advancements of the imaging have become allies in the management of JNA (Janakiram, Sharma and Paniker, 2016). Jorison (1996) described the limitations of endoscopic removal of such tumours. Kamel (1996), Tseng & Chao (1997) performed successful endoscopic excision of angiofibroma. Hazarika & Nayak, et al (2002) performed endoscopic resection of angiofibroma in 9 cases, assisted with KTP laser, where the tumour was confined to sphenopalatine foramen and nasopharynx, +/− sphenoid sinus. Endoscopic management of JNA is an ideal procedure to manage small to intermediate tumour (Nicoli, 2003). With improved skill and navigation support, larger tumours extending to critical areas, can be resected endoscopically.

Technique (Figs 22.2 and 25.5): The patient is induced with hypotensive general anaesethesia and kept on reversed Trendelenburg position. Nose is packed with cottonoid strip soaked with oxymetazoline solution or dilute adrenaline with saline for 10 minutes decongestion. The packs are removed and local infiltration 2% xylocaine with 1:200,000 adrenaline is injected on to the root of the middle turbinate, uncinate process and bulla. A partial resection of the middle turbinate is done followed by a type-2 medial maxillectomy for limited pterygopalatine (PTP) fossa and infratemporal fossa involvment and type-3 in extensive infratemporal fossa and superior extension as described under Chapter 22. The posterior bony wall of maxillary sinus is removed using angled Hajek-Koffler bone punch forceps or drill using diamond burr. The surface of the mass is cauterized with bipolar cautery or coblation to reduce vascularity. All secondary adhesions are released. If the tumour is too bulky, it can be resected partially with KTP532 or diode laser or bipolar forceps. In case of lateral extension, a gentle dissection is done to dissect the mass from the sphenopalatine fossa. In case of gross infratemporal fossa extension, modified

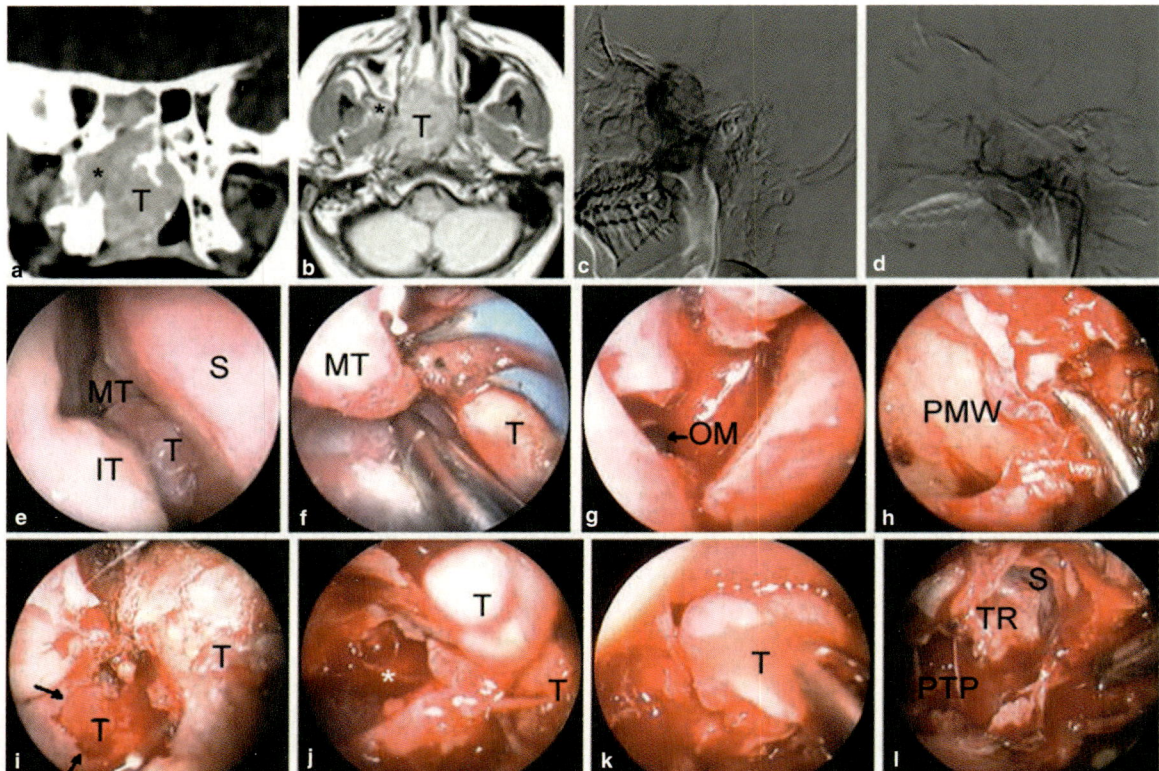

Fig. 25.5: a. Coronal CT showing tumour (T) extension to pterygopalatine fossa (*), sphenoid sinus and pterygoid recess, nasopharyngeal space, **b.** MRI showing tumour extending to left nasal cavity, pterygopalatine fossa (*) and entire nasopharynx, **c.** DSA showing the tumour blush, **d.** DSA after embolization showing disappearance of tumour blush, **e.** Endoscopic picture showing middle turbinate (MT), inferior turbinate (IT) tumour (T) extension to nasal cavity, **f.** Release of secondary adhesions of the tumour (T) from the middle turbinate (MT) and septum (S), **g.** Extended middle meatal antrostomy (Type-2 endoscopic partial maxillectomy), **h.** Bulging of posterior medial wall (PMW) due to tumour, exposure of sphenopalatine foramen and removal of posterior wall of maxilla with Hazek punch forceps, **i.** Exposure of tumour (T) after removal of posterior maxillary wall (black arrow), **j.** Tumour (T) is removed from the pterygopalatine fossa (white asterisk), **k.** Removal of tumour from the sphenoid sinus (S) and pterygoid recess (TR) after removal of the anterior wall, **l.** Posterolateral wall of sphenoid sinus and pterygoid recess, nasopharynx after complete tumour removal

Denker's approach (Fig. 25.6) is required to reach the lateral aspect of the tumour. The sphenopalatine vessels/internalmaxillary are cauterized or clipped to maintain haemostasis. In case of extension to the sphenoid sinus, the anterior wall is drilled and removed for better tumour exposure. The dissection is carried out in the subperiosteal plane especially from the septum and sphenoid avoiding direct contact reduces the intraoperative bleeding. Coblation plays a very important role in surface coagulation of the tumour by devascularization. In the absence of coblation, bipolar cautery can be used effectively (Fig. 25.4). If there is gross extension of the tumour to the opposite side, posterior part of the septum may have to be removed. If lateral recess of sphenoid sinus is present, then maxillary sinus medial wall is completely removed. Infraorbital nerve (an important landmark) is identified and drilling is done medially to expose the pterygoid bone and the anterior wall of the pterygoid is removed. Vidian canal is drilled, if there is tumour extension for exposure and removal (Chapter-22, Fig. 22.2 p&q). The tumour can be removed segment wise to facilitate more

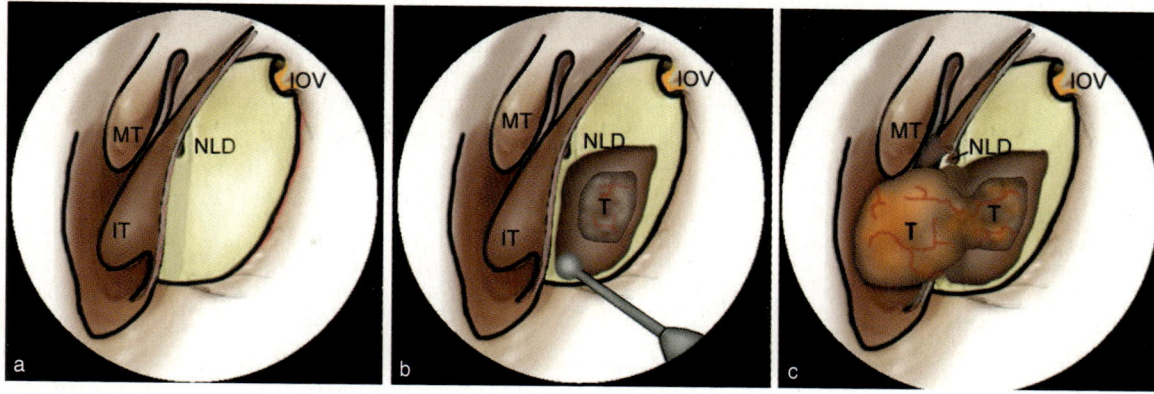

Fig. 25.6: Endoscopic modified Denker's approach: **a.** Exposure of anterolateral wall of maxilla up to the infraorbital vessel (IOV) and nerve and medial wall of maxilla till nasolacrimal duct (NLD). Posterior wall of maxilla is removed to expose the tumour (T), **b.** Removal of anterolateral wall and medial wall till NLD, **c.** Removal of medial wall of maxilla, inferior turbinate (IT) and division of NLD and remval of posterior medial wall to expose the tumour completely before mobilization and removal of tumour as shown in Fig. 25.5

working space and enabling complete removal of tumour. Tumour from the inferior orbital fissure (IOF) extension can be removed by gentle traction as JNA rarely is adherent to neurovascular structure. The tumour extension to superior orbital fissure (SOF), cavernous sinus and internal carotid artery should be removed as last step after clearing and removal of disease from other areas including nasopharynx. Use of Doppler is needed for safe removal of tumor from the carotid (Safadi, et al). Glad, et al. (2007) recommended preoperative embolization and found 60–70% blood loss during surgery, and minimized the blood transfusion required. Mishra and Verma (2017) observed the likelihood of residual disease being left following embolization and hence the importance of extended surgery for complete excision. The nasal cavity is irrigated with warm saline after excision of the tumour. Drilling is done with a diamond burr to smoothen and remove all sharp projection of bone. The nasal cavity is packed with surgicel.

BIBLIOGRAPHY

1. Abraham SC, Montgomery EA, Giardiello FM, *et al*. Frequent β-catenin mutations in juvenile nasopharyngeal angiofibromas. Am J Pathol 2001;158:1073–78.

2. Acuna, Tapia R. The nasopharyngeal fibroma and its treatment. Arch Otolaryngol 1956; 64: 451–55.

3. Andrews JC, Fisch U, Valavanis A, et al. The surgical management of extensive nasopharyngeal angiofibromas with the infratemporal fossa approach. Laryngoscope 1989;99(4):429–37.

4. Antonelli AR, Cappiello J, Di Lorenzo D, Donajo CA, Nicolai P, Orlandini A. Diagnosis, staging, and treatment of juvenile nasopharyngeal angiofibroma (JNA). Laryngoscope 1987;97(11): 1319–25.

5. Apostol JV, Frazell EL. Juvenile nasopharyngeal angiofibroma. A clinical study. Cancer 1965;18:869–78.

6. Barnes L, Weber CP, Karause J, et al. Angiofibroma—Aflow cytometric evaluation of 31 case. Skull Base 1992; 2(4):195–98.

7. Batsakis JG. Tumors of the Head and Neck: Clinical and Pathological Considerations. 2nd ed. Baltimore, Md: Williams & Wilkins; 1979: 296–300.

8. Bensch H, Ewing J. Neoplastic Disease. 4th edition, Saunders and Co., Philadelphia, 1941.

9. Bhatia ML, Mishra SC, Prakash J. Lateral extension of nasopharyngeal fibroma. J Laryng, 1967;81:99–06.

10. Biller HF, Sessions DG, Ogura JH. Angiofibroma– A treatment approach. Laryngoscope, 1974; 84(5):695–706.

11. Biller HF, Shugar JMA, Krespi YP. A new technique for wide field exposure of base skull. Arch Otolaryngol 1981;107(11):698–702.

12. Briant TDR, FiTzpatric PJ, Berman J. Naso-pharyngeal angiofibroma-A 20 year study. Laryngoscope 1978; 88: 1247–51.

13. Capps FCW, Irvine G, Timmis P. Four recent cases of juvenile fibroangioma of the postnasal space. J Laryng 1961;75:924–31.

14. Chen KT, Bauer FW. Sarcomatous transforma-tion of nasopharyngeal angiofibroma. Cancer 1992;49:369–71.

15. Coutinho-Camillo CM, Brentani MM, Nagai MA. Genetic alterations in juvenile naso-pharyngeal angiofibromas. Head Neck 2008; 30:390–400.

16. Dane WH. Juvenile nasopharyngeal fibroma in state of regression. Ann Otol 1954;63:997–1013.

17. Das C. Nasopharyngeal angiofibroma. Indian Journal of Otolaryngology, 1970;22:191–99.

18. Figi FA, Davis RE. The management of naso-pharyngeal fibromas. Laryngoscope 1950;60: 794–814. (Quoted by Das 1970)

19. Finerman WB. Juvenile nasopharyngeal angio-fibroma in the female. AMA Arch Otolaryngol 1951 Dec;54(6):620–23.

20. Fonseca AS, Vinhaes E, Boaventura V. Surgical treatment of non-embolized patients with nasoangiofibroma. Braz J Otorhinolaryngol 2008;74:583–87.

21. Girgis IH, Fahmy SA. Nasopharyngeal fibroma: Its histopathological nature. J Laryng 1973;87: 1107–23.

22. Glad H, Vainer B, Buchwald C, et al. Juvenile nasopharyngeal angiofibromas in Denmark 1981–2003: Diagnosis, incidence, and treatment. Acta Oto-Laryngologica. 2007;127(3):292–99.

23. Golabek W, Szymańska A, Szymański M, et al Juvenile angiofibroma with intracranial extension—diagnosis and treatment. Otolaryngol Pol, 2019 (73)6.

24. Gramann M, Wendler O, Haeberle L, Schick B. Expression of collagen type I-III in juvenile Angiofibroma. Cells Tissues Organs 2009;189: 403–09.

25. Gramann M, Wendler O, Haeberle L, Schick B. Prominent collagen types IV expression in juvenile angiofibromas. Histochem Cell Biol 2009 Jan;131(1):155–64.

26. Handousa FH, Farid H. Elwi AM; Naso-pharyngeal fibroma. J Laryng 1954;68: 647–66.

27. Harma RA. Nasopharyngeal angiofibroma. Acta Otolaryngologica, Suppl 1959;146:1–74.

28. Hazarika P, Nayak DR, Balakrishna R, et al. Endoscopic and KTP laser-assisted surgery for juvenile nasopharyngeal angiofibroma. Am J Otolaryngol. 2002 Sep-Oct;23(5):282–6.

29. Heinrich U, Brieger J, Gosepath J. Frequent chromosomal gains in recurrent juvenile Angiofibroma. Cancer Genetics 2007;175(2): 138–43.

30. Janeka IP, Chandra SN, Shekhar LN. Facial translocation—A new approach to cranial base. Otolaryngology—Head and Neck Surgery 1990; 103(3):413–19.

31. Jorissen M. The role of endoscopy in the management of paranasal sinus tumours. Acta Otorhinolaryngol Belg 1995;49:225–28.

32. Kamel RH. Transnasal endoscopic surgery in juvenile nasopharyngeal angiofibroma. J Laryngol Otol. 1996;110:962–68.

33. Karatay S, Karircioglu S, Erozden O. Significance of hormones in the pathogenesis of naso-pharyngeal angiofibroma. Acta Otolaryngol 1963;56:362–69.

34. Liu Z, Wang J, Wang H, et al. Hormone receptors and vascular endothelial growth factor in juvenile nasopharyngeal angiofibroma—immunohistochemical analysis and tissue microanalysis. Acta Otolaryngol 2015 Jan; 135(1):51–57.

35. Lorente JL, et al. Evolution in the treatment of angiofibroma. Acta Otorrinolaringol Esp Jul-Aug 2011;62(4):279–86.

36. Lund VJ, Stamberger H, Nicoli P, et al. European position paper on endoscopic management of tumours of the nose, paranasal sinuses and skull base. Rhinol Suppl. 2010;22:1–143.

37. Manglia AJ. Indication and technique of midfacial degloving—A 15 yrs experience. Arch Otolaryngol Head Neck Surg 1986 Jul;112(7): 750–52.

38. Maniglia AJ. Indications and techniques of midfacial degloving. A 15-year experience. Arch Otolaryngol Head Neck Surg. 1986 Jul;112(7):750–52.

39. Martin H, Ehrlich HE, Abels JC. Juvenile nasopharyngeal angiofibroma. Ann Surg 1948 March; 127(3): 513–36.

40. Mattei TA, Nogueira FG, Ramina R. Juvenile nasopharyngeal angiofibroma with intracranial extension. Otolaryngol Head Neck Surg 2011 Sep;145(3):498–504.

41. Maurice M, Milad M. Pathogenesis of juvenile nasopharyngeal fibroma. J Laryngol Otol 1981; 95(11)1121–26.

42. Mishra M, Verma V. Implication of embolization in residual disease in lateral extension of juvenile nasopharyngeal angiofibroma. *J Oral Biol Craniofac Res* 2019 Jan-Mar; 9(1): 115–18.

43. Misra RN, Shardana DS. The transpalatal surgical approach for removal of naso-pharyngeal fibromata. Indian J Otolaryngol 1956;8:1–15.

44. Nagai MA, Butugan O, Logullo A, Brentani MM. Expression of growth factors, proto-oncogenes, and p53 in nasopharyngeal angiofibromas. *Laryngoscope.* 1996;106(2):190–95.

45. Radkowski D, McGill T, Healy GB, Ohlms L, Jones DT. Angiofibroma. Changes in staging and treatment. Arch Otolaryngol Head Neck Surg 1996;122(2):122–29.

46. Ripel C, Plinkert P, Schick B, et al. Expression of members of the cadherin-/catenin-protein family in juvenile angiofibromas. Laryngo-Rhino-Otologie,2003; 82(5):353–57.

47. Roche PH, Paris J, Régis J. Management of invasive juvenile nasopharyngeal angiofibromas: The role of a multimodality approach. Neuro-surgery 2007;61:768–77.

48. Safadi A, Schreiber A, Fliss DM, Nicoli P. Juvenile angiofibroma current management strategies. J Neurol Surg B Skull Base 2018 Feb; 79(1): 21–30.

49. Sardana DS. Nasopharyngeal fibroma extension into cheeck. Archives of Otolaryngology 1965; 81:584.

50. Schick B, Brunner C, Praetorius M, et al. First evidence of genetic imbalance in angiofibroma. Laryngoscope 2002;112:397–401.

51. Schick B, Kahle G, Hässler R, Draf W. Chemo-therapy of juvenile angiofibroma—an alternative? HNO 1996;44(3):148–52.

52. Schick B, Veldung B, Wemmert S, et al. p53 and Her-2/neu in juvenile angiofibromas. Oncol Rep 2005 Mar;13(3):453–57.

53. Schiff, M. Juvenile nasopharyngeal angiofibroma: A theory of pathogenesis. The Laryngoscope, 1959;69:981–1016.

54. Scholtz AW, Appenroth E, Kammen-Jolly K, Scholtz LU, Thumfart WF. Juvenile naso-pharyngeal angiofibroma: management and therapy. Laryngoscope 2001;111:681–87.

55. Schuon R, Brieger J, Heinrich UR, Roth Y, Szyfter W, Mann WJ. Immunohistochemical analysis of growth mechanisms in juvenile nasopharyngeal angiofibroma. European Archives of Oto-Rhino-Laryngology 2007; 264(4): 389–94.

56. Singh R, Hazarika P, Nayak DR. Role of Le Forte Type-1 osteotomy approach in Juvenile nasopharyngeal angiofibroma. Int J Oral Maxillofac Surg 2011 Nov;40(11):1271–74.

57. Sternberg SS. Pathology of juvenile naso-pharyngeal angiofibroma: A Lesion of adolescent males. Cancer 1954;7:15–28.

58. Szymańska A, Szymański M, Czekajska-Chehab E, Szczerbo-Trojanowska M. Two types of lateral extension in juvenile nasopharyngeal angiofibroma: Diagnostic and therapeutic management. Eur Arch Otorhinolaryngol 2015; 272(01):159–66.

59. Tseng HZ, Chao WY. Transnasal endoscopic approach for juvenile nasopharyngeal angio-fibroma. Am J Otolaryngol. 1997;18:151–54.

60. Walike WW, MacKay B. Nasopharyngeal angiofibroma: Light and electron microscopic changes after stilbesterol therapy. Laryngo-scope 1970, 80(7):1109–21.

61. Wilson, Jol. Approach to Nasopharynx 1951; 65:738.

62. Witt TR, Saha JP, Stearnberg SS. Juvenile angiofibroma—a 30 years clinical review. Am J Surg 1983;146:521–25.

63. Zanation AM, Mitchell CA, Rose AS. Endoscopic skull base techniques for juvenile nasopharyngeal angiofibroma. Otolaryngol Clin North Am. 2012 Jun; 45(3):711–30, ix.

64. Zhang M, Sun X, Yu H, Hu L, Wang D. Biological distinctions between juvenile nasopharyngeal angiofibroma and vascular malformation: An immunohistochemical study. Acta Histochem. 2011;113:626–30. An immuno-histochemical study. Acta Histochem 2011;113: 626–30.

65. Janakiram TN, Sharma SB, Paniker VB. Endoscopic excision of non-embolized juvenile nasopharyngeal angiofibroma: Our technique. Indian Journal of Otolaryngology and Head and Neck Surgery 2016; 68:263–69.